CHILDHOOD CANCER

A Parent's Guide to Solid Tumor Cancers

D1369872

CHILDHOOD CANCER

A Parent's Guide to Solid Tumor Cancers

Honna Janes-Hodder & Nancy Keene

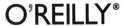

O'REILLY®

Beijing • Cambridge • Farnham • Köln • Paris • Sebastopol • Taipei • Tokyo

Childhood Cancer: A Parent's Guide to Solid Tumor Cancers
by Honna Janes-Hodder and Nancy Keene

Copyright © 1999 O'Reilly & Associates, Inc. All rights reserved.
Printed in the United States of America.

Published by O'Reilly & Associates, Inc., 101 Morris Street, Sebastopol, CA 95472.

Editor: Linda Lamb

Production Editor: Sarah Jane Shangraw

Printing History:

      August 1999: First Edition

Library of Congress Cataloging-in-Publication Data:

Janes-Hodder, Honna, 1966– .
    Childhood cancer: a parent's guide to solid tumor cancers / Honna Janes-Hodder and
       Nancy Keene.
      p.   cm.—(Patient-centered guides)
    Includes bibliographical references and index.
    ISBN 1-56592-531-9 (pbk.)
    1. Tumors in children—Popular works. I. Keene, Nancy.
II. Title. III. Series.
RC281.C4J36   1999
618.92'994—dc21

                         99-33120
                         CIP

Table of Contents

Foreword

Considerable progress has been made in the last 20 to 30 years in the cure of children with cancer. Currently, 70 to 75 percent of all children diagnosed with cancer can be cured, including those diagnosed with solid tumors. Nevertheless, having a child with cancer must be one of the most traumatic experiences one can imagine. This book was developed to help educate parents and caregivers of children with solid tumors in order to make the experience easier to endure. Indeed, a similar book has already been developed for the parents of children with leukemia (*Childhood Leukemia: A Guide for Families, Friends, and Caregivers,* by Nancy Keene).

For most people, it is easier to cope with a difficult situation if one has a better understanding of what is happening and why. This book will help parents gain a much better understanding of childhood cancer, its treatment, and their consequences. It also provides suggestions and guidelines to deal with the practical as well as the emotional aspects of this experience. The more parents understand about their child's disease, the more effectively they can participate in his care and the decisions about his treatment.

This book presents a comprehensive view addressing most aspects of the experience of having a child with cancer. Chapters address many of the common experiences of having a child with cancer: understanding clinical trials; general principles of surgery, radiation therapy, chemotherapy, and their side effects; bone marrow transplantation; novel approaches to therapy; choosing a (central venous) catheter; coping with procedures; and dealing with hospitalizations. These chapters can be extremely helpful in preparing for therapy. Nutrition can be a very important component in tolerating chemotherapy, and this is also addressed in considerable detail. There are also practical tips about record keeping and finances, as well as dealing with schools and addressing your child's educational needs.

Six chapters are devoted to the major solid tumors of childhood (excluding brain tumors): neuroblastoma, Wilms tumor, retinoblastoma, liver tumors, soft tissue sarcomas, and bone sarcomas. These chapters provide information about the origin and spread of these tumors, the signs and symptoms of disease, diagnosis and staging, prognostic indicators, treatment (surgery, chemotherapy, radiation, bone marrow rescue), and future directions. These chapters are organized in a very consistent manner, so information is easy to find. Furthermore, many points are illustrated with stories from the experiences of individual patients to make some of the information more accessible.

Finally, there are chapters dealing with more emotional and psychological components of the experience: the importance of siblings, family, and friends; other sources of support; dealing with feelings, behavior, and communication; anticipating the end of treatment and beyond; even preparing for the possibility of relapse or death. Again, these sections are generously illustrated with stories that provide examples from real life situations.

There are general themes that pervade this book that make it particularly valuable. For example, there is considerable empowerment in having a better knowledge base and understanding about the disease and its treatment. It is important for parents to participate in an active way in their child's care, and in the decision-making process. Also, it is important to be realistic but optimistic. Cancer is a serious and life-threatening illness, even in the best of circumstances. There are some cancers that can be cured reliably in the majority of cases, and others in which only a minority survive. Nevertheless, it is impossible to say with certainty at diagnosis if any individual patient will survive or not, so there is always reason for optimism. Indeed, the majority of children with solid tumors can be cured, but the chances of cure depend on the diagnosis, extent of disease, and certain other biological or genetic features that influence prognosis.

The rate of improvement in cure rates is plateauing, suggesting that current approaches are unlikely to offer hope of cure for the remaining 25 percent of children. We are encountering long-term effects of cancer and its treatment in the survivors. Nevertheless, this is also a time of great optimism. Laboratory studies of cancer cells have revealed a number of clues about what genetic changes are responsible for cells becoming malignant. These genes, proteins, and pathways represent unique features of cancer cells that should allow us to develop more specific approaches to therapy. These novel approaches should substantially improve the cure rates and have much less toxicity than with current approaches.

—Garrett M. Brodeur, MD
Audrey E. Evans Endowed Chair
Professor of Pediatrics
Chief, Division of Oncology
Children's Hospital of Philadelphia
Philadelphia, Pennsylvania

Introduction

We are all in the same boat, in a stormy sea,
and we owe each other a terrible loyalty.

—G. K. Chesterton

Honna's Story: My youngest child, Matthew, had been hospitalized for several weeks with mysterious bone pain. On July 12, 1993, Matthew's third birthday, we returned from some scans to find his hospital room full of gaily wrapped presents and his crib and IV pole festooned with colorful crepe paper. On this day, we were told that Matthew had stage IV neuroblastoma, and childhood cancer became part of our lives. A day that should have been filled with happiness instead marked the beginning of a long and difficult journey.

For a few weeks, I lived in a state of shock. However, once I accepted the reality of the situation, I began to ask questions. I had no medical training, but I had an inquisitive nature and a deep need to understand the fundamentals about the disease, the particulars of treatment, and the newest research. First, I purchased books about cancer from local bookstores, but was frustrated at how little information they contained on pediatric neuroblastoma. Next, I read medical books and journals from the library. I used this information to ask our oncologist innumerable questions. We often had lengthy conferences to go over my newest findings.

We live in the small community of Paradise, Newfoundland and Labrador. My family has always been close, so I was fortunate to have the support needed to sustain me, especially during the most difficult times. I also drew on the strength of my best friend, who stood by my side every step of the way. Frequent hospitalizations allowed me to get to know other parents of children with cancer. The nurses and technicians who took such good care of Matthew were sources of information and support, but soon became close friends as well.

As Matthew's treatment progressed, I continued my studies. I had a good knowledge of the fundamentals, and I felt it was important to stay current with the advances made in neuroblastoma treatment. I identified key researchers and I would often call them to discuss their work and learn of cutting edge treatments.

When my husband's parents gave me a computer for Christmas in 1995, a whole new world opened up for me. I had a wealth of information at my fingertips and ways to communicate efficiently with researchers all over the globe. I also met many parents of children with cancer who were searching for both information and support. This informal network grew into several Internet discussion groups with close to 700 members from sixteen countries—my extended family.

Nancy's Story: My life abruptly changed on Valentine's Day, 1992, when my three-year-old daughter was diagnosed with acute lymphoblastic leukemia (high risk). At the time, I was the full-time mother of two small daughters: Katy, three years old, and Alison, eighteen months.

The phone call from my pediatrician informing me of Katy's probable diagnosis began my transformation into a "hospital mom." On the two-hour trip to the nearest children's hospital, I naively thought that my background would equip me to deal with the difficulties ahead. I had a degree in biology, and had worked my way through the university in a series of hospital jobs. I had experience in the blood bank, the emergency room, the coronary care unit, and the IV (intravenous) team. After college, I was a paramedic with a busy rescue squad and for several years taught Emergency Medical Technician courses at the local community college. I understood the science and could speak the jargon; I thought I was prepared.

I was wrong. Nothing prepares a parent for the utter devastation of having a child diagnosed with cancer. My brain went on strike. I couldn't hear what was being said. I felt like I was trapped in a slow-motion horror movie.

I came home from Katy's first hospitalization with two shopping bags full of booklets, pamphlets, and single sheets containing information on a wide variety of topics. I didn't know how to prioritize what I needed to learn, so I started by researching everything that I could about leukemia. With the help of my wonderful family and hardworking friends, I began to rapidly fill several file cabinets with information on the medical aspects of the disease.

Emotionally, however, I felt lost. Since most of Katy's treatment was outpatient, I lived too far away to benefit from the hospital's support group. I knew no local parents whose child had cancer. I felt isolated. Then I discovered Candlelighters (see Appendix C, *Resource Organizations*). This marked a turning point in my ability to deal effectively with my daughter's disease. I began networking with other parents and made marvelous friends. I soon realized that we shared many of the same concerns and were dealing with similar problems. Advice from "veteran" parents became my lifeline.

My daughter was treated for over two years. During that time, my brother bought me my first computer, which I used to continue my scientific studies. I also discovered the first online support groups for adults with cancer. As the membership in the groups swelled, parents of children with cancer joined and networked. There I met Honna.

Why we wrote this book

When our children were on treatment, we each amassed not only a library of medical information, but scores of first-person accounts of how individual parents coped. It saddened us to think that most parents of children with cancer would, like us, expend precious time and energy to collect, assess, and prioritize information about their child's cancer. After all, parents are busy providing much of the treatment that their child receives. They make all appointments, prepare their child for procedures, buy and dispense medicines, deal with all of the physical and emotional side effects, and make daily decisions on when their child needs medical attention. In a sense, this book grew out of our concern that other overwhelmed parents should not have to duplicate our efforts to gather and organize information.

Although we are no longer in the trenches (parent slang for having a child on treatment), we are still very active in the patient community. We have a genuine desire to provide information that is accurate to newly diagnosed families. Misinformation is rampant.

What this book offers

This book is not intended to be autobiographical. Instead, we wanted to blend basic technical information in easy-to-understand language with stories and advice from many parents and survivors. We wanted to provide the insight and experiences of veteran parents, who have all felt the hope, helplessness, anger, humor, longing, panic, ignorance, warmth, and anguish of their children's treatment for cancer. We wanted parents to know how other children react to treatment, what to expect, and provide tips to make the experience easier.

Obtaining a basic understanding of topics such as medical terminology, common side effects of chemotherapy, and how to interpret blood counts can only improve the quality of life for the whole family suffering along with their child with cancer. Learning how to develop a partnership with your child's physician can vastly increase your family's comfort and peace of mind. Hearing parents describe their own emotional ups and downs, how they coped, and how they molded their family life around hospitalizations is a tremendous comfort. Just knowing that there are other kids on chemotherapy who refuse to eat anything but tacos or who have frequent rages makes one feel less alone. Our hope is that parents who read this book will encounter medical facts simply explained, will find advice that eases their daily life, and will feel empowered to be a strong advocate for their child.

The parent stories and suggestions in this book are true, although some names have been changed to protect children's privacy. Every word has been spoken by the parent of a child with cancer, a sibling of a child with cancer, or a childhood cancer survivor. They wanted to share with others what they learned.

How this book is organized

We have organized the book sequentially in an attempt to parallel most families' journey through treatment. We all start with diagnosis, try to cope with procedures, adjust to medical personnel, and deal with family and friends. We struggle to understand the disease and its treatment. We all seek out various methods of support, and deal with the strong feelings of our child with cancer and our other children. We try to work with our child's school to provide the richest and most appropriate education for our ill child. And, unfortunately, we must grieve, either for our child or for the child of a close friend we have made in our new community of cancer.

Because it is tremendously hard to focus on learning new things when you are emotionally battered and extremely tired, we have tried to keep each chapter short.

The first time that we introduce a medical term, we define it in the text. If you do not read the book sequentially and encounter an undefined term, it is also explained in the glossary at the end of the book.

Since approximately half of the children diagnosed with cancer are boys and half girls, we did not adopt the common convention of using only masculine personal pronouns. Because we do not like using he/she, we have alternated personal pronouns within chapters. This may seem awkward as you read, but it prevents half of the parents from feeling that the text does not apply to their child.

All of the medical information contained in this book is current for 1999. As treatment is constantly evolving and improving, there will inevitably be changes. However, many of the medicines now in use have been used for many years. Their use in combination and changes in dosages have accounted for the tremendous increase in treatment effectiveness in the last two decades. Scientists are currently studying some biological agents, however, that may dramatically improve treatment for childhood cancer. You will learn in this book how to discover the newest and most appropriate treatment for your child.

To meet some of the children you will read about in this book and to give you more places to find help for your cancer journey, we have included four appendices for reference: a photo gallery of children during and after treatment, blood counts and what they mean, resource organizations, and books and online sites. In addition, at the back of the book we have included an indispensable health record to be filled out at the end of treatment and copied and given to each subsequent caregiver for the rest of your child's life. This personal long-term follow-up guide will educate healthcare providers about the types of treatment your child had, and the follow-up schedule necessary to maintain optimal health.

How to use this book

While researching this book, we were repeatedly told by parents to "write the truth." Because the "truth" varies for each person, over one hundred parents, children with cancer, and siblings share portions of their experiences. This book is full of such snapshots in time, some of which may be hard to read, especially by families of children newly diagnosed. Here are our suggestions for a positive way to use the information contained in this book:

- Consider reading only sections that apply to the present or immediate future. Even if your child's prognosis indicates a high probability of cure, reading about relapse or death can be emotionally difficult.

- Realize that only a fraction of the problems that parents describe will affect your child. Every child is different; every child sails smoothly through some portions of treatment while encountering difficulties in others. The more you understand about the variability of cancer experiences, the better you will be able to cope with your own situation as well as be a good listener and helpful friend to other families you meet with differing diagnoses and circumstances.

- Take any concerns or questions that arise to your oncologist and/or pediatrician for answers (or more questions). The more you learn, the better you can advocate for your family and others.

- We have struggled to keep each chapter short and the technical information easy to read. If you want to delve into any topic in greater depth, Appendix D, *Books and Online Sites,* is a good place to start. It contains a list of pamphlets and books for parents as well as children of all ages. Reading tastes are an individual matter, so if something suggested in this appendix is not helpful or upsets you, put it down. You will probably find something else on the list that is more appropriate for you.

- Share the book with family and friends. Usually they desperately want to help and just don't know how. This book not only explains the diseases and treatments, but also offers dozens of concrete suggestions for family and friends.

Best wishes for a smooth journey through treatment and a bright future for the entire family.

Acknowledgments

This book is truly a collaborative effort for, without the help of many, it would simply not exist. Our heartfelt thanks to our families and friends who supported and encouraged us along the way. We will be forever grateful for your unwavering patience as we spent many months working on this book. We would especially like to thank our children—Matthew, Kristina, David, Kathryn, and Alison—for the unending joy they bring to our lives each day. Our deepest appreciation to our parents: Eugene and Muriel (Janes) Pretty, Uriel and Nathaniel Janes, and Bill and Doris Keene, for a lifetime of love, support, and encouragement. To our editor, Linda Lamb, whose creative instinct and gentle guidance was essential to the success of this book; to Carol Wenmoth, for her attention to detail and unfailing good cheer; and to Tim O'Reilly for his belief in and support of the patient-centered guides. The entire staff at O'Reilly & Associates has been not only knowledgeable and efficient, but dedicated in their effort to make this a comprehensive resource for those affected by pediatric solid tumors.

Many well known and respected members of the pediatric oncology community, and professionals in related fields, graciously carved time out of busy schedules to make invaluable suggestions and to ensure that the material in the book is factually correct. We especially appreciate the patient and thoughtful answers to our many phone calls and emails. This book grew out of a true collaboration of parents and professionals. Thank you: Clarke P. Anderson, MD; Peter C. Adamson, MD; D.M. Bass, MD; David Beele, LSW; Jean B. Belasco, MD; Garrett Brodeur, MD; Nancy J. Bunin, MD; Stan Calderwood, MD; William Carroll, MD; D. R. Chaulk, MD; Lynne Conlon, PhD; Max Coppes, MD, PhD; Ruth Daller, CRNP; Debra Ethier, RTT; Christina Falcone, Financial Counselor; Daniel Fiduccia, BA; Debra L. Friedman, MD; Joel W. Goldwein, MD; Mark Greenberg, MD; Stephan Grupp, MD, PhD; Jack Hand, MD; Bruce Himelstein, MD; Wendy Hobbie, RN, MSN, PNT; JoAnne Holdt, MA; Lawrence F. Jardine, MD; F. Leonard Johnson, MD; Anne E. Kazak, PhD; Beverly J. Lange, MD; Ann-Marie Leahey, MD; Susan J. Leclair, MS, CLS (NCA); John M. Maris, MD; Anna T. Meadows, MD; Grace Monaco, JD; Linn Murphree, MD; Ann Newman, RN; Mark Newman, MD; Cal Peddle, BSc, PhD; Greg Peddle, PhD; C. Patrick Reynolds, MD, PhD; Robert C. Seeger, MD; Hiro Shimada, MD; Steven Simms, PhD; Anne Spurgeon; Heidi Suni, MSW; Susan DiTaranto, RN, BSN; Ellen Tracy RN; David R. Ungar, MD; Judith G. Villablanca, MD; Daniel von Allmen, MD; and Richard B. Womer, MD.

More than words can express, we are deeply grateful to the parents, children with cancer, and their siblings, who generously opened their hearts and relived their pain while sharing their experiences with us. To all of you whose words form the heart and soul of this book, thank you: Brenda Andrews; Robin B.; Sheila Batten; LeeAnn Barnard; Mike and Kathy Blaker, parents of Adam; Patrice Boyle and Sean Boyle; Ted and Michele Bozarth; Sue Brooks; Noreen Burgess, Coley's mom; Dottie Bradford Buttafogo; Alicia Cauley; Naomi Chesler; Cathy and Tim Cooley; Allison E. Ellis; E. Engelmann; Dana Erickson; Mel Erickson; Kellie Espinoza; Donna Evans, Cienna's mommy; Art Farro; Rene Fernandez; Kate Foley, mom to Cameron, 4/25/94 to 5/31/98; Alana Freedman; Jenny Gardner; Sandra Gaynor; Judy Gelber; Shirley Enebrad Geller; Roxie Glaze; Lynn Goering; Kris H.; Lisa Hall; Erin Hall; Jessica Hargin; Linda Harrison; Kathryn G. Havemann; Douglas L. Herstrom; Connie Higbee-Jones; David Hodder; Ruth Hoffman; Chris Hurley; David and Esther Hurst; the Jordan Family; Erin A. Jordan; Fr. Joseph; Peggy Kaiser; Susan Kalika; Beth Karanicola; Winnie Kittiko; Lisa Korenko; Missy Layfield; Susanne Lehrman; Elinor Lemky; the Peter G. Lewis Family; Pam Lim; Gail and John Lindekugel, parents of Levi; Dierdre McCarthy-King; Sara McDonnall; Lori Michelle Miller; Marilyn Brodeur Morin; Wendy Mitchell; Amanda Moodie; Jean Morris; Leslee Morris; Laura Myer; Carolyn Nordberg; M. Clare Paris; Jeff Pasowicz; Jennifer Peterson; Donna Phelps; Laura Randall, RN, mother of Matthew; Mary Riecke; Lynne A. Rief; Wendy Rigden McCurley; Jennifer E. Rohloff; Steve and Shirlene S.; Carole Schuette; Sharon Schuster; Janice Scott; Susan Sennett; Erin Shanahan; Lynnette Shanahan; Lori Shipman; Lorrie Simonetti; Cathi Smith; Carl and Diane Snedeker; Anne Spurgeon; Jenni Swink; Leeann T.; Iris Taylor; T. Terwilliger; Wendy Thompson; Marie Thomsen; Gigi N. Thorsen; Lisa Tignor; Sarah, Tim, and John Allen Tinkel; Michael and Cheryl Tobias; Shoshana Tobias; Laura Todd-Pierce; Michele Trieb; Cathy Tschumy; Susan E. Tuccio; Kathleen Tucker; Bridget Tuxen; Dina Van Yperen; Annie Walls; Ralene Walls; Kimbra Suzanne Wilder; Jean Wilkerson; the Yantis Family; Lise Yasui; Cheryl Zeichner; Ellen Zimmerman; and those who wish to remain anonymous.

Thank you to Patty Feist-Mack for allowing us to include the CHILDCANCER list included under "Signs and symptoms" in Chapter 1, *Diagnosis*.

Thanks also to Mitzi Waltz. Some of the material in Chapter 22, *School*, was adapted from her book *Pervasive Developmental Disorders: Finding a Diagnosis and Getting Help* (O'Reilly, 1999).

Despite the inspiration and contributions of so many, any errors, omissions, misstatements, or flaws in the book are entirely our own.

Diagnosis

A journey of a thousand leagues
begins with a single step.

—Lao-tzu

CANCER IS A WORD THAT evokes many images and emotions. To hear this word used in the same sentence as your child's name is terrifying. From that point forward, life will never be the same. Families are forced into the childhood cancer realm, a world often described as an emotional roller coaster ride in the dark. Once the initial shock of diagnosis has passed, however, the reality that most children with cancer are cured provides strength and hope.

Signs and symptoms

Cancer begins with the transformation of a single cell. The malignant changes that occur in these renegade cells can cause several signs and symptoms, many of which mimic common childhood illnesses.

Most cases of childhood cancer are diagnosed based on symptoms. Parents are usually the first to notice that something is wrong with their child. Occasionally, a diagnosis of cancer is based on chance findings during well baby visits to the pediatrician. Rarely, it is discovered accidentally on an x-ray done for other reasons.

Any deviation from the child's normal behavior or health that persists or is not easily explained gives reason for further investigation by the pediatrician. The following are some of the signs and symptoms which may indicate the presence of childhood cancer:

- Continued, unexplained weight loss
- Headaches, often with early morning vomiting
- Increased swelling or persistent pain in bones, joints, the back, or legs
- Lump, especially in the abdomen, neck, chest, pelvis, or armpits
- Development of excessive bruising or bleeding

- Constant infections
- A whitish color behind the pupil
- Nausea which persists or vomiting without nausea
- Constant tiredness or noticeable paleness
- Eye or vision changes which occur suddenly and persist
- Recurrent or persistent fevers of unknown origin

> *The day that I took Cassandra (age five) to the pediatrician, I had assumed she would be sent home on antibiotics for some type of infection. She had been complaining of pain in her left knee and had developed a large lump on her left buttock. Instead, we left with instructions for her to eat nothing, since she was going to be sedated the following morning for some scans at the hospital. From that point on, things happened very fast. I remember only bits and pieces of those first few days at the hospital. I was told that Cassandra had rhabdomyosarcoma, that the following day they would do a biopsy and implant a central catheter, and that chemotherapy would be started as soon as possible.*

Most parents react to their concerns by taking their child to a doctor. Usually, the doctor performs a physical exam and may order a complete blood count (CBC) or x-rays. Sometimes the diagnosis is not as easy and fast as Cassandra's.

> *When Hailee was a baby, we noticed that sometimes her eye appeared white and sometimes it looked reddish. We were worried, but the pediatrician said that she was healthy. He eventually gave us a referral to see an ophthalmologist when we insisted. Since he didn't feel it was an emergency, it took three months to see the eye specialist, who diagnosed her unilateral retinoblastoma. By that time, Hailee's retina was detached, and her eye had to be enucleated. I remember feeling completely shocked when the specialist said that she had a disease that would kill her if left untreated. We were angry, because for several months we had been taking her to the pediatrician, and even told him about a picture that had been taken of Hailee that showed an odd white reflex in her eye. Still, he felt that there was nothing wrong. If it had been diagnosed sooner, we might have been able to save her eye.*

Where should your child receive treatment?

After a tentative diagnosis of childhood cancer, most physicians refer the child for further tests and treatment to the closest major medical center with expertise in treating children with cancer. Every child with cancer should be treated at a facility that uses a team approach, including pediatric oncologists/hematologists, specialized surgeons and pathologists, pediatric nurse practitioners, radiologists, pediatric surgeons, rehabilitation specialists, education specialists, and social workers. State-of-the-art treatment is provided at these institutions, offering your child the best chance for remission (disappearance of disease in response to treatment) and, ultimately, cure.

Physical responses

Many parents become physically ill in the weeks following diagnosis. This is not surprising, given that most parents stop eating or grab only fast food, normal sleep patterns are a thing of the past, and staying in the hospital exposes them to all sorts of illnesses. Every waking moment is filled with excruciating emotional stress, which makes the physical stress so much more potent.

The second week in the hospital I developed a ferocious sore throat, runny nose, and bad cough. Her counts were on the way down, and they ordered me out of the hospital until I was well. It was agony.

．．．．．

That first week, every time my son threw up, so did I. I also had almost uncontrollable diarrhea. Every new stressful event in the hospital just dissolved my gut; I could feel it happening. Thank God this faded away after a few weeks.

Parental illness is a very common event. To attempt to prevent its occurrence, it is helpful to try to eat nutritious meals, get a break from your child's bedside to take a walk outdoors, and find time to sleep. Care needs to be taken not to overuse drugs or alcohol. Whereas physical illnesses usually end after a period of adjustment, emotional effects continue throughout treatment.

Emotional responses

The shock of diagnosis results in an overwhelming number of intense emotions for the child and the parents. The length of time people experience each of these feelings differs greatly, depending on pre-existing emotional issues and coping ability. Many of these emotions reappear at different times during the child's treatment. Some of the feelings that parents experience are described below. Children and teens' emotional responses to diagnosis are discussed in Chapter 24, *Feelings, Communication, and Behavior*.

Confusion and numbness

In their anguish, most parents remember only bits and pieces of the doctor's early explanations about their child's disease. This dreamlike state is an almost universal response to shock. The brain provides protective layers of numbness and confusion to prevent emotional overload. This allows parents to examine information in smaller, less threatening pieces. Oncologists understand this phenomenon and are usually quite willing to repeat information as often as necessary. It is sometimes helpful to write down instructions, record them on a small tape recorder, or ask a friend to help keep track of all the new and complex information.

> When I left the doctor's office, I was a mass of hysteria. I couldn't breathe and felt as if I was suffocating. Tears were flowing nonstop. I had lost total control of myself and had no idea of how to stop my world from turning upside down.

. . . . .

> When the doctor said mass or tumor, I still didn't connect it to cancer or realize the seriousness of her situation.

. . . . .

> For a brief moment I stared at the doctor's face and felt totally confused by what he was explaining to me. In an instant that internal chaos was joined with a scream of terror that came from some place inside me that, up until that point, I never knew existed.

Denial

In the first few days after diagnosis, many parents use denial to shield themselves from the reality of the situation. They simply cannot believe that their child has a life-threatening illness. In order to convince themselves that the diagnosis is not a mistake, some parents find comfort in seeking a second opinion (see Chapter 4, *Forming a Partnership with the Medical Team*). Denial may serve as a useful method to survive the first few days after diagnosis, but a gradual acceptance must occur so that the family can begin to make the necessary adjustments to cancer treatment. Life has dramatically changed. Once parents accept the doctor's encouraging optimism, push their fears into the background, and begin to believe that their child can survive, they will be better able to provide support for their child and their family.

> *I walked into the empty hospital playroom and saw my wife clutch-ing Matthew's teddy bear. Her eyes were red and swollen from crying. I had no idea what had happened. A minute later the doctor came into the room with several residents (doctors who are receiving specialized training). He told me that Matthew had cancer and that he was very sick. I remember thinking that there had to have been a mistake. Maybe he was reading the wrong chart? My initial reaction was that it was physi-cally impossible for one of my children to have cancer. Cancer is a dis-ease of the elderly. Kids don't get cancer!*

Guilt

Guilt is a common and normal reaction to childhood cancer. Parents feel that they have failed to protect their child, and blame themselves. It is especially difficult because the cause of their child's cancer, in most instances, cannot be explained. There are questions: How could we have prevented this? What did we do wrong? How did we miss the signs? Why didn't we bring her to the doctor sooner? Why didn't we insist that the doctor do blood work? Did he inherit this from me? Why didn't we live in a safer place? Maybe I shouldn't have let him drink the well water. Was it because of the fumes from painting the house? Why? Why? Why? It may be difficult to accept, but parents need to remember that nothing they consciously did caused their child's illness.

Nancy Roach describes some of these feelings in her booklet *The Last Day of April*:

> Almost as soon as Erin's illness was diagnosed, our self-recrimination began. What had we done to cause this illness? Was I careful enough during pregnancy? We knew radiation was a possible contributor; where had we taken Erin that she might have been exposed? I wondered about the toxic glue used in my advertising work or the silk screen ink used in my artwork. Bob questioned the fumes from some wood preservatives used in a project. We analyzed everything—food, fumes, and TV. Fortunately, most of the guilt feelings were relieved by knowledge and by meeting other parents whose...children had been exposed to an entirely different environment.

> $\bullet \quad \bullet \quad \bullet \quad \bullet \quad \bullet$

> Knowing that I shouldn't feel guilty doesn't help. Knowing that there probably wasn't anything I could have done to protect my adorable little girl doesn't help. Even if it could be proven that those caustic chlorine fumes and that huge coal pile had nothing to do with her cancer, it wouldn't help.

Fear and helplessness

A diagnosis of childhood cancer strips parents of control over their child's daily life. Previously, parents established routines and rules which defined family life. Children woke up, washed and dressed, ate breakfast, perhaps attended day care or school, played with friends, and performed chores. Life was predictable. Suddenly, the family is thrust into a new world populated by an ever-changing cast of characters (interns, residents, fellows, oncologists, IV teams, nurses, social workers) and containing a new language (medical terminology): a new world full of hospitalizations, procedures, and drugs.

Until adjustment begins, parents sometimes feel utterly helpless. Physicians whom they have never met are making life or death decisions for their child. Even if parents are comfortable in a hospital environment, feelings of helplessness may develop because there is simply not enough time in the day to care for a very sick child, deal with their own emotions, begin to educate themselves about the disease, notify friends and family, make job decisions, and restructure the family to deal with the crisis.

Parents also experience different levels of anxiety, including fear and panic. Many parents have trouble sleeping and feel overwhelmed by fears of what the future holds. Their world has turned inside out—they have gone from adults in control of their lives to helpless people who cannot protect their child.

Many parents state that helplessness begins to disappear when a sense of reality returns. They begin to make decisions, study their options, learn about the disease, and grow comfortable with the hospital and staff. However, feelings of fear, panic, and anxiety periodically erupt for many parents at varying times throughout their child's treatment.

> *It's not a nice way to have to live. What's waiting around the next corner? That's a scary question. One of my biggest fears is the uncertainty of the future. All that we can do is the best we can and hope that it's enough.*

· · · · ·

> *Sometimes I would feel incredible waves of absolute terror wash over me. The kind of fear that causes your breathing to become difficult and your heart to beat faster. While I would be consciously aware of what was happening, there was nothing I could do to stop it. It's happened sometimes very late at night, when I'm lying in bed, staring off into the darkness. It's so intense that for a brief moment, I try to comfort myself by thinking that it can't be real, because it's just too horrible. During those moments, these thoughts only offer a second or two of comfort. Then I become aware of just how wide my eyes are opened in the darkness.*

Anger

Anger is a universal response to the diagnosis of cancer.

> *Life isn't fair, but yet the sun still comes up each morning. To be angry because your child has cancer is normal. The question is where to direct that anger. Sometimes I feel as if I'm angry with the entire world. In my heart, though, my outrage is directed solely at each and every cancer cell feeding on my child.*

Expressing anger is normal and can be cathartic. Attempting to internalize this powerful emotion is usually not possible at the moment of diagnosis. It is nobody's fault that children are stricken with cancer. Since parents cannot direct their anger at the cancer, they target doctors, nurses, spouses, siblings, and sometimes even the ill child. Because anger directed at other people can be very destructive, it is necessary to devise ways to express the anger. Some suggestions from parents for managing anger follow.

Anger at healthcare team:

- Try to improve communication with doctors
- Discuss feelings with one of the nurses
- Discuss feelings with social workers
- Talk with parents of other ill children

Anger at family:

- Physical exercise
- Do yoga or relaxation exercises
- Keep a journal or tape-record feelings
- Cry in the shower or pound the walls
- Listen to music
- Read other people's stories about cancer
- Talk with friends
- Talk with parents of other ill children
- Join or start a support group
- Improve communication within family
- Try individual or family counseling
- Live one day at a time

Anger at God:

- Discuss feelings with spouse or close friends
- Discuss feelings with clergy or church members
- Re-examine faith
- Trust in God
- Pray

It is important to remember that angry feelings are normal and expected. Discovering healthy ways to vent anger is a vital tool for all parents.

Loss of control

Parents sometimes feel overwhelmed by the sudden loss of control after their child is diagnosed with cancer. This is especially true for parents who are used to having a measure of power and authority in the workplace or the home.

> My husband had a difficult time after our son was diagnosed with neuroblastoma. We have a traditional marriage, and he was used to his role as provider and protector for the family. It was hard for him to deal with the fact that he couldn't fix everything.

Parents can regain some control over the situation by learning about their child's disease and its treatments. This knowledge can be used to advocate for their child. However, parents should recognize that attempting to completely control their child's treatment can impede the child's medical care. For more information, see Chapter 4.

Sadness and grief

Parents feel an acute sense of loss when their child is diagnosed with cancer. They feel unprepared to cope with the possibility of death, and fear that they may simply not be able to deal with the enormity of the problems facing the family. Parents describe feeling engulfed by sadness. Grieving for the child is common, even when the prognosis is good. Parents grieve the loss of normalcy, the realization that life will never be the same. They grieve the loss of their dreams and aspirations for their child. Shame and embarrassment are also felt by some parents. Cultural background, individual coping styles, basic temperament, and family dynamics all affect the type of emotions experienced.

> I have an overwhelming sadness and, unfortunately for me, that means feelings of helplessness. I wish I could muster up a fighting spirit, but I just can't right now.

· · · · ·

> While I have moments of deep sadness and despair, I try not to let them turn into hours and certainly not days. I am too aware of the fact that I may have the rest of my life to grieve.

Parents travel a tumultuous emotional path where overwhelming emotions subside only to resurface later. All of these are normal, common responses to a catastrophic event. For the majority of parents, these strong emotions begin to fade as hope grows.

Hope

After being buffeted by illness, anger, fear, sadness, grief, and guilt, most parents welcome the growth of hope. Hope is the belief in a better tomorrow. Hope sustains the will to live and gives the strength to endure each trial. Hope is not a way around, it is a way through. The majority of children conquer childhood cancer and live long and happy lives. There is reason for hope.

Twenty-five years ago, very few children with cancer were cured. Over the last few decades, due to research and participation in clinical trials (see Chapter 5, *Clinical Trials*), the majority of children are cured. In another twenty-five years, perhaps all children diagnosed with cancer will be cured.

Many families discover a renewed sense of both the fragility and beauty of life after the diagnosis. Outpourings of love and support from family and friends provide comfort and sustenance. Many parents speak of a renewed appreciation for life and consider each day with their child as a precious gift.

The immediate future

It is important for you to know that you are not alone. Many have traveled the childhood cancer path before you, and, unfortunately, many will follow after you. While it is sad to know that others are forced into this terrifying journey, you can take some small solace from knowing that you are not the only parents to experience these feelings.

The next several chapters will provide specific disease-related information: how to get the best doctors and treatment plan, what type of catheter to choose, whether your child should be enrolled in a clinical study, and various forms of cancer treatment. Veteran parents will explain what choices they made, how they adjusted, learned, and became active participants in their children's treatment. Sharing experiences with parents and survivors of childhood cancer may help your family develop its own unique strategy for coping with the challenges ahead.

A Mother's View

Memory is a funny thing. I'd be hard pressed to remember what I had for dinner last night, but like many people, the day of the Challenger explosion and, even further back, the day of John Kennedy's death are etched in my mind to the smallest detail.

And like a smaller group of people, the day of my child's cancer diagnosis is a strong and vivid memory, even seven years later. Most of the time, I don't dwell on that series of images. It was, after all, a chapter in our lives, and one that is now blessedly behind us. But early each autumn, when I get a whiff of the crisp smell of leaves in the air, it brings back that dark day when our lives changed forever.

Many of the memories are painful and, like my daughter's scars, they fade a little more each year, but will never completely disappear. While dealing with the medical and physical aspects of the disease, my husband and I also made many emotional discoveries. We sometimes encountered ignorance and narrow-mindedness, which made me more sad than angry. Mistakes were made, tempers were short, and family relations were strained. But we saw the other side, too. Somehow, our sense of humor held on throughout the ordeal, and when that kicked in, we had some of the best laughs of our lives. There was compassion and understanding when we needed it most. And people were there for us like never before.

I remember two young fathers on our street, torn by the news, who wanted to help but felt helpless. My husband came home from the hospital late one night to find that our lawn had been mowed and our leaves had been raked by them. They had found a way to make a small difference that day.

Another time, a neighbor came to our house bearing a bakery box full of pastries and the message that his family was praying for our daughter nightly around their supper table. The image of this man, his wife, and his eight children joining in prayer for us will never leave me.

A close friend entered the hospital during that first terrible week we were there, to give birth to her son. I held her baby, she held me, and we laughed and cried together.

Sometimes, when I look back at that time, I feel as though everything that is wrong with the world and everything that is right are somehow distilled in one small child's battle to live. We learned so very much about people and about life.

Surely people who haven't experienced a crisis of this magnitude would believe that we would want to put that time behind us and forget as much of it as possible. But the fact is, we grew a little through our pain, like it or not. We see through new eyes. Not all of it is good or happy, but it is profound.

I treasure good friends like never before. I view life as much more fragile and precious than I used to. I think of myself as a tougher person than I was, but I cry more easily now. And sure, I still yell at my kids and eagerly await each September when they will be out of my hair for a few hours each day. But I hold them with more tenderness when they hop off the school bus into my arms. And I like to think that some of the people around us, who saw how suddenly and drastically a family's life can change, hold their children a little dearer as well.

Do I want to forget those terrible days and nights seven years ago? Not on your life. And I hope the smell of autumn leaves will still bring the memories back when I'm a grandmother, even if I can't remember what I had for dinner last night.

—Kathy Tucker
CURE Childhood Cancer Newsletter

CHAPTER 2

Coping with Procedures

*Forewarned, forearmed; to be prepared is
half the victory.*

—Cervantes
Don Quixote

THE PURPOSE OF THIS chapter is to prepare both child and parent for several common procedures by providing detailed descriptions of each. Since many procedures are repeated, frequently during the treatment for childhood cancer, it is important to establish a routine that is comfortable for your child. The procedure itself may cause discomfort, but a well prepared, calm child fares far better than a frightened one.

Planning for procedures

Procedures are needed to make diagnoses, check for spread of disease, give treatment, and monitor response to treatment. Interventions range from figuring out the best way for your child to take numerous pills to having multiple and time-consuming body scans. Some procedures are pain-free and the family merely needs clear explanations about what to expect. Others can cause both physical and psychological distress. These reactions can be avoided or minimized by medication and/or good coping skills.

A family-centered approach works best when planning and implementing procedures. The procedures are often as (or more) frightening for parents as for patients. Memories of them can be long lasting. For this reason, children, parents, and staff should work together toward planning for and coping with procedures.

As soon as possible after your child's diagnosis, find out if the hospital has a child life program or other such team (of nurses, psychologists, social workers) that helps prepare families for procedures. The purpose of these programs is to minimize psychological trauma, promote optimal development, and maintain, as much as possible, normal living patterns during hospitalizations. They attempt to minimize the child's stress by giving the child developmentally appropriate explanations of the reasons for procedures and hospital routines.

> Matthew was in sixth grade when he was diagnosed, and he was worried about the surgery for implanting the port. He didn't know what the scar would look like and he was concerned about AIDS, because it had been in the news a lot that year. The child life specialist came in and really helped. She showed him what a port looked like, then they explored the pre-op area, the actual surgery room, and post-op. She showed him on a cloth doll exactly where the incision would be and how the scar would look. Then she introduced him to "Fred," the IV pump. She said that Fred would be going places with him, and that Fred would keep him from getting so many pokes. She told Matthew that he could bring something from home to hang on Fred. Of course, he brought in a really ugly stuffed animal. Throughout treatment, she really helped his fears and my feelings about losing control over my child's daily life.

Many child life specialists or other team members accompany children to and provide support during procedures. They establish relationships with children based on warmth, respect, empathy, and understanding of developmental stages. They also communicate with the other members of the healthcare team about the psychosocial needs of children and their families.

Your response, as well as your child's, depends on temperament, age, previous medical or dental experiences, and other factors. Discuss with the child life professional or social worker when and how to prepare your child for upcoming procedures. Usually, parents need to experiment with how much advance notice to give younger children about procedures. Some children do better with several days to prepare, while others worry themselves sick. Sometimes, needs change over the course of treatment, so good communication and flexibility are essential.

> I started giving my four-year-old daughter two days notice before procedures. But she began to wake up every day worried that "something bad was going to happen soon." So we talked it over and decided to look at the calendar together every Sunday to review what would happen that week. She was a much happier child after that.

Try to schedule procedures so that the same person does the same procedure each time. Although it may not always be possible, try to arrange for the same doctor to do each of your child's procedures, the same nurse to access the Port-a-cath (catheter described in Chapter 6, *Catheters*), and the same technician for blood work. Call ahead to check for unexpected changes to prevent any surprises. Repetition can provide comfort and reassurance to children.

Parents can ask for the medical professional with the most experience to perform procedures, such as spinal taps. In the hospital hierarchy, attending physicians are above fellows and residents. However, at some large teaching facilities, attending physicians may not do these procedures very often. Many times, the fellow or resident (and in states where it is allowed, the nurse) is more skilled, because they do the vast majority of these procedures.

Parents should have a choice whether to be present or not during a medical procedure. Parents set the tone. A calm parent and a well-prepared child give the best chance for a quick, peaceful procedure. If you find that you are unable to be of help to your child during procedures, ask the child life specialist or other member of the healthcare team to be present solely to comfort your child.

> We decided from the very beginning that, even though it's no fun to have a bone marrow or a spinal, we were going to make something positive out of it. So we made it a party. We'd bring pizza, popcorn, or ice cream to the hospital. We helped Kristin think of the nurses as her friends. We'd celebrate after a procedure by going out to eat at one of the neat little restaurants near the hospital.

Giving children some control over what happens helps tremendously.

> Katy and I wrote down her requests for each procedure that first week in the hospital. For example, during spinal taps she wanted me (not a nurse) to hold her in position, she wanted lidocaine to be given with a needle, not the pneumatic gun, and she had a rigid sequence of songs that I sang.

Oncology clinics usually have a special box full of toys for children who have had a procedure. It sometimes helps for the child to have a treat to look forward to afterward. Some parents occasionally bring a special gift to sneak into the box for their child to find.

Pain management

The goal of pediatric pain management should be to minimize discomfort while performing the procedure. The two methods to achieve this goal are psychological (using the mind) and pharmacological (using drugs). These two methods can be used together to provide an integrated mind/body approach.

Psychological method

Preparation for every procedure is essential. Unexpected stress is more difficult to cope with than anticipated stress. If children understand what is going to happen, where it will happen, who will be there, and what it will feel like, they will be less anxious and better able to cope. Methods to prepare children are:

- Verbally explain each step in the procedure.

- If possible, meet the person who will perform the procedure.

- Tour the room where the procedure will take place.

- Small children can "play" the procedure on dolls.

- Older children can observe a "demonstration" on a doll.

- Adolescents may observe a videotape describing the procedure.

- Encourage discussion and answer all questions.

> For my child, playing about procedures helped release many feelings. Parents can buy medical kits at the store or simply stock their own from clinic castoffs and the pharmacy. We had IV bottles made from empty shampoo containers, complete with tubing and plastic needles. Several dolls had accessed ports, and many stuffed animals in our house fell apart after being speared by the pen during countless spinal taps. Katy's younger sister even ran around sometimes with her own pretend port taped onto her chest.

· · · · ·

> My daughter (three years old) took an old stuffed animal to the clinic with her. Having the nurse and doctor perform the procedure first on "bear" helped her immensely.

Hypnosis is a well documented method for reducing discomfort during painful procedures. If performed by a qualified healthcare professional (psychologist, physician, nurse, social worker, or child life specialist), hypnosis can help your child control painful sensations, release anxiety, and diminish pain. The professional helps guide children or teens into an altered state of consciousness that helps focus or narrow attention. To locate a qualified practitioner, call the American Society of Clinical Hypnosis at (837) 297-3317.

Imagery is a way to deliberately create a mental image of sights, sounds, tastes, smells, and feelings. Imagery is an active process that helps children or teens feel as if they are actually entering the imagined place. Focusing on pleasant images allows the child to shift attention from the pain. It can also allow the child to actually alter the experience of pain, which simultaneously gives the child control and diminishes pain. Ask if the hospital has someone to teach your child this very effective technique.

The following description of using imagery was written by Jennifer Rohloff when she was seventeen years old, and is reprinted from the *Free to Be Yourself* newsletter of Cancer Services of Allen County, Indiana.

My Special Place

Many people had a special place when they were young—a special place that they still remember. This place could be an area that has a special meaning for them, or a place where they used to go when they wanted to be alone. My special place location is over the rainbow.

I discovered this place when I was twelve years old, during a relaxation session. These sessions were designed to reduce pain and stress brought on by chemotherapy. This was a place that I could visualize in my mind so that I could go there anytime that I wanted to—not only for pain, but when I was happy, mad, or sad.

It is surrounded by sand and tall, fanning palm trees everywhere. The blue sky is always clear, and the bright sun shines every day. It is usually quiet because I am alone, but often I can hear the sounds of birds flying by.

Every time I come to this place I like to lie down in the sand. As I lie there, I can feel the gritty sand beneath me. Once in a while I get up and go looking for seashells. I usually find some different shapes and sizes.

The ones I like the best are the ones that you can hear the sound of the ocean in. After a while I get up and start to walk around. As I walk, I can feel the breeze going right through me, and I can smell the salt water. It reminds me of being at a beach in Florida. Whenever I start to feel sad or alone or if I am in pain, I usually go jump in the water because it is a soothing place for me. I like to float around in the water because it gives me a refreshing feeling that nobody can hurt me here. I could stay in this place all day because I do not worry about anything while I am here.

To me this place is like a home away from home. It is like heaven because you can do anything you want to do here. Even though this place may seem imaginary or like a fantasy world to some people, it is not to me. I think it is real because it is a place where I can go and be myself.

Distraction can be used successfully with all age groups, but it should never be used as a substitute for preparation. Babies can be distracted by colorful, moving objects. Parents can help distract preschoolers by showing picture books or videos, telling stories, singing songs, or blowing bubbles. Many youngsters are comforted by hugging a favorite stuffed animal. School-age children can watch videos or TV, or listen to music. Several institutions use interactive videos to help distract older children or teens.

Matthew had many bone marrow aspirations, all but two performed without the aid of sedation. Through a little bit of trial and error, I learned that it was best for me to not make him aware that the procedure would be needed until a few hours before it was actually performed. We developed a ritual that helped him a great deal. I would place a finger puppet on one of my fingers and tell him that he could squeeze the puppet as hard as he felt was necessary. I asked him to try and keep eye contact with me at all times, and we would practice deep breathing during the aspiration. I also told him it was okay to cry or scream as loud as he wanted to if he felt like it. The oncologist would always tell Matthew that he was sorry that it hurt so much. I remember once, Matthew reached up from the treatment table and put his arms around his doctor's neck. "That's okay," he said. "I know you didn't want to hurt me."

Other adjunctive therapies that are used successfully to help deal with medical treatments are relaxation, biofeedback, massage, and acupuncture. Ask the hospital's child life specialist, psychologist, or nurse to discuss and practice different methods of pain management with your child.

Pharmacological method

Most pediatric oncology clinics offer the option of sedation and/or anesthesia for painful procedures. Sometimes anesthesia is available only for infants or overwhelmingly anxious children. If you find that your child is distressed by painful procedures (bone marrow aspiration and lumbar puncture, for example), it is reasonable to explore all available options for pain relief.

One father, a doctor just completing his anesthesia residency, explained:

> That first bone marrow was horrible. To have my little three year old look up at me with tears in her eyes and ask, "What else are you going to let them do to me, daddy?" was just too much. It was the worst day of my life.

His wife, a nurse, said:

> We really made waves by insisting that Meagan be sedated for her spinal taps and bone marrows. It was mostly a logistical problem, but we held firm, and now it has become much more routine for many other kids as well.

The ideal pain relief drug for children should be easy to administer, predictable in effect, provide adequate pain relief, have a short duration, and have minimal side effects. There are three topical anesthetics in wide use for pediatric procedures. EMLA cream is a cream put on the skin one to two hours prior to the painful procedure. Numby Stuff also uses a cream anesthetic, but a mild electrical current helps it penetrate the skin in just a few minutes. Ethyl chloride spray is used immediately before the procedure to anesthetize the surface of the skin. For more information, see Chapter 15, *Chemotherapy.*

Drugs for sedation and/or general anesthesia are given intravenously. Some facilities take the child into the operating room (OR) for the procedure, while others use a preoperative area or clinic sedation room and allow the parent to be present the entire time.

Drugs used for pediatric anesthesia during procedures include:

- **Valium or Versed plus morphine or fentanyl.** Valium and Versed are sedatives, which are used with pain relievers such as morphine or fentanyl. These drugs can be given in the clinic, but due to the possibility of slowed breathing, expert monitoring is required and emergency equipment should be present. The combination of a sedative and a pain reliever will result in your child's being awake but sedated. The child may move or cry, but will not remember the procedure. Often, EMLA or lidocaine are also used to ensure that the procedure is pain-free.

- **Propofol.** A milky liquid given by IV, propofol has rapid onset with a rapid recovery. Administration and monitoring by an anesthesiologist (doctor who specializes in giving anesthetics) are required. Propofol, a general anesthetic, will cause your child to lose consciousness. At low doses, propofol prevents memory of the procedure, but may not relieve all pain, so it is often used with EMLA or lidocaine.

- **Ketamine.** Ketamine needs expert monitoring. It has a much longer recovery time than the drugs listed above, and upon awakening, up to 30 percent of children may become confused and/or hallucinate. For these reasons, ketamine is no longer in wide use for pediatric sedation for procedures.

There are many types of drugs and several methods used in administering them, from very temporary (ten minute) mild sedation to full general anesthesia in the operating room. Discuss with your oncologist and anesthesiologist which method will work best for your child.

> Let's face it, kids don't care about lab work or protocols, they just want to know if they are going to be hurt again. I think that one of our most important jobs is to advocate, strongly if necessary, for adequate pain control. If the dose doesn't work and the doctor just shrugs her shoulders, say you want a different dosage or drug used. If you encounter resistance, ask that an anesthesiologist be consulted. Remember that good pain control and/or amnesia will make a big difference in your child's state of mind during treatment.

Since treatment for childhood cancer can take many months, some children build up a tolerance for sedatives and pain relievers. Often, over time, doses may need to be increased or drugs changed. If your child remembers the procedure or feels pain, advocate for a change in drug and/or dosage. It is reasonable to request that an anesthesiologist be present to ensure adequate pain relief.

> My five-year-old has been very hard to sedate for medical procedures such as spinal taps. His oncologist experimented with the commonly used drugs, Versed and fentanyl, to find a combination that would work. For some recent procedures, he was premedicated with Ativan.

Then he was given Versed and Pentobarb instead of fentanyl. I think we've got it right now, since the last sedation went very well. He still has a full 24 hours of vomiting and headache afterwards (even when he receives antinausea drugs), but at least we don't have to hold him down during spinal taps anymore.

All sedation can result in complications, primarily to the airway. It is imperative that sedation occur under the care of trained, experienced personnel and that the child is monitored until fully recovered from the anesthesia.

Procedures

Understanding what will occur during a procedure and what other parents do to prepare their children will arm you with essential information. Knowing what to expect will lower the anxiety level of both parent and child and lay the foundation for months of tolerable tests. The descriptions of procedures in the rest of the chapter may not exactly mirror your experience. Practices vary by hospital and practitioner and this variability should be expected. What should be the same, however, is your comfort in asking questions and getting the support and help you need to prepare for and cope with your child's procedures.

Questions to ask before procedures

Parents need information prior to procedures in order to prepare themselves and their child. Some suggested questions to ask the physician are:

- Why is this procedure necessary for my child and how will it affect her treatment?
- What information will it provide?
- Who will perform the procedure?
- Will it be an inpatient or outpatient procedure?
- Please explain the procedure in detail.
- Is there any literature available that describes it?
- Is there a child life specialist on staff who will help prepare my child for the procedure?
- If not, are there parents who can come talk to me about how to prepare my child?

- Is the procedure painful?
- What type of anesthetic or sedation is used?
- What are the risks, if any?
- What are the common and rare side effects?
- When will we get the results?

Audiogram

Some of the chemotherapy drugs that children receive for cancer treatment can cause hearing loss. Your child's doctor may order a hearing test, called an audiogram, to monitor for possible hearing problems.

During the audiogram, your child will be placed in a soundproof room to prevent outside noises from interfering with the test. You should be allowed to remain with your child during this procedure. Earphones will be placed on his ears, through which sounds, such as beeps and tones, are relayed. Your child will be asked to signal when he has heard the sound by either raising his hand or pressing a button. Each ear will be tested separately. The results of the audiogram are then usually displayed in the form of a graph. The amount of hearing loss is measured in decibels.

> Matthew experienced some high-frequency hearing loss from the cisplatin he received as part of his treatment for neuroblastoma. He would have periodic audiograms performed at various stages of his treatment protocol. They were never a big deal for him, and in fact, he found them to be fun in many ways. The audiologist had a knack for making him feel comfortable. I think to Matthew, stepping into the soundproof booth and putting on his headset was somewhat like a game. The first few audiograms were done with me sitting in the booth beside him. Eventually, he reached a point where he felt he could do this test on his own, and so I would sit with the audiologist, watching him through the window. I think I might have messed the test up a few times with all those funny faces I was making at him. Fortunately for us, the audiologist had a sense of humor!

Blood draws

Frequent blood draws are a part of life during cancer treatment. Blood specimens are primarily used for three purposes: to obtain a CBC, evaluate blood chemistries, or culture the blood to check for infection. A CBC measures the types and numbers of cells in the blood. It tells the physician how effective the drugs are and how susceptible to infection the child is. Blood chemistries measure substances contained in the blood plasma to determine if the liver and kidneys are functioning properly. Blood cultures help evaluate whether the child is developing a bacterial or fungal infection. For a list of normal blood counts, see Appendix B, *Blood Counts and What They Mean*.

If only a CBC is needed, a finger poke will provide enough blood. Blood chemistries or cultures require one or more vials of blood obtained from a vein in the arm or the right atrial catheter.

Blood is usually drawn from the large vein on the inside of the elbow using a procedure similar to starting an IV, except that the needle is removed rather than left in the arm. The advice in the section "Starting an IV," later in this chapter, also applies to drawing blood from the arm.

Children with catheters usually have blood drawn from the catheter rather than the arm or finger. These procedures are described in Chapter 6.

Blood transfusions

Treatment for cancer can cause severe anemia (a low number of oxygen-carrying red blood cells). Many children require transfusions of red cells periodically throughout treatment.

> *Whenever my son needed a transfusion, I brought along bags of coloring books, food, and toys. The number of VCRs at the clinic was limited, so I tried to make arrangements for one ahead of time. When anemic (hematocrit below 20 percent), he didn't have much energy, but by the end of the transfusion, his cheeks were rosy and he had tremendous vitality. It was hard to keep him still. After one unit (bag) of red cells, his hematocrit usually jumped up to around 30.*

One bag (or unit) of red cells takes approximately two to four hours to administer and is given through an IV or catheter. If your child develops chills and/or fever during a transfusion, the nurse should be notified so that the transfusion can be stopped immediately.

There are some risks of infection from red cell transfusions. Since new tests have been devised to detect the AIDS virus, the risk of exposure is minuscule, less than 1 in 450,000. Although there are excellent tests for the various types of hepatitis, exposure to this disease is still possible, although the risk is less than 1 in 4,000. The cytomegalovirus is also a concern. These risks are the reason transfusions are given only when absolutely necessary.

> *My daughter received several transfusions at the clinic in Children's Hospital with no problems. After we traveled back to our home, she needed her first transfusion at the local hospital. Our pediatrician said to expect to be in the hospital at least eight hours. I asked why it would take so long when it only took four hours at Children's. He said he had worked out a formula and determined that she needed two units of packed cells. I mentioned that she only was given one unit each time at Children's. He called the oncologist, who said it was better to give the smaller amount. We went to the hospital where a unit of red cells was given. Then a nurse came in with another unit. I questioned why he was doing that and he said, "Doctor's orders." I asked him to verify that order, as we had already discussed it with the doctor. He went into another room to call the doctor, and came back and said the pediatrician thought she needed 30 cc more packed cells. I called Children's and they said she didn't need more, so I told them not to give the second unit. It just wasn't worth the risk of hepatitis to get 30 cc of blood. Even though I was pleasant, the nurses were angry at me for questioning the doctor.*

Bone marrow aspiration

Some current protocols designed to treat children with cancer require bone marrow aspirations, a process by which bone marrow is sucked out with a needle from the cavity of the bone. Unless sedated, many children and teens describe bone marrow aspirations as uncomfortable to unbearable. EMLA cream, a topical anesthetic, can be applied one to two hours prior to the aspiration to help numb the area. Many institutions sedate children and teens for this procedure.

The purpose of the first (diagnostic) aspiration is to determine if cancerous cells have spread to the bone marrow. Some protocols require bone marrow aspirations to be performed on several occasions, taking place at specific times during the course of treatment.

To obtain a sample of the bone marrow, doctors usually use the iliac crest of the hip (the top of the hip bone in back or front). This bone is right under the skin and contains a large amount of marrow. In some instances, marrow is collected from other sites, such as the sternum (breast bone) or tibia (bone in lower leg).

If the sample is to be taken from the back hip bone, the child lies face down or on his side on a table, sometimes on a pillow to elevate the hip. The doctor will feel the site, then wipe it several times with an antiseptic to eliminate any germs. Sterile paper is placed around the site, and the doctor will wear sterile gloves. Then an anesthetic (usually lidocaine) is sometimes injected into the skin and a small area of bone. This causes a burning and stinging sensation that passes quickly. The physician usually rubs the area to allow the drug to fully anesthetize the area. The physician then pushes a hollow needle (with a plug inside) through the skin into the bone, withdraws the plug, and attaches a syringe. The liquid marrow is then aspirated (sucked out) through the syringe. Then these cells are looked at under a microscope by a pathologist to determine if disease is present.

> Melissa (age five) has had several bone marrow aspirations since her diagnosis of stage IV neuroblastoma in 1995. We always use propofol (which I refer to as the "milk of human kindness," because of its milky appearance) before the procedure. After the aspiration is over, Melissa wakes up from a very deep sleep and has felt no pain whatsoever. She's usually hungry and ready to go ASAP. Propofol has worked exceptionally well for her.

Bone scan

A bone scan is a special test that is performed in nuclear medicine to assess the status of a particular bone or the entire skeletal system. It is often used when the oncologist suspects that there is cancer present, either in the form of a primary bone sarcoma or when there is suspicion of metastatic disease.

Your child will be given an injection of a radioactive material, called technetium, that will travel through the blood to the bones. Approximately two hours later, the scan will be performed. You should be allowed to stay with your child during this procedure.

> Mikey (age four) had numerous full body bone scans which would pinpoint hot spots after injection of radioactive isotopes. He also had MRIs of his legs, as well as CT scans and x-rays, but the bone scans were the scary ones for me. I suppose it was because it would outline his whole skeleton, and I could see those glowing areas.

Computed tomography (CT)

Computed tomography (CT) is also called "CAT" for computerized axial tomography. CT is a complex, computer enhanced procedure for obtaining x-ray images of the body. The machine looks very much like a big donut, and your child will be placed in the hole in the middle. Instead of having a fixed x-ray directed at one part of the body, during a CT scan an x-ray tube rotates around the body generating hundreds of images as it moves. These images are called "slices." CT imaging allows the doctor to see soft tissue structures in great detail.

Before the procedure begins, your child may have to remove some items of clothing or jewelry that may interfere with the CT scan. Sometimes your child will be asked to wear a hospital gown. Your child may need to receive a liquid dye, called a contrast agent, prior to or during the scan. The contrast agent may be given intravenously and/or orally. The technologist will position your child in a manner so that the area being imaged will be inside the opening of the CT machine. The technologist does not stay in the room while the images are being taken.

> Rachel, unfortunately, is very familiar with CT scans. From the beginning we've looked for ways to get her to lie still. The way we accomplished this was by me standing next to her and holding her hand. The parent must wear a shield in order to do this. The CT scanner at our hospital does not make that much noise, and they just got a new one that looks like a donut with a hole in it that moves around her so she doesn't have to change positions. Anyway, they had a tape player and I would always bring one of her favorite tapes and set the tape player right next to her during the whole thing. Also, they would let her have her blankie and baby with her. They were very accommodating.

If you plan to remain with your child, you will need to wear a lead apron to protect your body from unnecessary exposure to radiation. Sometimes, if the site being imaged is the chest area, your child may be asked to breathe in and hold his breath for several seconds. It is important that your child remain still during the CT scanning process. Small children who are unable to remain motionless for several minutes at a time may be sedated before the procedure. You are usually asked to stay in the department until the images have been reviewed by the technologist to ensure that they are adequate.

My son handled CT scans like a little trooper. Even at the age of three, he never needed sedation to help him remain perfectly still. He had so many of them, he was able to lip-sync along with the recording that was asking him to "breathe in and hold your breath." The only part he strongly disliked was having to drink the contrast material before the scan. We experimented with this until we found something that was palatable for him. We mixed the contrast with orange juice, which made it much easier for him to drink.

Conventional x-ray

When a doctor suspects that a child has cancer, she may order an x-ray of the site. X-rays, a type of electromagnetic radiation, provide the doctor with a quick and simple method of viewing organs and structures inside your child's body. Pictures are taken and then displayed on a film or a computer screen.

Before the x-ray is taken, your child will be asked to remove any items of clothing or jewelry that could interfere with the pictures. The child is then positioned by the technologist in a manner that will make it easiest to get the images that are needed. Sometimes, such as in the case of chest x-rays, your child may be asked to breathe in, hold his breath, and remain perfectly still for a few seconds. The technologist leaves the room during the time that the x-rays are taken. As with CTs, if you are planning to stay with your child, you will be asked to wear a lead apron to protect you from radiation. Your child may also have to wear a lead apron or lead shield to protect specific areas of his body. Pregnant women should not be present in the room when x-rays are being taken.

Echocardiogram

Several drugs used to fight cancer can damage the muscle of the heart, decreasing its ability to contract effectively. Many protocols require a baseline echocardiogram to measure the heart's ability to pump before any chemotherapy drugs are given. Echocardiograms are then given periodically during and after treatment to check for heart muscle damage.

An echocardiogram uses ultrasound waves to measure the amount of blood that leaves the heart each time it contracts. This percentage (blood ejected during a contraction compared to blood in the heart when it is relaxed) is called the ejection fraction.

The echocardiogram is performed by a technician, nurse, or doctor. The child or teen lies on a table and has conductive jelly applied to the chest. Then the technician puts a transducer (which emits the ultrasound waves) on the jelly and moves the device around on the chest to obtain different views of the heart. Pressure is applied on the transducer and can sometimes cause discomfort. The test results are displayed on a videotape and photographed for later interpretation.

> Meagan used to watch a video during the echocardiogram. Sometimes she would eat a sucker or a popsicle. She found it to be boring, not painful.

Finger pokes

Finger pokes are different from blood draws in several ways. First, EMLA can be used successfully. Put a blob of EMLA on the tip of the middle finger. Cover the fingertip with plastic wrap, and tape it on the finger. Another method is to buy long, thin balloons with a diameter a bit wider than your child's finger. Cut off the open end, leaving only enough balloon to cover the finger up to the first knuckle. Fill the tip of the balloon with EMLA and slide it on the fingertip. EMLA needs to be applied an hour before a finger poke to be effective. At the laboratory, remove the plastic wrap or balloon, wipe off the EMLA, and ask for a warm pack. Wrapping this heated pack around the finger for a few minutes opens the capillaries to allow the blood to flow out more readily. Now your child is ready for a pain-free finger poke.

The technician will hold the finger and quickly stick it with a small sharp instrument. Blood will be collected in narrow tubes or a small container. It is usually necessary for the technician to squeeze the fingertip to get enough blood. If EMLA is not used, the squeezing part is uncomfortable and the finger can ache for quite a while.

> Even though we use EMLA, Katy (five years old) still becomes angry when she has to have a finger poke. I asked her why it was upsetting if there was no pain, and she replied, "It doesn't hurt my body anymore, but it still hurts my feelings."

Gallium scan

Gallium scans are performed in the nuclear medicine department. Prior to the scan, your child will be injected with a radiopharmaceutical, called gallium citrate. Usually the scan will be performed 24 to 48 hours after the injection. Gallium localizes at sites of infection and malignancy. You should be allowed to stay with your child during this procedure.

Gastronomy

A gastronomy is a feeding tube placed through the abdominal wall into the stomach. Gastronomy tubes are often placed so that nutrition can be provided directly in a child's stomach. This is appropriate for children who cannot eat normally because of chronic swallowing problems or long-term pain in the mouth or throat, or for children who have lost their normal appetite for a prolonged period due to disease or treatment. The stomach end of the feeding tube has a small balloon which prevents it from being accidentally pulled all the way out.

A skilled gastroenterologist can perform the procedure in about ten minutes. Most children have general anesthesia for the procedure and remain in the hospital for one to two days postoperatively to receive pain medication and make sure that they tolerate feedings through the tube. Care of the tube is simple, and after two to three months the tube may be replaced with an unobtrusive skin level device called a "button." After a short recovery, children may play, bathe, and swim normally.

The tube is used for liquid feedings and medications as long as the child requires. If a child no longer requires the tube, it is removed and a bandage is placed over the site. The wound closes spontaneously in a day or two.

Intravenous pyelogram (IVP)

Your child's doctor may order an IVP if she feels that there is an abnormality involving the urinary tract. Your child may need to fast after midnight or for an appropriate length of time before the procedure. Prior to the IVP, your child will have a contrast material injected into the bloodstream through an IV. The X-rays are taken as the contrast material is collected and excreted by the kidneys. The process usually takes about an hour. Children with an allergy to iodine should not have this test. You should be allowed to stay with your child while the IVP is being performed.

Magnetic resonance imaging (MRI)

MRI uses a magnetic field to create two-dimensional images of a cross section of an internal organ. Before the procedure begins, your child may have to remove some items of clothing or jewelry that may interfere with the MRI. Sometimes your child will be asked to wear a hospital gown. Your child may need to receive a liquid dye, called a contrast agent, prior to or during the scan. The child lies on a platform that slides into a long tube. Inside the tube is a donut-shaped magnet. A special device, called a surface coil, is then placed around the area of the body that is to be imaged, and then it is positioned inside the MRI.

> During the first year of getting scans, Cassandra (age five) would have to be anesthetized to have the MRI done, since it scared her to be in that tube for so long. It was difficult for her to come out of the anesthesia and she would be crabby for the rest of the day. One day she decided, at my prodding, that she would try to do it without being asleep if I would stay with her and hold her hand. She has done it this way ever since. She listens to music and usually falls asleep, while I am stretched out, holding her hand inside the tube for up to an hour. To celebrate having the scans finished, Cassandra and I go shopping for something special afterwards— for awhile it was different colored Converse high tops. On those evenings, my husband, the girls, and I go out for a special dinner to celebrate the cancer still being gone!

The technologist does not stay in the room while the MRI is being performed. The MRI machine will make a loud knocking noise as the images are being taken. Your child may need to wear special ear plugs to help block out this sound. Young children, or any child with a fear of closed-in spaces (claustrophobia), may need to be sedated for the MRI procedure.

MIBG

Children who have neuroblastoma may require a special nuclear medicine scan called 131 I-meta-iodobenzylguanidine, which is also referred to as MIBG. Your child will be injected with radioactive material 48 hours prior to having the scan. MIBG accumulates in neuroblastoma cells, which then appear on the scan as a "hot spot." Usually, the day prior to the injection, and for three to five days after, she will need to take an oral medication, called potassium iodide, to protect her thyroid gland.

During the scan, the technician will place your child on a scanning bed, and two special cameras, one above and one below the bed, take images from head to foot. You should be permitted to stay with your child during this procedure. MIBG scans usually take much longer than other imaging techniques, and the child must remain very still during the procedure. Some young children will need to be sedated while the test is being done.

> One of the scans that Matthew disliked most of all was the MIBG scan. Not because there was anything painful involved, but because he found it to be so incredibly boring. He knew if we were making a visit to nuclear medicine for that particular test, it meant spending the next few hours lying motionless on the scanning bed. Fortunately, Matthew developed a very good relationship with the technicians who performed the procedure. They were wonderful to him, and he came to love them all very much. It certainly made things a lot easier for both of us. In the many times he required an MIBG scan, he never once needed to be sedated—very impressive for a child diagnosed at the age of three with neuroblastoma. I think this was because of his attitude and because of how he was treated by the technicians.

Parents often notice obvious hot spots during the MIBG scan. It is important to bear in mind that MIBG is excreted in the urine, and rare false positive results can appear in the groin area (for example, urine-soaked diapers or underwear). False positive results are also possible if the radiopharmaceutical leaks around the central line or IV used for injection of the material.

MUGA scan

A multiple-gated acquisition (MUGA) scan tests cardiac function. Prior to having a MUGA scan, children are sometimes given a sedative to help them relax and stay perfectly still for the fifteen to twenty minute test. An injection of red cells or proteins tagged with a mildly radioactive substance (called technetium) is given through an IV. The child lies on a table with a large movable camera above. This special camera records sequential images of the technetium as it moves through the heart. These pictures of the heart's function allow doctors to determine how efficiently the heart muscle is pumping and if any damage to the heart has occurred.

> My three-year-old daughter had a MUGA scan before she received any chemotherapy. They gave her an injection, and she fell asleep. They

laid her on her back on a big table and moved a huge contraption around
her to take pictures of her heart beating. We watched on a screen, and
they printed out a copy on paper for the doctors.

If either the echocardiogram or MUGA scan show heart damage, the oncologist may reduce the dosage or remove the drug causing the damage from the child's protocol.

Needle aspiration biopsy

Needle aspiration biopsies are sometimes used to obtain a sample of cells from a mass of unknown origin. Prior to the biopsy, children need to fast for several hours. The doctor will first use ultrasound, CT, or fluoroscopy images to determine the exact location to be biopsied. Once your child has been anesthetized, a needle is guided into the mass and a sample is removed. The sample is then sent to a pathologist who will view the cells under a microscope. Your child will need to stay in bed for the next several hours with vital signs closely monitored to ensure there is no bleeding.

> *Eric (age sixteen) had a fine-needle biopsy of some lesions appearing*
> *on his brain. His oncologist thought that his osteosarcoma had metasta-*
> *sized. I was with him as he was sedated in the CT room, standing right*
> *beside him, holding his hand when he fell asleep. I saw the medication*
> *being injected and knew it was coming, although Eric didn't. Since his*
> *Port-a-cath was already accessed, it was easy to put him to sleep with IV*
> *drugs. The biopsy was guided by the CT pictures and a metal frame*
> *which had been "screwed" into his skull. Because of the sedation, Eric*
> *didn't feel any pain.*

Platelet transfusions

Platelets are an important component of the blood. They help form clots and stop bleeding by repairing breaks in the walls of blood vessels. A normal platelet count for a healthy child is 150,000/mm^3 to 420,000/ mm^3. Chemotherapy severely depresses the platelet count for most children. If a transfusion is not given, uncontrollable bleeding can result. Many centers require a transfusion when the child's platelet count goes below 10,000 to 20,000/ mm^3, and sometimes repeat transfusions are required every two or three days until the marrow recovers.

> *Justin had a platelet reaction which caused profuse sweating and dif-*
> *ficulty breathing. They stopped the transfusion immediately, and he got*
> *over it.*

· · · · ·

> *Three-year-old Matthew had countless platelet transfusions, and*
> *only once did he have a reaction. It was an awful thing to watch, but the*
> *nurse that was monitoring him was very calm and professional, which*
> *helped both of us. Matthew was always premedicated for his platelet*
> *transfusions with Benadryl, which made him very drowsy. Most often he*
> *would sleep through the entire transfusion.*

Infections transmitted by platelets are identical to those of other blood products: hepatitis, cytomegalovirus, and HIV (the virus that causes AIDS). The
chance of contracting these infections is very small. Because uncontrollable
bleeding can be life threatening, prevention is paramount.

Pulmonary function test

Some of the chemotherapy drugs that children receive can damage the
lungs. Your child's doctor may order a pulmonary function test to evaluate
her respiratory status. The basic pulmonary function test is called a spiro-
gram. Your child will be asked to blow into the machine, which will measure the air that is being inhaled and exhaled. The respiratory technician
who administers the test will coach and instruct your child throughout the
procedure to ensure that she is giving her maximum effort. The test will be
administered at least three times to ensure that the results are reliable. You
should be permitted to stay with your child while this test is being performed.

> *Our son didn't like having pulmonary function tests. On the outside,*
> *it looks so simple. But blowing into the spirogram was hard for him. He*
> *was usually a little tired after the test was complete. We would always*
> *make a trip to the hospital gift shop afterwards, because we felt he*
> *deserved a special treat for working so hard.*

Spinal tap (lumbar puncture or LP)

Due to the blood-brain barrier, systemic chemotherapy sometimes cannot
destroy cancer cells present in the central nervous system (brain and spinal

cord). Chemotherapy drugs may then have to be directly injected into the cerebrospinal fluid in order to kill any cancer cells present. For certain diseases, spinal taps are used to monitor response to treatment.

Some hospitals routinely sedate children for spinal taps, and others do not. If the child is not sedated, EMLA cream is usually prescribed. This anesthetic cream is applied to the spinal tap site one to two hours prior to the procedure to anesthetize deep into the tissue and prevent some or all of the pain associated with the procedure. For more information about EMLA, see "Starting an IV."

To perform a spinal tap, the physician or nurse practitioner will ask the child to lie on her side with her head tucked close to the chest and knees drawn up. A nurse or parent usually helps hold the child in this position. The doctor will feel the designated spot in the lower back, and will swab it with antiseptic several times. The antiseptic feels very cold on the skin. A sterile sheet will drape the area, and the doctor will wear sterile gloves. One or two shots of an anesthetic (usually lidocaine) may be injected into the skin and deeper tissues. This causes a painful stinging or burning sensation that lasts about a minute. If EMLA was used, the doctor may still inject anesthetic into the deep tissues. A few minutes wait is necessary to ensure that the area is fully anesthetized.

> During spinals, Brent listens to rock and roll on his walkman, but he keeps the volume low enough so that he can still hear what is going on. He likes me to lift up the earpiece and tell him when each part of the procedure is finished and what's coming next.

It is essential that the child hold very still for the rest of the procedure. The doctor will push a fine, hollow needle between two vertebrae into the space where cerebrospinal fluid (CSF) is found. The CSF will begin to drip out of the hollow needle into a container. After a small amount is collected, a syringe is attached to the needle in the back and the medicine is slowly injected, causing a sensation of coldness or pressure down the leg. The needle is then removed and the spot bandaged. The CSF is sent to the laboratory to see if any cancer cells are present and to measure glucose and protein. Occasionally, older children and teenagers get severe headaches from spinal taps. These can sometimes be prevented by lying still for up to an hour after the procedure.

Starting an IV

Some children with cancer have a permanent right atrial catheter implanted in their chest within a week after diagnosis (see Chapter 6) to avoid the pain of multiple IV sticks. However, there may be instances when your child will need an intravenous line started, as well.

Many pediatric hospitals have teams of technicians who specialize in starting IVs and drawing blood. The IV technician will generally use a vein in the lower arm or hand. First, a constricting band is put above the site to make the veins larger and easier to see and feel. The vein is felt by the technician, the area is cleaned, and the needle is inserted. Sometimes a needle is left in place and sometimes it is withdrawn leaving only a thin, plastic tube in the vein. The technician will make sure that the needle (or tube) is in the proper place, then cover the site with a clear dressing, and secure it with tape.

Some methods that help when having an IV started are:

- Stay calm. The body reacts to fear by constricting the blood vessels near the skin surface. Small children are usually more calm with a parent present; teenagers may or may not desire privacy. Listening to music, visualizing a tranquil scene (mountains covered with snow, floating in a pool), or using the same technician each time can help.

- Use EMLA cream or Numby Stuff. EMLA—a cream anesthetic—is applied to the skin one to two hours prior to the procedure to prevent pain. In some cases, it can constrict the veins, so experiment to see if it works for your child. Numby Stuff—a needle-free anesthetic—delivers a cream anesthetic through the skin using a mild, low-level electric current. EMLA cream and Numby Stuff are not recommended when giving medications that can burn the skin if leakage occurs (for example, vincristine).

- Keep warm. Cold temperatures cause the surface blood vessels to constrict. Wrapping your child in a blanket and putting a hot water bottle on the arm can enlarge the veins.

- Drink lots of fluids. Dehydration decreases the fluid in the veins, so encourage lots of drinking.

- Let gravity help. If your child is lying in bed, have her hang her arm down over the side to increase the size of the vessels in the arm and hand.

- **Let your child be in control.** If your child has a preference, let him pick the arm to be stuck. If he is a veteran of many IVs, let him point out the best vein. Good technicians know that patients are quite aware of their best bet for a good vein.

- **Stop if problems develop.** The art of treating children is spending lots of time on preparation and not much time on procedures. If a conflict arises between your child and technician, take a time-out and regroup. Children can be remarkably cooperative if their needs are respected and they are given some control over the situation.

> *You'll think I'm crazy, but I'll tell you this story anyway. After getting stuck constantly for a year, my daughter (five years old) lost it one day when she needed an IV. She started screaming and crying, just flew into a rage. I told the tech, "Let's let her calm down. Why don't you stick me for a change?" She was a sport and started a line in my arm. I told my daughter that I had forgotten how much it hurt and I could understand why she was upset. I told her to let us know when she was ready. She just walked over and held out her arm.*

Subcutaneous injections

Some children require medications given by subcutaneous injection during their treatment. For example, Neupogen (G-CSF) a colony-stimulating factor that is often used to boost the white blood cell count, is usually given by subcutaneous injection.

To minimize pain caused by subcutaneous injections, apply EMLA cream one to two hours before administration. Parents can also reduce pain by rubbing ice over the site to numb the area prior to injection.

> *We always used EMLA cream before our son needed a subcutaneous injection. I think part of the benefit to him was pharmacological, and part of it was psychological. He just seemed to be more at ease with the injections when he knew the EMLA was applied a few hours before the needle was given.*

Taking pills

Over the course of your child's treatment for cancer, it will be necessary to administer pills and/or liquid medications on a regular basis. When giving oral medications, it is essential to get off to a good start and establish cooperation early. In the following suggestions from veteran parents, you may find one technique that works well for your child.

> To teach Brent (six years old) to swallow pills, when we were eating corn for dinner I encouraged him to swallow one kernel whole. Luckily, it went right down and he got over his fear of pills.

. . . . .

> I wanted Katy (three years old) to feel like we were a team right from the first night. So I made a big deal out of tasting each of her medications and pronouncing it good. Thank goodness I did because the pill was nauseating—bitter, metallic, with a lingering aftertaste. I asked the nurse for some small gel caps, and packed them with the pills which I had broken in half. I gave Katy her choice of drinks to take her pills with and taught her to swallow gel caps with a large sip of liquid.

Gel caps come in many sizes. Number 4s are small enough for a three or four year old to swallow. Many pills can be chewed or swallowed whole without taste problems. Just remember that children develop different taste preferences and aversions to medications, and gel caps are useful for any medication that bothers them.

> After much trial and error with medications, Meagan's method became chewing up pills with chocolate chips. She's kept this up for the long haul.

. . . . .

> I always give choices such as, "Do you want the white pill or the six yellow pills first?" It gives her a little control in her chaotic world.

For younger children, many parents crush the pills in a small amount of pudding, applesauce, jam, frozen juice concentrate, or other favorite food.

> Jeremy was four when he was diagnosed, and we used to crush up the pills and mix them with ice cream. This worked well for us.

. . . . .

> Carrie Beth was two when diagnosed. She hated the taste of the pills, so I would submerge them in teaspoonfuls of pure maple syrup. The next year when she just decided she didn't want to cooperate about taking pills, I'd say to her and her two older sisters, "Strawberry gum for everybody

as soon as Carrie Beth finishes her pills." Then I would leave, and the
older kids encouraged her to swallow the pills.

Some children receiving cancer treatment take SMZ-TMP (sulfamethoxazole and trimethoprim), Bactrim, or Septra two to three times a week to prevent pneumonia. It comes in liquid or pill form, and is produced by several different manufacturers. Ask your pharmacist for a kid taste test. Letting your child choose a medicine that appeals to him encourages compliance.

Whenever my son had to take a liquid medicine, such as antibiotics,
he enjoyed taking it from a syringe. I would draw up the proper amount,
then he would put it in his mouth and push the plunger.

Issues for teenagers about taking pills are completely different from those of young children. The problems with teens revolve around autonomy, control, and feelings of invulnerability. It is normal for teenagers to be noncompliant. Teenagers cannot be forced to take pills if they choose to not cooperate. Trying to coerce teens fuels conflict and tends to frustrate everyone. If you need help, ask for an assessment by the psychosocial team at the hospital to work out a plan for adherence to treatment. Everyone will need to be flexible to reach a favorable outcome.

I think the main problem with teens is making sure that they take the
meds. Joel (fifteen years old) has been very responsible about taking his
nightly pills. I've tried to make it easy for him by having an index card for
the week and he marks off the med as he takes it. I also put the meds on a
dry erase board on the fridge as a reminder. As he takes the med, he
erases it. That way it's easy for him (and me) to see at a glance if he's
taken his stuff. The index card alone wasn't working because he couldn't
find a pen or forgot to mark it off.

One of the biggest concerns with teens is noncompliance. I think it's a
delicate balancing act to allow the teen to be responsible for taking his
own meds and yet have some supervision of the process. Our meds are
kept in a small plastic basket on the kitchen counter. All meds are taken
there. I'd never want him to keep his meds in his room where I would
have no idea if he had taken them or not.

Taking a temperature

During the period in which a child is treated for cancer, fever becomes an enemy because it is often the first sign of infection. Parents take hundreds of temperatures, especially when their child is not feeling well. Temperatures can be taken under the tongue, under the arm, or in the ear using a special type of thermometer. Rectal temperatures are not recommended due to the risk of tears and infection. Here are a few suggestions that might help, especially when blood counts are depressed.

- Use a glass thermometer under the tongue.

- Digital thermometers can be purchased at any drug store. Some have an alarm that beeps when it is time to remove the thermometer.

    We bought a digital thermometer that we only use under his arm. It has worked well for us.

- Tympanic thermometers measure infrared waves and are very easy to use.

    When my in-laws asked at diagnosis if there was anything that we needed, I asked them to try to buy a tympanic (ear) thermometer. The device cost over a hundred dollars then, but it worked beautifully. It takes only one second to obtain a temperature. You can even use it when she is asleep without waking her. They are now sold at pharmacies and drug stores, and cost much less.

Before you leave the hospital, you should know when to call the clinic because of fever. Usually, parents are told not to give any medication for fever and to call if the fever goes above 101°F (38.5°C). This allows the doctors to make a judgment on whether it is an infection that requires treatment. It is especially important for parents of children with implanted catheters to know when to call the clinic, as an untreated infection can be life-threatening.

Ultrasound imaging

Ultrasound provides the doctor with a quick and radiation-free tool for imaging internal organs. The ultrasound involves placing a small device called a transducer against the skin of the child in the area that needs to be examined. The transducer sends inaudible sound waves into the body, which bounce off the internal organ being imaged and return to the transducer. The ultrasound machine uses these sound waves to form an image of the organ.

Before the procedure begins, your child may have to remove some items of clothing or jewelry that could interfere with the ultrasound. Sometimes your child will be asked to wear a hospital gown. The technologist will position your child on the examination table, and a clear gel will be applied to the area to be imaged. The technologist will move the transducer over the surface of the skin while the child remains still and relaxed. After the images have been taken, you may need to wait until the pictures are reviewed before you can leave the department.

Urine specimens

Chemotherapy requires frequent urine specimens. One way to help obtain a sample is to encourage lots of drinking the hour before or ask the nurse to increase the drip rate on the IV. Explain to your child why the test is necessary. Ask the nurse to show how the dip sticks work (they change color, so they are quite popular with preschoolers). Use a "hat" under the toilet seat. This is a shallow plastic bucket that fits under the seat and catches the urine.

> Turn on the water while the child sits on the toilet. I don't know why it works, but it does.

As all parents learn, eating and elimination are areas that the child controls. If she just can't or won't urinate in the hat, go out, buy her the largest drink you can find, and wait.

> Meagan is scheduled to go off therapy this May. She's doing well, and is very happy. A father at our support group was reminding a new set of parents to remember to view life from the child's perspective; he said that, especially with little ones, parents sometimes agonize more than the child. He said that at the end of the first year of treatment he and his wife were reflecting on how much misery their child had endured, and then she piped up and said, "This has been a great year for me!" Meagan is the same. When I have bad days and get preoccupied with the uncertain future, I see Meagan skipping along and saying as she frequently does, "I'm such a happy girl."

CHAPTER 3

Family and Friends

Shared joy is double joy, shared sorrow is
half sorrow.

—Swedish proverb

THE INTERACTIONS BETWEEN the parents of a child with cancer and their extended family and friends are complex. Potential exists for loving support and generous help, as well as for bitter disappointment and disputes. The diagnosis of cancer creates a ripple effect first touching the immediate family, then extended family, friends, coworkers, schoolmates, church members, and the entire community. Parents are usually surprised at the diversity of coping abilities exhibited by relatives and friends.

This chapter discusses some of the experiences the family might encounter, as well as scores of ideas for helpful things that family and friends can do. To prevent possible misunderstandings between family members and friends, veteran parents also share ideas on things that do not help.

The extended family

Extended family—aunts, uncles, cousins, grandparents—can cushion the shock of a cancer diagnosis by loving words and actions. Extended family members sometimes drop their own lives to rush to the side of the child with cancer, and often remain steadfast for the years of treatment. Regrettably, family members may not be helpful, either from ignorance of what is helpful or simply because they are overwhelmed by events in their own lives. The following sections explore how some families notified extended family members, kept the lines of communication open, and dealt with grandparents.

Notifying the family

Notifying relatives is one of the first painful jobs for the parent of a child diagnosed with cancer. In times of crisis, family is refuge, and the news is usually quickly shared. Here are some ways parents have told their relatives:

I called my sister and asked her to take care of telling everyone. She called my other sister, and together they told my frail mother.

. . . . .

I don't know if I will ever be able to completely forgive myself for the unbelievably cruel way I told my mother that Matthew had cancer. We were in-patient at the time, and she had been with me all day helping to provide care. When the doctor asked to see me in another room, I left Matthew in terrible pain lying in her arms. Since we were just in the next room, she could hear my screams when the doctor said it was cancer. But because she was holding Matthew, she couldn't come to find out what was wrong. All she could do was sit there holding him, listening to my screams. I remember walking back into his room, where she sat with a look of terror on her face. I told her that Matthew had been diagnosed with cancer, and that I didn't want her falling apart in front of him. And then I left the room to scream some more. I can only imagine the hurt she was feeling at that moment.

Paradoxically, the family members who may provide the greatest support may also be sources of added stress. Some extended families and even entire communities rally around the stricken family, while support never materializes for others. Several factors affect the strength of support: well-established community ties, good communication within extended family, physical proximity to extended family, and clear exchange of information on needs of the affected family. If any of these elements are missing, support may evaporate.

We had just moved 3,000 miles away from family and friends for my husband to accept a new job. So each family member and some close friends used their vacation time to fly out and take two-week shifts at our new house to help out.

Some families have support throughout treatment.

Shortly after Jesse relapsed, I was praying with my Bible study group. With four children aged one to nine, I just didn't know how we would manage with one parent 100 miles away at the hospital and one parent working. The group decided to collect enough money to allow my sister to quit her job and move in to take care of the other three children while I was at the hospital with Jesse. She stayed for eight months. It was such a wonderful thing. They didn't even ask us; they just said they would support her financially so that she could care for my children and keep the household running.

Staying in touch

The most important first step for families is to set up clear communication over what truly will help. Sometimes, the child is too sick or too fatigued for company, and this needs to be expressed. Establishing a telephone chain is a good way to keep family informed of the child's progress. One family member can be delegated as communicator, and this person will relay the information to another person who will then phone another. Some families leave updates on their telephone answering machines. When visits are welcome, make them brief and cheerful. Not only do long visits distress sick children, but they can also overtax a tired parent.

There were many days I wanted to hide in bed and pull the covers over my head. I know everyone was well meaning and genuinely cared, but the constant stream of people through the house and phone ringing added to the stress we were already under. We already had a home care nurse coming five days a week, a physical therapist coming three days a week, in addition to constant phone calls to follow up on blood work and tests, appointments to schedule, and family members to keep track of. Bubba, our dog, loved all the commotion, but the rest of us tired quickly.

Helpful things for family to do

Families differ in what is truly helpful for them. The suggestions in this chapter are snapshots of what some families appreciated. True listening and working on maintaining the relationship is paramount. Connections can be made in many different, unique, and personally meaningful ways:

- Be sensitive to the emotional state of both child and parent. Sometimes parents want to talk about the cancer; sometimes they just need a hand to hold.

- Encourage all members of the family to keep in touch through visits, calls, mail, videotapes, audiotapes, or pictures.

- Be understanding if the parents do not want phone calls in the hospital. Remember that the child can hear all phone conversations when parents talk on the phone in the room.

> *The first three days in the hospital I spent much of my time crying on the phone when talking to friends and relatives. Then I realized how frightening this must be to my two-year-old. So I just took the phone off the hook and left it there. Now, each time Jennifer is hospitalized, I call one friend and have her spread the news, then I take the phone off the hook again and concentrate on my daughter.*

- A cheerful hospital room really boosts a child's spirits. Encourage sending balloon bouquets, funny cards, posters, toys, or humorous books. Be aware that some hospitals do not allow rubber balloons, only mylar. Rubber balloons can be a choking hazard. Flowers are also not allowed in children's rooms since they can increase risk of infection.

> *We plastered the walls with pictures of family and friends and so many people sent balloons that the ceiling was covered. It was a lovely sight.*

- Laughter helps heal the mind and body, so send funny videotapes or arrive with a good joke if you think it's appropriate.

> *My brother Bill and his wonderful girlfriend Cathy created an exciting "trip" for my four-year-old daughter. She was bald, big-bellied, and her counts were too low to leave the house, but her interest in fashion was as sharp as ever. Bill and Cathy bought ten outfits, rigged up a dressing room, and with Cathy as saleswoman, turned Katy's bedroom into a fashion salon. She tried on outfits, discussed all of their merits and shortcomings, and had a fabulous time. It was a real high point for her.*

- Puzzles, games, picture books, coloring books, age-appropriate computer games, and crafts are welcome. Remember that attention spans are sometimes shortened by treatment, so keep it simple.

A friend who was a nurse came to my son's room shortly before Christmas and brought an entire gingerbread house kit, including confectioner's sugar for the icing. We had a very good time putting it together.

- Offer to give the parent a break from the hospital room. A walk outside, shopping trip, haircut, dinner with a spouse, or just a long shower can be very refreshing.

- Donate frequent flyer miles to distant family members who have the time but not the money to help.

A close friend (who lived three thousand miles away) had just lost her job and wished she could be there for us. My parents gave her their frequent flyer miles. She flew in for three weeks during a hard part of treatment and helped enormously.

- If you don't hear from a family member, call. Often silence means that he doesn't know what to do or say.

Grandparents

Grandparents grieve deeply when a grandchild is diagnosed with cancer. They are concerned not only for their grandchild, but for their own child (the parent) as well. Cancer wreaks havoc with grandparents' expectations, reversing the natural order of life and death. Grandparents frequently say, "Why not me? I'm the one who is old." Parents express anguish at having to tell the grandparents the grim news. Cancer in a grandchild is a major shock to bear.

In researching this book, descriptions of grandparents' reactions tended to fall into two categories: pillars of strength or additional burdens.

Many parents reported that the grandparents responded to the crisis with tremendous emotional, physical, and financial support.

Our parents did a lot of caretaking. They helped with meals, babysitting, cleaning, washing clothes, etc. They also stayed with Jeremy in the hospital when we were not able to.

• • • • •

My mother was a rock. She put her busy life on hold to come help. She took care of the baby and kept the household running when I was living at the hospital with my very ill daughter. She was strong, and it gave me strength.

Some parents express tremendous gratitude for the role played by the grandparents in providing much-needed stability to the family rocked by cancer. Caring for the siblings and running the household allow the parents to care for the sick child and return to work.

> We were very fortunate when Sean (age three) was diagnosed with neuroblastoma, because my parents live just twenty minutes from my house. Although it was difficult for them, they were extremely supportive and we included them in the discussions with the oncologist. While my parents didn't have any answers for us, they did help to keep us grounded. When Sean had his bone marrow transplant, my mom was able to take six weeks off work to help out. She would stay with Sean in the hospital so I could work part-time.

> Two years after Sean was diagnosed he suffered a relapse. By this time, my dad had retired and was able to help by taking Sean to his chemotherapy treatments twice a week. Not only was this a big help to me, but it provided some very special bonding time for Sean and his grandfather. I don't know how we could have gotten through without the help of my parents.

Other families are not so fortunate. Many grandparents are too old, too ill, or simply unable to cope with a crisis of this magnitude. Some simply fall apart.

> My mother became hysterical when my daughter was diagnosed. She called every day, sobbing. Luckily, she lived far away and this minimized the disruption. We had to ask her not to come because we couldn't handle the catastrophe at home and her neediness too. It hurt her feelings, but we just couldn't cope with it.

Other grandparents allow pre-existing problems with their adult child to color their perceptions of what the family needs. Sometimes cancer allows grandparents to renew criticism of the way grandchildren are being raised:

> While we stayed at the hospital the grandparents moved into our house to care for our eight-year-old daughter. They decided that this was their chance to "whip her into shape, teach her some manners, and get her room cleaned up." Our daughter was in tears, and we ended up saying, "We appreciate your help, but we will take over."

Sometimes grandparents try to blame the parents for the cancer or make other kinds of hurtful comments. Disagreements can also arise if grandparents try to take charge. Criticizing parents' choice of doctors, hospitals, or treatment can be very disruptive and further stress the family's resources. Some grandparents simply cannot cope and withdraw from the situation.

> I will never, ever be able to forget how my mother let me and my son down. She never came to the hospital, saying, "He's too sick for company." I told her he would love to see her, that his little face just would light up when he had visitors. But she never came. She never offered to help at home when he was so ill. She just disappeared.

It is hard to predict how anyone will react to the diagnosis of childhood cancer. Grandparents are no exception. Some respond with the wisdom gleaned from decades of living, others become needy, and some withdraw. It is natural in a time of grave crisis to look to your parents for support and help, but it is important to remember that grandparents' ability to respond also depends on events in their own lives. If problems develop, help can be obtained from hospital social workers or through individual counseling.

Friends

Like family, friends can cushion the shock of diagnosis and ease the difficulties of treatment with their words and actions.

> Brenda had been my best friend since we were both little girls. After we received the diagnosis, she continued to be there for me in every way possible. She was willing to listen when I was angry at the world, to cry with me if I needed a good cry, to give me space when she knew I needed to be alone with my thoughts, and she was comfortable with the silence when I didn't feel like talking at all. She will always be my best friend.

Notifying friends

The easiest way to notify friends is to delegate one person to do the job. Calling and asking one neighbor or close friend to do this prevents numerous tearful conversations. Most parents are at their child's bedside and want to avoid more emotional upheaval, especially in front of the child. Parents need to recognize that friends' emotions will mirror their own shock, fear, worry, or helplessness. Since most friends want to help but don't know what to do or say, giving cues of what would be helpful are welcome.

> *I wish that I had designated an intermediary to relay information between me and the rest of the world. As it was, I had to repeat information about Elizabeth's condition over and over again every day. By the end of the day, I would be exhausted and near hysteria all over again. If I had one person that I could relay information to, and they in turn would tell everyone else, I think I would have been a lot stronger emotionally and everyone else would have been assured of getting all of the information that was available.*

Helpful things for friends to do

It is a given that the family of a newly diagnosed child is overwhelmed. The list of helpful things to do is endless, but here are some suggestions from veteran parents.

Household

- Provide meals.

> *One of the nicest things that friends did was to bring us a huge picnic basket full of food to the hospital. We spread a blanket on the floor, Erica crawled out of bed, and the entire family sat down together and ate. Most people don't realize how expensive it is to have to eat every meal at the hospital cafeteria, so the picnic was not only fun, but helped us to save a few dollars.*

- Take care of pets or livestock.
- Mow grass, shovel snow, rake leaves, weed gardens.

> *We came home from the hospital one evening right before Christmas, and found a freshly cut, fragrant Christmas tree leaning next to our door. I'll never forget that kindness.*

- Clean house.

> *My husband's cousin sent her cleaning lady over to our house. It was so neat and such a luxury to come home to find the stove and windows sparkling clean.*

- Grocery shop (especially when the family is due home from the hospital).
- Do laundry or drop off and pick up dry cleaning.
- Provide a place to stay near the hospital.

One of the ladies from the school where I worked came up to the ICU waiting room where we were sleeping and pressed her house key into my hand. She lived five minutes from the hospital. She said, "My basement is made up, there's a futon, there's a TV, you are coming and staying at my house." I hardly knew her, but we accepted. Every day when we came in from the hospital, there was some cute little treat waiting for us like a bowl of cookies, or two packages of hot chocolate and a thermos of hot milk.

Siblings

- Babysit whenever parents go to clinic, emergency room, or for a prolonged hospital stay.
- When parents are home with a sick child, take sibling(s) to the park, sports event, or a movie.
- Invite sibling(s) over for meals.
- If you bring a gift for the sick child, bring something for the sibling(s), too.

Friends from home sent boxes of art supplies to us when the whole family spent those first ten weeks at a Ronald McDonald house far from our home. They sent scissors, paints, paper, colored pens. It was a great help for Carrie Beth and her two sisters. One friend even sent an Easter package with straw hats for each girl, and flowers, ribbons, and glue to decorate them with.

- Offer to help sibling(s) with homework.
- Drive sibling(s) to lessons, games, or school.
- Listen to how they are feeling and coping. Siblings' lives have been shattered, they have limited time with their parents, and they need support and care.

Psychological support

- Call frequently, and be open to listening if the parents want to talk about their feelings.

   What I wished for most was that friends and family had been able to call more often to see how we were doing; that someone could have handled my confidence on the good days and my tears on the bad days. It somehow took too much emotional energy to make a call myself, but I valued any phone call I received.

- Call to talk about topics that are not related to cancer.

- If one parent had to leave work to stay in the hospital with the sick child, co-workers can send messages by mail or tape.

   One very neat thing that was an emotional boost was that my friends and former co-workers from Kansas faxed us messages and pictures and things to Meagan while we were in the hospital. It was very nice to get such fresh messages—it really shortened the miles.

- If you think the family might be interested, call Candlelighters, the American Cancer Society, or the social worker at the local hospital to find out if there are support groups for parents and/or kids in your area.

- Offer to take the children to the support groups, or go with the parents. For most families, the parent support group becomes a second family with ties of shared experience as deep and strong as blood relations.

- Drive parents and child to clinic visits.

- Buy books (uplifting ones) for the family if they are readers.

- Send cards or letters.

   Word got around my parents' hometown, and I received cards from many high school acquaintances, who still cared enough to call or write and say we're praying for you, please let us know how things are going. It was so neat to get so many cards out of the blue that said, "I'm thinking about you."

- Babysit the sick child so that the parents can go out to eat, exercise, take a walk, or just get out of the hospital or house.

- Ask parents if you could enroll them in Candlelighters and other helpful organizations.

- Donate blood. Your blood will not be used specifically for the ill child, but will replenish the general supply, which is depleted by children with cancer.

- Send the family a gift certificate for professional photographs.

My daughter wanted her picture taken several months into treatment. She was bald, sick, and frightened of strangers. I called Donnette Studio, asked to speak to the photographer who was best with kids, and explained the situation. I told him that how the pictures looked didn't matter, I wanted it to be a fun experience. He scheduled one and one half hours for the appointment, and he played with her the majority of that time. They did puppets, chased each other around, and just had a ball. She had a glorious smile on her face for the pictures, and we go back every six months to see Donny.

- Ask "What needs to be done?" and then do it.

A close friend called and asked what she could do. So I asked if she could drive our second car the 100 miles to the hospital so that my husband could return in it to work. She came with her family to the Ronald McDonald House with two big bags containing the following: snack foods, a large box of stationery, envelopes, stamps, books to read, a book handmade by her three-year-old daughter containing dozens of cut-out pictures of children's clothing pasted on construction paper (which my daughter adored looking at), and a beautiful, new, handmade, lace-trimmed dress for my daughter. It was full length and baggy enough to cover all bandages and tubing. She wore it almost every day for a year. It was a wonderful thing for my friend to do.

- Give lots of hugs.

Grandpa Fred is a 71-year-old retiree who has been visiting pediatric oncology patients at Children's for almost twelve years. He begins his day at 9:30 every morning on the teens ward, then he moves on to visit the younger patients, the playroom, and the clinic. Grandpa Fred always takes pictures of his young friends, very good ones, and has filled twenty-three photo albums with them. Fred has two prints made of each picture he takes and gives one to the families. He also helps Santa on Christmas and visits on Halloween. He has been the camp manager at Camp Good

Times every summer for eight years. Fred feels that a hug is more impor-
tant than anything he can say to someone. "Listening and giving a hug,"
he says, "that's the best I can do."

Financial support

Helping families avoid financial disaster can be the next greatest gift after the life of the child and the strength of the family. It is estimated that even fully insured families spend 25 percent or more of their income on co-payments, travel, motels, meals, and other uncovered items. Uninsured or under-insured families may lose their savings or even their house. Even families with full health insurance, such as those in Canada, have additional expenses that are not covered. Most families need financial help. Here are some suggestions:

- Start a support fund.

    A friend of mine called and asked very tentatively if we would mind if she started a support fund. We felt awkward, but we needed help, so we said okay. She did everything herself, and the money she raised was very, very helpful. We did ask her to stop the fund when people started calling us to ask if they could use giving to the fund as an advertisement for their business.

- Share leave. Governments and some companies have leave banks that permit persons who are ill or taking care of someone who is ill to use other co-workers' leave so they won't have their pay docked.

    My husband's co-workers didn't collect money, they did something even more valuable. They donated sick leave hours, so that he was able to be at the hospital frequently during those first few months without losing a paycheck.

- Job share. Some families work out job-share arrangements in which a co-worker donates time to perform part of one job to enable one parent to spend time at the hospital. Job sharing allows the job to get done, keeps peace at the job site, and prevents financial losses for the family. Another possibility would be for one or more friends with similar skills (e.g., word processing, filing, sales, etc.) to rotate through the job on a volunteer basis to cover for the parent of the ill child.

- Collect money at church or work to give informally.

The day my daughter was diagnosed, my husband's co-workers passed the hat and gave us over $250. I was embarrassed, but it paid for gas, meals, and the motel until there was an opening in the Ronald McDonald House.

• • • • •

Finances were a main concern for us because I wanted to cut back on work to be at home with Meagan. Sometimes my co-workers would pool money and present it with a card saying, "Here's a couple of days' work that you won't have to worry about."

• Collect money by organizing a bake sale, dance, or raffle.

Co-workers of my husband held a Halloween party for us and charged admission. We were very uncomfortable with the idea at first, but they were looking for an excuse to have a party, and it helped us out.

• Keeping track of medical bills is time-consuming, frustrating, and exhausting. If you are a close relative or friend, you could offer to review, organize, and file (or enter into a computer) the voluminous paperwork. Making the calls and writing the letters over contested claims or errors in billing are very helpful.

Help from schoolmates

• Encourage visits (if appropriate), cards, and phone calls from classmates.
• Ask the teacher to send the school newspaper and other news along with assignments.
• Classmates can sign a brightly colored banner to send to the hospital.

Brent's kindergarten class sent a packet containing a picture drawn for him by each child in the class. They also made him a book. Another time they sent him a letter written on huge poster board. He couldn't wait to get back to school.

• • • • •

Leeann's elementary school was very understanding and helpful. She had been in a program for gifted children after spending her first three years at the school in a mainstream program. I had done extensive volunteer work at the school in the classroom and on the PTA, so we had established a presence where a lot of people knew us. A good friend pulled together a fundraiser at the school in addition to bringing food by the house and many offers of help with Leeann's brothers.

Religious support

- If the family goes to church, contact the clergy.
- Arrange for the pastor, rabbi, priest, or church members to visit the hospital, if that is what the family wants.
- Arrange prayer services for the sick child and the family.
- Have the child's Sunday school class (or whatever class is appropriate for the family's denomination) send pictures, posters, letters, balloons, or tapes to the sick child.

> The day our son was diagnosed, we raced next door to ask our wonderful neighbors to take care of our dog. The news of his diagnosis quickly spread, and we found out later that five neighborhood families gathered that very night to pray for Brent.

Accepting help

One father's thoughts on accepting help:

> I had always been considered the provider in our family. I think I did a very good job with that, too. But nothing prepared me for the nightmare that Matthew's cancer brought into our lives. It took me some time to realize it, but I came to the conclusion that it was impossible for me to do this on my own.

One mother's thoughts on accepting help:

> The most important advice I received as the parent of a child newly diagnosed with cancer came from a hospital nurse whom I turned to when I was overwhelmed with all the advice being offered by family and friends. This wise nurse said, "Don't discount anything. You're going to need all the help you can get." I think it is very important for families to remain open and accept the help that is offered. It often comes when least expected and from unlikely sources. I was totally unprepared at diagnosis for how much help I would need, and I'm glad that I remained open to offers of kindness. This is not the time to show the world how strong you are.

What to say

The following are some suggestions for family and friends on what to say and how to offer help. Of course, much depends on the type of relationship that already exists, but a specific offer can always be accepted or graciously declined.

• I am so sorry.

• I didn't call earlier because I didn't know what to say.

• Our family would like do your yardwork. It will make us feel as if we are helping in a small way.

• We want to clean your house for you once a week. What day would be convenient?

• Would it help if we took care of your dog (or cat, or bird)? We would love to do it.

• I walk my dog three times a day. May I walk yours, too?

• The church is setting up a system to deliver meals to your house. When is the best time to drop them off?

• I will take care of Jimmy whenever you need to take John to the hospital. Call us anytime, day or night, and we will come pick him up.

Things that do not help

Out of ignorance, people sometimes say hurtful things to parents of children with cancer. If you are a family member or friend of a parent in this situation, please do not say any of the following:

• "God only gives people what they can handle." (Some people cannot handle the stress of childhood cancer.)

• "I know just how you feel." (Unless you have a child with cancer, you simply don't know.)

• "You are so brave," or "so strong," etc. (Parents are not heroes; they are normal people struggling with extraordinary stress.)

• "They are doing such wonderful things to save children with cancer these days." (Yes, the prognosis may be good, but what parents and children are going through is not wonderful.)

- "Well, we're all going to die one day." (True, but parents do not need to be reminded of this fact.)

- "It's God's will." (This is just not a helpful thing to hear.)

- "At least you have other kids," or "Thank goodness you are still young enough to have other children." (A child cannot be replaced.)

> *A woman whom I worked with, but did not know well, came up to me one day and out of the blue said, "When Erica gets to heaven to be with Jesus, He will love her." All I could think to say was, "Well, I'm sorry, but Jesus can't have her right now."*

Parents also make the following suggestions of things to avoid doing:

- Do not say, "Let us know if there is anything we can do." It is far better to make a specific suggestion.

> *Many well-wishing friends always said, "Let me know what I can do." I wish they had just "done," instead of asking for direction. It took too much energy to decide, call them, make arrangements, etc. I wish someone would have said, "When is your clinic day? I'll bring dinner," or "I'll babysit Sunday afternoon so you two can go out to lunch."*

- Do not make personal comments in front of the child: when will his hair grow back in, she's lost so much weight, he's so pale, etc.

- Do not do things that require the parent to support you (for example, repeatedly call up crying).

- Do not talk continually about the cancer; some normal conversations are welcome.

- Do not ask "what if" questions: What if he can't go to school? What if your insurance won't cover it? What if she dies? The present is really all the parents can deal with.

- Stories of children you know who have survived cancer and are doing fine are welcome. Stories of those who have died or who have long-term side effects should not be shared.

Losing friends

It is an unfortunate reality that most parents of children with cancer lose friends. For a variety of reasons, some friends just can't cope and either suddenly disappear or gradually fade away. Many times this can be prevented by calling them to keep them involved, but sometimes, they just can't handle the stress.

> *Except for one good friend, none of my friends called when I was home. It seemed that after the initial three-month crisis, they removed themselves from the situation, as often happens.*

· · · · · ·

> *I had a friend who really thought herself to be empathetic, except that she just couldn't "deal with" hospitals. She said that they made her uncomfortable, so she wouldn't visit. I also got tired of her talking about the silver lining of the dark cloud that has been hanging over my head. I have a really hard time dealing with that.*

· · · · ·

> *Friends? What friends? They disappeared, family, too. No one knew what to say to us.*

Restructuring family life

Childhood cancer does not strike only families with brave children and heroic parents. In the United States, the popular press has responded to people's fear of cancer by churning out story after story of people who faced the diagnosis with almost superhuman hope and strength. Families rally round, the community cheers, and human will triumphs over the evil of cancer. This simply is not always the case. Cancer strikes all types of families: single-parent families, those with two parents in the home, financially secure families, those with no insurance, families with strong community ties, those who have just moved to a new community, families of every size, type, and color. Most parents do find unexpected reserves of strength to deal with the crisis. They survive the years of stress and pain, emerging different and sometimes stronger. Still, expectations of heroism are not appropriate.

Keeping the household functioning

Every family of a child with cancer needs massive assistance. It is important for families to recognize this early and learn not only to accept aid gracefully but also to ask for help when needed. As discussed earlier in the chapter, most family members, friends, neighbors, and church members want to help, but they need direction from the family on what is helpful but not intrusive.

In families where both parents are employed, decisions must be made about the jobs. It is better, if possible, to use all available sick leave and vacation days prior to deciding whether one parent needs to terminate employment. Parents need to be able to evaluate their financial situation and insurance availability. This requires time and clarity of thought, both of which are in short supply in the weeks following diagnosis.

> *I was eight months pregnant when my two-year-old son, Carl, was diagnosed. I went on maternity leave, but we needed to make arrangements quickly with my husband's employer to allow him time off to care for Carl in the hospital after I had the baby. Even worse, I knew I would have to deliver by caesarian section. Carl's protocol required him to be in the hospital for one week, then home for one week from September through January. My husband worked out a schedule in which he worked 70 hours the week Carl was home, then was off work the week Carl was hospitalized. He then only needed to use ten hours of leave, and was able to stay with Carl in the hospital.*

Family and Medical Leave Act

In August 1993, the Family and Medical Leave Act (FMLA) became federal law in the US. FMLA protects job security of workers in large companies who must take a leave of absence to care for a seriously ill immediate family member. It also covers employees who are unable to work because of their own medical condition, as well as when a child is born, adopted, or placed in foster care. The Family and Medical Leave Act:

- Applies to employers with 50 or more employees who work for at least twenty work weeks within a 75-mile radius.

- Provides twelve weeks of unpaid leave during any twelve-month period to care for a seriously ill spouse, child, or parent. In certain instances, the employee may take intermittent leave by reducing his or her normal work schedule's hours or taking leave in blocks of time.

- Requires employer to continue to provide benefits, including health insurance, during the leave period.

- Requires employer to return employee to the same or equivalent position upon return from the leave. Some benefits, such as seniority, need not accrue during periods of unpaid FMLA leave.

- Requires employee to give 30-day notice of the need to take FMLA leave when the need is foreseeable.

- Is enforced by complaints to the Wage and Hour Division, US Department of Labor, or by private lawsuit. The nearest office of the Wage and Hour Division may be located by looking in the US Government pages of your telephone directory.

In Canada, a parent may be entitled to benefits under the Employment Insurance Act. Consideration is provided in the act for a parent having to leave work to provide care for an ill child. Entitlement to benefits is made on a case by case basis. Should a parent qualify, benefits are determined by the number of hours the parent has worked prior to making the claim. For further information, parents should contact the nearest Human Resources Development Canada office listed in the Government of Canada pages of the telephone directory.

Marriage

Cancer treatment places enormous pressure on a marriage. Couples may be separated for long periods of time, emotions are high, and coping styles differ. Initially, family life is shattered. Couples must simply survive the first few overwhelming weeks, then work together to rearrange the pieces in a new pattern. Here are parents' suggestions and stories about how they managed:

- Share medical decisions.

> *My husband and I shared decision-making by keeping a joint medical journal. The days that my husband stayed at the hospital, he would write down all medicines given, side effects, fever, vital signs, food consumed, sleep patterns, and any questions that needed to be asked at the next rounds. This way, I knew exactly what had been happening. Decisions were made as we traded shifts at our son's bedside.*

· · · · ·

> *I made most of the medical decisions. My husband did not know what a protocol was, nor did he ever learn the names of the medicines. He came with me to medical conferences, however, and his presence gave me strength.*

- Take turns staying in the hospital with the ill child.

We took turns going in with our son for painful procedures. The doctors loved to see my husband come in because he's a friendly, easygoing person who never asked them any medical questions. We shared hospital duty, also. I would be there during any crisis because I was the person better able to be a strong advocate, but he went when our son was feeling better and needed entertaining company. It worked out well.

• • • • •

My husband fell apart emotionally when our daughter was diagnosed, and he never really recovered. He stayed with her once in the hospital and cried almost the whole time. She never wanted him to go again, so I did all hospital duty.

• • • • •

Whenever Brent was in the hospital, we both wanted to be there. We were able to be there most of the time because our children have a wonderful aunt and uncle who stayed with them when needed. During Brent's second extended stay in the hospital, we both let go a little, and we each took turns sleeping at the Ronald McDonald House. That way we each got a decent night's sleep (or some sleep) every other night.

• • • • •

My wife took care of most of the medical information gathering because she had a scientific background. But my work schedule was more flexible, so I took my son for almost all of his treatments and hospitalizations. I cherish my memories of those long hours in the car and waiting room, because we were always so very close.

- Share responsibility for home care.

My husband worked long hours, and therefore I had to do almost all of the home care. It was very hard on me, especially in the beginning when she was so ill and needed so many medications. I felt like I was doing all the horrible things to her; I wish that he could have done some of it.

• • • • •

We had a traditional relationship in which I took care of the kids and he worked. I didn't expect him to cook or clean when I was staying at the hospital, it was all he could do to ferry our daughter to her various activities and go to work.

*We both worked full time, so we staggered our shifts. He worked 7 to
3, I worked 3 to 11. He did every single dressing change for the Hickman
catheter—584 changes, we counted them up. Wherever I left off during
the day, he took over. He was great, and it really worked out well for us.
We shared it all.*

· · · · ·

*My husband really didn't help at all. I couldn't even go out because
he wouldn't give the pills. He kept saying that he was afraid that he would
make a mistake.*

- Accept differences in coping styles.

*We both coped differently, but we learned to work around it. I didn't
want to deal with "what if" questions, but he was a pessimist and constantly asked the fellow questions about things that might happen. I felt
that it was a waste of energy to worry about things that might never happen. I didn't want to hear it and felt that it just added to my burden. It
was all I could do to survive every day. We worked it out by going to conferences together, but I would ask my questions and then leave. He stayed
behind to ask all of his questions.*

· · · · ·

*My husband didn't have the desire to read as much as I did. How-
ever, whenever I read something that I felt he should read, he always took
the time to do so and then we discussed it.*

· · · · ·

*My husband and I have always been a team. We complement the
strengths and weaknesses of each other and I think that was the reason we
managed to hold everything together. When I was down, he would bring
me up. When he was down, I would do the same for him. With the exception of the initial trauma when our son was diagnosed, we handled things
in that manner throughout treatment.*

- Seek counseling.

*I went for counseling because I couldn't sleep. At night, I got stuck
thinking the same things over and over and worrying. I ended up spending two years on antidepressants, which I think really saved my life. They*

helped me sleep and kept me on an even keel. I'm off them now, my son is off treatment, and everything is looking up.

· · · · ·

My husband and I went to counseling to try to work out a way to split up the child rearing and household duties because I was over-whelmed and resenting it. I guess it helped a little bit, but the best thing that came out of it was that I kept seeing the counselor by myself. My son wanted to go to the "feelings doctor," too. I received a lot of very helpful, practical advice on the many behavior problems my son developed. And my son had an objective, safe person to talk things over with.

Some marriages survive and some don't. It is usually marriages with serious pre-existing problems that are further strained by cancer treatment.

My husband had a lot of problems that really brought my daughter and me down. The cancer really opened my eyes to what was important in life. We stayed together through treatment, but we divorced after the bone marrow transplant. I just realized that life is too short to spend it in a bad relationship.

· · · · ·

My husband went to work rather than with us to Children's when our son was diagnosed. It went downhill from there. He started using drugs and mistreating us, so we divorced.

Siblings

It takes an entire chapter to deal with the complex feelings that siblings confront when their brother or sister has cancer. Chapter 23, *Siblings*, provides an in-depth examination of the issues from the perspective of both siblings and parents.

People can be thoughtless. I think that a lot of people are afraid of upsetting us by talking about cancer and possibly saying the wrong thing. They also feel vulnerable because they suddenly realize it could happen to them. One of the stupidest questions I've ever had asked of me was "How did he get it?" If I knew that, he wouldn't have it! I've been tempted to say, "He has eaten too many Peanut M&Ms!" They don't realize how insensi-

tive they are. When I first told a good friend and neighbor about Evan's tumor, that was the first thing that she said. I needed sympathy and a shoulder to cry on, not a dumb question. Needless to say, there was no support from her, and she never called to ask about Evan after his surgery or during his radiation, which was tough for him. We spent the whole summer 110 miles away from home and family. I understand what was behind the question, fear that her girls would get it, but it still hurt. Her daughter was one of my son's best friends, but after surgery and radiation when he had too much pain to run and play, she wouldn't have anything to do with him. That really hurt him. Now that he can run and play again, she is calling for Evan to play, but Evan refuses. This is what my Nana called a fair-weather friend, and who needs them?

On the other hand, our next-door-neighbors have been wonderful. Their daughter will play with Evan no matter what he's physically capable of, whether it's just watching a movie or riding bikes. Her dad and mom have cut our grass, pulled our weeds, and waged a losing war against the chipmunk eating all my spring bulbs. What a difference with true friends!

CHAPTER 4

Forming a Partnership with the Medical Team

It is our duty as physicians to estimate
probabilities and to discipline expectations;
but leading away from probabilities there are
paths of possibilities, toward which it is our
duty to hold aloft the light, and the
name of that light is hope.

—Karl Menninger
The Vital Balance

IT IS VITALLY IMPORTANT THAT parents and the healthcare team establish and maintain a relationship based on excellent medical care, good communication, and caring. In this partnership, trust is paramount. Unlike many other diseases, children with cancer spend months or years being treated on an inpatient and outpatient basis. Physicians rely on parents to make and keep appointments, give the proper medicines at the appropriate times, prepare the child for procedures, and be vigilant in noticing any illness or drug side effect. Parents rely on physicians for medical knowledge, expertise in performing procedures, good judgment, caring, and clear communication.

A climate of cooperation and respect between the healthcare team and parents allows children to thrive. This chapter will explore ways to create and maintain that environment.

The hospital

After diagnosis, a steady parade of anonymous faces enters the life of a child with cancer. To understand who is responsible for the child's treatment, an explanation of hospital pecking order is necessary.

The doctors

A medical student is a college graduate who is attending medical school. Medical students often wear white coats, but do not have MD after the name on their name tags. They are not doctors.

An intern (also called a first year resident) is a graduate of medical school who is in her first year of postgraduate training.

A resident is a graduate of medical school in his second or third year of postgraduate training. Most of the residents at pediatric hospitals will be pediatricians upon completion of their residencies.

After residency, if the pediatric resident wishes to further specialize in oncology (the study of cancer), he applies for a fellowship in pediatric oncology. Fellows work only at academic centers with fellowship programs, not all pediatric oncology centers. A fellow who treats children with cancer is a doctor who has completed four years of medical school, one year of internship, two to three years of residency in pediatrics, and is taking additional specialty training in pediatric oncology. In the US, pediatric residency is three years. In Canada, it is four years, however, there is no internship.

Above fellows in the hospital hierarchy are attending physicians (called simply "attendings"). These well-established doctors are hired by the medical center to provide and oversee medical care and to train interns, residents, and fellows. They are frequently also professors on the staff of the medical school.

> *Our medical team was wonderful. They always answered our questions and spent the time with us that we needed. We had a group of doctors who were all working together for the patients. I always felt that we were known by each doctor, and that they were on top of Paige's treatment.*

When a child arrives at a teaching hospital, he will be assigned an attending. This physician will provide continuous care throughout treatment. The physician in charge of your child's care should be board certified or have equivalent medical credentials. This means that she has taken rigorous written and oral tests by a board of examiners in her specialty, and meets a high standard of competence. You can call the American Board of Medical Specialties at (800) 776-2378 to find out if your child's physician is board certified.

While an inpatient, your child will see a large number of other doctors. Residents usually rotate to different services every four weeks, so they are an ever-changing group. If questions arise about your child's illness or treatment that the resident cannot answer, you should ask the fellow or attending assigned to your child.

If your family is insured by a health maintenance organization (HMO), you probably will be sent to the affiliated hospital, which will have one or more pediatric oncologists on staff.

The nurses

An essential part of the hospital hierarchy is the nursing staff. The following explanations will help you understand which type of nurse is caring for your child.

An LPN is a licensed practical nurse. LPNs complete a vocational training program and have a narrow scope of practice; for example, they usually do not start IVs or give IV medications.

An RN is a registered nurse who obtained an associate or bachelor's degree in nursing, and then passed a licensing examination. These medical professionals give medicines, take vital signs (heart rate, breathing rate, blood pressure), monitor IV machines, change bandages, and care for patients in hospitals, clinics, and doctors' offices.

> At our hospital, each of our nurses is different, but each is wonderful. They simply love the kids. They throw parties, set up dream trips, act as counselor, best friend, stern parent. They hug moms and dads. They cry. I have come to respect them so much because they have such a hard job to do, and they do it so well.

A nurse practitioner or clinical nurse specialist is a registered nurse who has completed an educational program that has taught her advanced skills. For example, in some hospitals and clinics, nurse practitioners perform procedures such as spinal taps.

The head or charge nurse is the supervisor of all the nurses on the floor for one shift. If you have any problems with a nurse, your first step in resolving them would be to talk to the nurse involved. If this does not work, a discussion with the charge nurse is necessary.

The clinical nurse manager is the administrator for an entire unit such as an oncology floor or oncology clinic. She is in charge of all of the nurses on the unit.

Finding an oncologist

Parents do not have the luxury of time in choosing a pediatric oncologist. At diagnosis, the family is usually referred to the nearest pediatric center of excellence. The young patient may be assigned the fellow or attending who happens to be on call at the time of diagnosis.

During treatment, your child may see myriad doctors. A permanent assignment should be made for all outpatient treatment. Often the assigned oncologist is a good match, and the family finds the doctor competent, caring, and easy to communicate with. If the medical facility allows you to choose your child's oncologist, here are several traits to look for:

- Board certified in the field of pediatric oncology
- Establishes good rapport with child
- Communicates clearly and compassionately
- Skillful in performing procedures
- Answers all questions
- Consults with other doctors on complex problems
- Uses language that is easy to understand
- Makes the results of all tests available
- Willing to let parents participate in the decision-making process
- Respects parents' values
- Able to deliver the truth with hope

If you don't develop a good rapport with the physician assigned to you, ask to be assigned to a different physician whom you have met on rounds or during clinic visits. Most parents are accommodated, for hospitals realize the importance of good communication between family and physician. You will, however, still see different physicians, because many institutions have rotating physicians on call.

Choosing a hospital

At diagnosis, if your family is not initially referred to a specific hospital, or if there are several excellent pediatric hospitals in the area to choose from, it may be necessary to choose where you would like your child to be treated. Parents can obtain a free referral to an accredited center from either the National Cancer Institute, (800) 4-CANCER, or the offices of the Children's Cancer Group, the Pediatric Oncology Group, the National Wilms Tumor Study Group, or the Intergroup Rhabdomyosarcoma Study Group:

Children's Cancer Group
P.O. Box 60012
Arcadia, CA 91066
(626) 447-0064
(800) 458-6223 (US and Canada)

Pediatric Oncology Group Operations Office
645 N. Michigan Avenue, Suite 910
Chicago, IL 60611
(312) 482-9944

National Wilms Tumor Study Group
Fred Hutchinson Cancer Research Center
1100 Fairview Avenue, N
Seattle, WA 98109
(206) 667-4842

Intergroup Rhabdomyosarcoma Study Group (IRSG) Operations Office
Mayo 930E, Mayo Clinic
200 First Street, SW
Rochester, MN 55905

Types of relationships

There are primarily three types of relationships that develop between physicians and parents:

- **Paternal.** In a paternal relationship, the parent is submissive, and the doctor assumes a fatherly role. The problem with this dynamic is that although medical personnel never intend harm; they are human, and mistakes occur. If parents are not monitoring drugs and treatments, these mistakes may go unnoticed. In addition, parents are the experts on their own child and his reactions to drugs and treatments. A surprising number of parents are intimidated by doctors and express the fear that if they question the doctors their child will suffer. This type of behavior robs the child of an adult advocate who speaks up when something seems wrong.

- **Adversarial.** Some parents adopt an "us against them" attitude that is counterproductive. They seem to feel that the disease and treatment are the fault of medical staff, and they blame staff for any setbacks that occur. This attitude undermines the child's confidence in his doctor, a crucial component for healing.

> *I knew one family who just hated the children's hospital. They called it the "house of horrors" or the "torture chamber" in front of their children. Small wonder that their children were terrified.*

- **Collegial.** This is a true partnership in which parents and doctors are all on the same footing and they respect each other's domains and expertise. Here the doctor recognizes that the parents are the experts on their own child and are essential in ensuring that the protocol is followed. The parents respect the physician's expertise and feel comfortable discussing various treatment options or concerns that arise. Honest communication is necessary for this partnership to work, but the effort is well worth it. The child has confidence in his doctor, the parents have reduced their stress by creating a supportive relationship with the physician, and the physician feels comfortable that the family will comply with the treatment plan, giving the child the best chance for a cure.

> *We had a wonderful relationship with the oncologist assigned to us. He blended perfectly the science and the art of medicine. His manner with our daughter was warm, he was extremely well qualified professionally, and he was very easy to talk to. I could bring in articles to discuss with him, and he welcomed the discussion. Although he was busy, he never rushed us. I laughed when I saw that he had written in the chart, "Mother asks innumerable appropriate questions."*

Another mother relates a different experience:

> *We tried very hard to form a partnership with the medical team but failed. The staff seemed very guarded and distant, almost wary of a parent wanting to participate in the decisions made for the child. I learned to*

use the medical library and took research reports in to them to get some help for side effects and get some drug dosages reduced. Things improved, but I was never considered a partner in the healthcare team; I was viewed as a problem.

Communication

Clear and frequent communication is the lifeblood of a positive doctor/parent relationship. Doctors need to be able to explain clearly and listen well, and parents need to feel comfortable asking questions and expressing concerns before they grow into grievances. Nurses and doctors cannot read parents' minds, nor can a parent prepare her child for a procedure unless it has been explained well. The following are parent suggestions on how to establish and maintain good communication:

- Tell the staff how much you would like to know.

    I told them the first day to treat me like a medical student. I asked them to share all information, current studies, lab results, everything, with me. I told them, in advance, that I hoped they wouldn't be offended by lots of questions, because knowledge was comfort to me.

- Inform staff of your child's temperament, likes, and dislikes.

    Whenever my daughter was hospitalized, I made a point of kindly reminding doctors and nurses that she was extremely sensitive, and would benefit from quiet voices and soothing explanations of anything that was about to occur, such as taking temperatures, vital signs, or adjustments to her IV.

- Encourage a close relationship between doctor, nurse, and child. Insist that all medical personnel respect the young person's dignity. Do not let anyone talk in front of the child as if she is not there. The relationship between the child and the medical staff is important. If a problem persists, you have the right to ask the offending person to leave. Marina Rozen observes in *Advice to Doctors and Other Big People*:

    The best part about the doctor is when he gives me bubble gum. The worst part is when he's in the room with me and my mom and he only talks to my mom. I've told him I don't like that, but he doesn't listen.

- Many children's hospitals assign each patient a primary nurse who will oversee all care. Try to form a close relationship with your child's nurse. Nurses usually possess vast knowledge and experience about both medical and practical aspects of cancer treatment. Often, the nurse can rectify misunderstandings between doctor and parents.

- Children and teenagers should be included as part of the team. They should be consulted about treatments and procedures and be given age-appropriate choices.

- Cooperate. If your hometown pediatrician will handle all of your child's outpatient treatment, find ways to facilitate communication between oncologist and pediatrician.

Leeann's doctor here in town has been great. She doesn't usually treat children, but knows how to talk to them without talking down to them. She would take the time during her hospital rounds to help Leeann with her homework and laugh at all of our stupid jokes. A good sense of humor was a must for all of us.

- Go to all appointments with a written list of questions. This prevents the exhausted parent from forgetting something important and saves the staff from numerous follow-up phone calls.

- Ask for definitions of unfamiliar terms. Repeat back the information to ensure that it was understood correctly. Writing down answers or tape recording conferences are both common practices.

We found that sitting down and talking things over with the nurses helped immensely. They were very familiar with each drug and its side effects. They told us many stories about children who had been through the same thing and were doing well years later. They always seemed to have time to give encouragement, a smile, or a hug.

- Some parents want to read their child's medical chart to obtain more details on their child's condition and to help in formulating questions for the medical team. Often, the doctor or nurse will let the parents read it in the child's hospital room or in the waiting room at the clinic. Most states/provinces have laws that allow patient access to all records. However, you may have to write to the doctor asking to review the chart and pay any photocopy costs.

- If you have questions or concerns, discuss them with the resident. If she is unable to provide satisfactory answers, ask the child's assigned fellow or attending physician.

- The medical team includes many specialists: doctors, nurses, physical therapists, nutritionists, x-ray technicians, radiation therapists, and more. At training hospitals, many of these persons will be in the early stages of their training. If a procedure is not going well, you have the right to tell the person to stop and to request a more skilled person to do the job.

> At our hospital, family practice residents rotate through, and are often assigned to do procedures. My son was on a protocol that required a rescue drug to be administered at a certain time. Once, the resident tried for an hour to do a spinal tap, and just couldn't do it. My son was very late getting the rescue drug, and I was worried. Later, I requested a conference with the oncologist and asked him to perform all the procedures in the future. He agreed, but I didn't intervene that first time and I felt very guilty.

- Know your rights. Legally, your child cannot be treated without your permission. If a procedure is proposed that you do not feel comfortable with, keep asking questions until you feel fully informed. You have the legal right to refuse the procedure if you do not think that it is necessary. However, if the hospital feels that you are wrongfully withholding permission for treatment (i.e., you reject standard treatment in favor of an unproven remedy, or you are so concerned about side effects that you are endangering the child's chance for cure), they can take you to court. The child is the important person in this equation, and both the hospital and the parents have input once you step into the legal arena.

- Don't let problems build up into a long laundry list of grievances.

- Use "I" statements. For example, "I feel upset when you won't answer my questions" rather than, "You never listen to me."

- If it helps you feel more comfortable, keep track of your child's treatments to check for mistakes.

> Few children were on the high-risk protocol at the time my daughter was being treated. The attendings always knew exactly what was supposed to be done, but the fellows sometimes made mistakes. I was embar-

rassed to correct them, but I just kept reminding myself that they had dozens of protocols to keep track of, and I had only one.

- Be specific and not confrontational when describing problems. Allow room for the staff to save face. For example, "My daughter has to go to radiation after this bone marrow aspiration. I want it to go smoothly, so I would appreciate it if Dr. Smith, the attending, does the procedure instead of the intern," rather than, "I'm not going to let that intern near my daughter again." Another example is, "My son gets very nervous the longer we wait for our appointment. We have waited over two hours for our last two appointments. Could we call ahead next time to see if the doctor is on schedule?" rather than "Do you think your time is more valuable than mine?"

Noah was five months old and receiving radiation treatment for a small tumor located adjacent to the optic nerve. I felt very strongly that an infant should be able to wake up to his mother (and that not having the mother present was emotionally damaging to the baby). I was upset that the anesthesia team was not honoring this concern, and I was simply told, "He won't remember." I made the point that "He may not remember here," pointing to my head, but that "He does remember here," pointing to my heart. I arranged to be called to the treatment room shortly before he awakened from anesthesia.

- If you have something to discuss with the doctor that will take some time, request a conference. These are routinely scheduled between parents and physicians, and should allow enough time for a thorough discussion. Grabbing a busy doctor in the hallway is not fair to her, and may not result in a satisfactory answer for you.

- Do not be afraid to make waves if you are right or to apologize if you are wrong.

- Show appreciation.

I sent thank you notes to three residents after my daughter's first hospitalization. The notes were short but sweet. I wanted them to know how much we appreciated their many kindnesses.

· · · · ·

Early in my daughter's treatment, we changed pediatricians. The first was aloof and patronizing, and the second was smart, warm, funny, and caring. He was a constant bright spot in our lives through some dark times. So every year during my daughter's treatment, she and her younger sister put on their Santa hats and brought homemade cookies to her pediatrician and nurse. This year was the first time she was able to walk in, and she looked them in the eye and sang, "We Wish You a Merry Christmas." Her nurse went in the back room and cried, and her doctor got misty-eyed. I'll always be thankful for their care.

In his book *Head First: The Biology of Hope,* Norman Cousins shares portions of his commencement talks at the medical schools of UCLA, Harvard, George Washington University, and Baylor University:

> *There are qualities beyond pure medical competence that patients need and look for in doctors. They want reassurance. They want to be looked after and not just looked over. They want to be listened to. They want to feel that it makes a difference to the physician, a very big difference, whether they live or die. They want to feel that they are in the doctor's thoughts. The physician holds the lifeline. The physician's words and not just his prescriptions are attached to that lifeline.*

> *This aspect of medicine has not changed in thousands of years. Not all the king's horses and all the king's men—not all the tomography and the thallium scanners and two-D electrocardiograms and medicinal mood modifiers—can preempt the physician's primary role as the keeper of the keys to the body's own healing system.*

> *I pray that you will never allow your knowledge to get in the way of your relationship with your patients. I pray that all the technological marvels at your command will not prevent you from practicing medicine out of a little black bag. I pray that when you go into a patient's room you will recognize that the main distance is not from the door to the bed, but from the patient's eyes to your own—and that the shortest distance between those two points is a horizontal straight line—the kind of straight line that works best when the physician bends low to the patient's loneliness and fear and pain and the overwhelming sense of mortality that comes flooding up out of the unknown, and when the physician's hand on the patient's shoulder or arm is a shelter against the darkness.*

> *I pray that, even as you attach the highest value to your science, you will never forget that it works best when combined with your art, and,*

indeed, that your art is what is most enduring in your profession. For,
ultimately, it is the physician's respect for the human soul that determines
the worth of his science.

Getting a second opinion

Conscientious doctors welcome consultations and encourage second opinions. Because there are many gray areas in medicine where judgment and experience are as important as knowledge, consultations are frequent. Many insurance companies require second opinions. If, after discussions with the doctor, you are still uneasy about any aspect of your child's medical care, you should not hesitate to seek another opinion.

There are two ways to get a second opinion: see another specialist or ask the child's physician to arrange a multidisciplinary second opinion. Many parents seek a second opinion at the time of diagnosis. Do not do this in secret. Explain to your child's oncologist that before proceeding you would like a second opinion, and ask for his recommendation. The Childhood Cancer Ombudsman Program (see Appendix C, *Resource Organizations*), with dozens of participating board certified pediatric oncologists, will review your child's treatment plan and offer second opinions without charge. To allow for a thorough analysis, arrange to have copies of all records sent ahead to the physician(s) who will give the second opinion.

Multidisciplinary second opinions incorporate the views of several different specialists. Parents who would like to get various viewpoints can ask to have the child's situation discussed at a tumor board, which usually meets weekly at major medical centers. These boards include medical, surgical, and radiation oncologists, as well as fellows and residents. Your child's oncologist will present the facts of your child's case for discussion. Ask him to tell you what was said at the meeting.

Doctors informally seek second opinions all the time. Residents confer with their fellow for complicated situations; fellows confer with the attending when unusual drug reactions or responses to treatment occur. Parents should feel free to ask their physician if he has conferred with other staff members to gain additional viewpoints.

> *Brent developed a seizure disorder after a rare drug reaction so he*
> *was on anticonvulsant medications as well as chemotherapy for two*
> *years. We were worried about the interaction of all the drugs, as well as*

the advisability of his continuing on the more aggressive arm of the proto-
col. We asked the fellow to arrange a care conference, and she met with
the clinic director as well as Brent's neurologist to discuss how to best
manage his care.

Parents often fear seeking a second opinion because they are afraid of offending the doctor or creating antagonism. Conscientious doctors do not resent a parent seeking a second opinion. If she does resist, consider changing doctors. Cancer is life or death, and you won't have a second chance.

Two opinions that agree are all that parents should require before proceeding. Treatment for cancer should begin within days of diagnosis. Parents who drag their child from doctor to doctor are denying the gravity of the situation; they hope that someone will give them more favorable news. But the longer they delay treatment, the worse the possible outcome.

Conflict resolution

Conflict is a part of life. In a situation where a child's life is threatened, such as childhood cancer, the heightened emotions and constant involvement with the medical bureaucracy guarantee conflict. Clashes are inevitable and resolving them is of paramount importance. As Henry Ford once said, "Don't find fault, find a remedy."

Here are some suggestions from parents on how to resolve problems:

- Treat the doctors with respect, and expect respect from them.

    I always wanted to be treated as an intelligent adult, not someone of
    lesser status. So I would ask each medical person what they wished to be
    called. We would either both go by first names or both go by titles. I did
    not want to be called mom.

- Expect a reasonable amount of sensitivity from the staff.

    One of the things that I didn't appreciate was constantly being told
    that we were lucky and Elizabeth had the "good cancer." One nurse actu-
    ally told me that they call Wilms the "spit and rub" cancer because it is so
    easy to get rid of.

- Treat the staff with sensitivity. Recognize that you are under enormous stress, and so are the doctors and nurses. Do not blame them for the disease or explode in anger. Be an advocate, not an adversary.

- If a problem develops, state the issue clearly, without accusations, and then suggest a solution.

  I found out late in my daughter's treatment that short-acting, safe sedatives were being used for many children at the clinic to prevent pain and anxiety during treatments. Only parents who knew about it and requested it received this service. I felt that my daughter's life would have been incredibly improved if we had been able to remove the trauma of procedures. I was angry. But I also realized that although I thought that they were wrong not to offer the service, I was partially at fault for not expressing more clearly how much difficulty she had the week before and after a procedure. I called the director of the clinic and carefully explained that I thought that poor staff/parent communication was creating hardships for the children. I suggested that the entire staff meet with a panel of parents to try to improve communication and to educate the doctors on the impact of pain on the children's daily life. They were very supportive and scheduled the conference. This is a classic example of how something good can come out of a disagreement, if both parties are receptive to solving the problem.

- Recognize that it is hard to speak up, especially if you have never had to be assertive before. But it is very important to solve the problem before it grows and poisons the relationship.

- Most large medical centers have social workers and psychologists on staff to help families. One of their major duties is to serve as mediators between staff and parents. Ask their advice on problem solving.

- Monitor your own feelings of anger and fear. Be careful not to dump on staff inappropriately. On the other hand, do not let a physician or nurse behave unprofessionally toward you or your child. We all have bad days, but we should not take it out on each other.

- Do not fear reprisal for speaking up. It is possible to be assertive without aggression or argument.

- There are times when no resolution is possible, but expressing one's feelings can be a great release.

  My son and I waited in an exam room for over an hour for a painful procedure. When I went out to ask the receptionist what had caused the delay, she said that a parent had brought in a child without an appointment. This parent frequently failed to bring in her child for treatment, and consequently, whenever she appeared, the doctors dropped everything to take care of the child. When the doctor finally came in, one and one half hours later, my son was in tears. The doctor did not explain the delay or apologize, he just silently started the procedure.

After it was finished, I went out of the room, found the doctor, and said, "I am so angry. You just left us in here for hours and traumatized my son. Our time is valuable, too." He told me that I should have more compassion for the other mother because her life was very difficult. I replied that he encouraged her to not make appointments by dropping everything whenever she appeared. I added that it wasn't fair to those parents who played by the rules; she was being rewarded for her irresponsibility. After we had each stated our position, we left without resolution.

Changing doctors

Changing doctors is not a step to be taken lightly, but it can be a great relief if the relationship has deteriorated beyond repair. It is a good policy to exhaust all possible remedies prior to separating, or the same problems may arise with the new doctor. Communication, verbal or written, and mediation, using the social service staff, can sometimes resolve the issues and prevent the disruption of changing doctors.

Although there are many reasons for changing doctors, some of the most common are:

* Grave medical error(s) made
* Inability to communicate or answer questions
* Serious clash of philosophy—for example, a paternalistic doctor and a parent who wishes to be informed and share in the decision-making

It is one of life's great struggles to face cancer. If you have a physician whom you trust, can rely on for the best medical treatment, feel comfortable with, communicate freely with, and can count on for advice and support, the struggle is greatly eased. If, on the other hand, the doctor adds to your discomfort rather than reducing it, change.

Do not change doctors because you're searching for a better diagnosis. If two reputable physicians, or a tumor board, have agreed on the diagnosis and treatment, it is best for the child to immediately begin treatment.

Many parents choose to continue with a physician in whom they have no confidence, due to fears of reprisals. This simply doesn't happen at large centers of excellence. While there may be lingering bitterness or anger between parents and doctors, the child will continue to benefit from the best-known treatment. Children may actually suffer more from the additional family stress caused by a poor doctor/parent relationship than from changing doctors.

Once the decision is made, parents must be candid. Either verbally or in writing, an explanation should be given for the change and a formal request made to transfer records to the new physician. Physicians are legally required to transfer all records upon written request.

Minna Nathanson, in a statement presented to the President's Commission for the Study of Ethical Problems in Medicine and Biomedical and Behavioral Research, stated:

> And, finally, I wish that professional care team members would all accept and allow questioning, so that parents would feel more comfortable being participants in the decisions about their child's treatment and assistants in their child's care, and that there would be an understanding that parents who show symptoms of stress are reacting normally, not pathologically. Every parent I have ever talked to about their child's illness and hospitalization—whether it be for childhood cancer, cystic fibrosis, spinal bifida, or even a one-shot surgery—has confirmed that most parents are experts on their own child and as extra eyes and ears can help to avoid mistakes in treatment and aid in keeping the child more comfortable and emotionally better prepared for treatment. If there are medical care staff who would say that this is the opposite of what they find, I would ask them to search deeply to see if they are treating parents as intruders in the decision-making and caretaking processes.

CHAPTER 5

Clinical Trials

*The challenge in pediatric oncology remains
clear: to strive for the cure and health of all
children through the development of more
effective yet less damaging treatment for our
young patients.*

—Daniel M. Green, MD and
Giulio J. D'Angio, MD
*Late Effects of Treatment for
Childhood Cancer*

WITHIN DAYS OF ARRIVING at a major pediatric medical center with a child newly diagnosed with cancer, parents may be asked to enroll their child in a clinical trial. A clinical trial is a research study that uses human volunteers to answer specific scientific questions. Pediatric clinical trials are all directed toward improving existing treatments. Clinical trials test approaches that are thought to be promising. They can also fine-tune existing treatments, improve the results or reduce the toxicity of known treatments, or develop new ways to discern response to treatments. More than half of all children with cancer in North America are enrolled in clinical trials during their experience with cancer.

Making an informed judgment on whether to participate is crucial, as it will determine what treatment your child will receive in the months to come. This chapter will explain the terms *clinical trial* and *protocol* and will give examples of how different parents made decisions on this important issue.

Why are children enrolled in clinical trials?

The enormous improvements in treating childhood cancer have been the direct result of clinical trials. In order to accurately evaluate any new treatment, large numbers of patients are needed in each clinical trial.

Because clinical trials offer the most up-to-date treatment available, children who participate in a clinical trial may benefit from the newest research. Most parents derive comfort from knowing that the knowledge gained will make an important contribution to medical science, and may help other children with cancer.

What is standard treatment?

Standard treatment is the best treatment known for a specific type of cancer. As results from ongoing and completed clinical trials are analyzed, more knowledge is accumulated, and standard treatments evolve. However, for some diseases there is no standard treatment.

Most clinical trials divide patients into two or more groups (arms). One arm of the trial is the standard treatment, and the other arms are the experimental portions, which scientists hope will prove to be more effective or less toxic than the standard treatment. Each arm is based on preliminary, but not conclusive, information that it will be beneficial and is carefully reviewed by experts in the field before implementation.

What is randomization?

Some scientific studies require a process called randomization. This means that after parents agree to enroll their child in a clinical trial, a computer will randomly assign the child to one arm of the study. If there are three arms, the parents will not know which of the three (one standard, two experimental) their child will receive until the computer assigns one. One group of patients (the control group) always receives the standard treatment to provide a basis for comparison to the experimental arms. Because neither the physician nor the parents choose the treatment option, a comparable mix of patients is assured.

At the time the clinical trial is designed, there is no conclusive evidence to indicate which arm will prove to be superior. It is not possible to predict if your child will benefit from participating in the study. Most arms incorporate standard therapy and only a small portion of the arm contains the experimental agents. "Experimental" drugs have usually been used previously, but their efficacy in a given circumstance may not be known.

We had a hard time deciding whether to go with the standard treatment or to participate in the study. The "B" arm of the study seemed, on intuition, to be too harsh for her because she was so weak at the time. We finally did opt for the study, hoping we wouldn't be randomized to "B." We chose the study basically so that the computer could choose and we wouldn't ever have to think "we should have gone with the study." As it turned out, we were randomized to the standard arm, so we got what we wanted while still participating in the study.

Who designs clinical trials?

In the United States and Canada, there are four primary pediatric research groups: Children's Cancer Group (CCG), Pediatric Oncology Group (POG), National Wilms Tumor Study Group (NWTSG), and Intergroup Rhabdomyosarcoma Study Group (IRSG). Most large pediatric medical centers work in close cooperation with one of these groups, although there are some centers which design their own clinical trials. Experts from many institutions usually collaborate in the design of clinical trials.

In July 1998, a Pediatric Intergroup Summit was held by the leaders of the four pediatric cancer clinical trials cooperative groups (CCG, POG, NWTSG, and IRSG). A decision was made to form a single pediatric cancer clinical trials organization. Unification of these groups will have advantages for children with cancer as well as pediatric cancer researchers. It will pool the intellectual resources of all four groups, allowing research that had not been previously possible. Large population-based studies and coordinated treatment trials will help researchers gather data that will be generalizable to the entire North American population of children with cancer. It is hoped that integration of these groups will be complete by the year 2002.

Who supervises clinical trials?

The ethical and legal codes ruling medical practice also apply to clinical trials. In addition, most research is federally funded or regulated, with rules to protect patients (this includes all CCG, POG, NWTSG, and IRSG trials). CCG, POG, NWTSG, and IRSG also have review boards which meet at prearranged dates for the duration of a clinical trial to ensure that the risks of all parts of the trial are acceptable relative to the benefits. If one arm of the trial is causing unexpected or unacceptable side effects, that portion will be terminated, and the children enrolled will be given the better treatment. If one of the arms appears to be less effective than the standard, it will be terminated. Conversely, if one arm is better than the standard, the trial will also be terminated. Whenever a treatment is proven to be superior, all children receive it.

All institutions that conduct clinical trials also have an Institutional Review Board (IRB) or an ethics committee which reviews and approves all research taking place there. These boards, whose purpose is to protect patients, are made up of scientists, doctors, sometimes clergy, and often citizens from the community.

What questions should parents ask about clinical trials?

To fully understand the clinical trial that has been proposed for your child, here are some important questions to ask the oncologist:

- What is the purpose of the study?
- Who is sponsoring the study? Who reviews it? How often is it reviewed? Who monitors patient safety?
- What tests and treatments will be done during the study? How do these differ from standard treatment?
- Why is it thought that the treatment being studied may be better than standard treatment?
- What are the possible benefits?
- What are all possible disadvantages?
- What are the possible side effects or risks of the study? What are the side effects of the study compared to those of standard treatment?
- How will the study affect my child's daily life?
- What are the possible long-term impacts of the study compared to those of the standard treatment?
- How long will the study last? Is this shorter or longer than standard treatment?
- Will the study require more hospitalization than standard treatment?
- Does the study include long-term follow-up care?
- What happens if my child is harmed as a result of the research?

- Compare the study to standard treatment in terms of possible outcomes, side effects, time involved, costs, and quality of life.

- Have insurers been reimbursing for care under this protocol?

When discussing the clinical trial with the oncologist, it is perfectly reasonable to ensure that the information will be available for later review. Many parents bring a tape recorder or a friend to take notes. Some parents write down all of the doctor's answers for later reference.

What is informed consent?

Informed consent requires full disclosure and discussion, and may be handled in four stages. First, all the treatments available to the child must be laid on the table and discussed—not just the treatment available at your hospital or through your doctor, but all the treatments that could be beneficial, wherever they are given. Second, the parents and, to the extent possible, the child, should discuss these options and decide that they want to consider one of them. Next, the option selected is thoroughly discussed, with all its benefits and risks clearly explained. Finally, those aspects of the study that are considered experimental and those that are standard need to be clearly described. A fully informed medical decision weighs the relative merits of a therapy after full disclosure of benefits, risks, and alternatives.

During the discussions between the doctor(s) and family, all questions should be answered in language that is clearly understood by the parents, and there should be no pressure to enroll the child in the study. The objective of the informed consent process is to ensure the participants are comfortable with their choice and can comply with it.

> We had many discussions with the staff prior to signing the informed consent to participate in the clinical trial. We asked innumerable questions, all of which were answered in a frank and honest manner. We felt that participating gave our child the best chance for a cure, and we felt good about increasing the knowledge that would help other children later.

> · · · · ·

> Sean missed the deadline when he was diagnosed for enrolling in a clinical trial. However, when he relapsed we did enroll him. The particular trial he was in was a randomized computer trial that decided if he

was getting one or two chemotherapy agents. We felt if we enrolled him in the trial, maybe the results would help other children.

The form that parents sign will have language similar to the following: "The study described above has been explained to me, and I voluntarily agree to have my child participate in this study. I have had all of my questions answered, and understand that all future questions that I have about this research will be answered by the investigators listed above."

> *Paige (age four) took part in a clinical trial to treat her stage IV neuroblastoma. Her oncologist was the principal investigator, and he presented it to us as the best treatment plan for her. I have a stepsister who is a pediatric oncology nurse/researcher, and we discussed the treatment plan with her. Once all our questions were answered to our satisfaction, we decided to agree to the clinical trial.*

Parents are experts on their children, but no matter how much reading they do, they are not experts on cancer. By the time a study is published in the literature, doctors on the cutting edge of treatment are two to four years into improving that treatment or learning of its shortcomings. For this reason, it is best to make decisions in partnership with knowledgeable medical caregivers, rather than in isolation.

No matter how comfortable you are with your child's treating oncologist, it is sometimes helpful to have another medical caregiver help sort out your options. Often, that person will be the family's pediatrician or family doctor. Second opinions can also be arranged through the Childhood Cancer Ombudsman Program, which uses volunteer specialists to provide free help to families considering the range of treatment options and informed consent process. (See Appendix C, *Resource Organizations*, for contact information.)

What is a protocol?

A protocol, also known as a "road map," is a recipe for treating cancer. Just like a recipe for baking a cake, it has ingredients that go in at certain times and in certain ways in order for the recipe to have the best chance for success. The protocol document lists the drugs, dosages, and tests for each segment of treatment. If your child is enrolled in a clinical trial, the protocol will outline the treatment for each arm.

The clinical trial that my child was enrolled in had three arms—A, B, and C. He was in the A portion, so we only referred to the A section of the protocol, which clearly outlined each procedure and drug to be given for the duration of the trial. It also listed the follow-up care required by that particular clinical trial.

· · · · ·

When Matthew was diagnosed, he was started on a protocol that was designed to answer two questions. After the induction portion of the protocol, the first question was to determine if bone marrow transplantation improved survival for children with high risk neuroblastoma. He was to receive either a transplant or several additional months of consolidation therapy. The second question was designed to answer whether or not 13 cis-retinoic acid improved the event-free survival rate. This was done through a randomization process. We hoped that Matthew would get that opportunity, and as it turned out, he was randomized to get the drug.

The protocol may be 5 to 100 pages long, and the family may also be given an abbreviated version (1 to 2 pages) to provide quick and easy reference on a daily basis. Parents and teenage patients should review these documents carefully with the oncologist so that all portions are understood. It will be the parent's responsibility to make the appropriate appointments and give oral medications at the correct times.

Many parents express anguish when discussing their child's protocol, primarily because they misunderstand that the protocol is merely a guideline. Therapy frequently needs to be modified depending on each child's response to treatment.

It took me a long time to get over my hang-up that things needed to go exactly as per protocol. Any deviations on dose or days was a major stress for me. It took talking to many parents, as well as doctors and nurses, to realize and feel comfortable with the fact that no one ever goes along perfectly and that the protocol is meant as the broad guideline. There will always be times when your child will be off drugs or on half dose because of illness or low counts or whatever. It took a long time to realize that this is not going to ruin the effectiveness, that the child gets what she can handle without causing undue harm.

· · · · ·

I didn't know what a protocol was when Preston was diagnosed, and I understood from the doctors that this was the "exact" regime which must be followed to cure Preston. It frightened me whenever changes were made in the protocol. After a time, I came to view the protocol as merely a guideline which is individualized for each patient according to his tolerance and reaction to the drugs.

Should parents receive the entire trial document?

The clinical trial protocol described earlier is actually a very small portion of an extensive document describing all aspects of the clinical study. The entire document often exceeds 100 pages and covers the following topics: study hypothesis, experimental design, scientific background and rationale with relevant references from the scientific literature, patient eligibility and randomization, therapy for each arm of the study, required observations, pathology guidelines, radiation therapy guidelines (if applicable), supportive care guidelines, specific information about each drug, relapse therapy guidelines, statistical considerations, study committee, record keeping, reporting of adverse drug reactions, and consent form.

Parents are sometimes not aware that this lengthy document exists. Admittedly, for some parents the full protocol could be overwhelming or boring. There are many parents, however, who throw themselves into research to better understand their child's illness. These parents may benefit from having a copy of the study document for several reasons. First, it provides a description of the clinical trials that preceded the present one and explains the reasons the investigators designed this particular study. Second, it provides detailed descriptions of drug reactions, which comforts many parents who worry that their child is the only one exhibiting extreme responses to some drugs. Third, motivated parents who have only one protocol to keep track of occasionally prevent serious errors in treatment. Physicians treat scores of children on dozens of protocols and sometimes make mistakes. And finally, for parents who are adrift in the world of cancer treatment, it can provide a bit of control over their child's life. It gives the parents a job to do: monitor their child's treatment.

Since knowledge is comfort for me, I really wanted to have the entire clinical trial document, despite its technical language. Whereas the brief protocol that I had listed day, drug, dose, the expanded version listed the potential side effects for each drug, and what actions should be taken should any occur. I learned the parameters.

Parents have a right to review all literature and information related to their child's treatment. There are no moral or ethical restrictions that come into play. If you wish to read all of the details of the study, simply insist that a copy be provided to you.

What happens if parents say no?

Parents have the right to say yes or no to a proposed clinical trial. If the family chooses standard treatment rather than a clinical trial, the decision will be respected. The child will be given the best known treatment for his type of cancer.

Our son's doctor gave us the paperwork on the clinical trial to read and told us that it was our decision and that he would not pressure us. We really decided not to join the study for financial reasons. My husband was a student and we had no health insurance. One of the parts of the study required more clinic visits, and we just couldn't afford it.

Can parents remove their child?

Yes. If parents have questions or concerns about any aspect of the trial, they should talk it over with their doctor. If the problem is not resolved, parents have the right to remove their child at any time from a clinical trial. This decision will not be held against the parent, and the child will still receive the best available care for her type of cancer. On the consent form signed by the parent, there will be language similar to this: "You are free to not have your child participate in this research or to withdraw your child at any time without penalty or jeopardizing future care."

Jesse was enrolled in a clinical trial to assess long-term consequences of radiation. The testing was free, and we were glad to participate. Unfortunately, the billing department of the hospital continually billed us in error. We tried to correct the problem, but it became such a hassle that we withdrew from the study.

Pros and cons of clinical trials

Pros of clinical trials are:

- Patients receive either state-of-the-art investigational therapy or the best standard therapy available.

- Clinical trials can provide an opportunity to benefit from a new therapy before it is generally available.

- Information gained from clinical trials will benefit children with cancer in the future.

- Children enrolled in clinical trials may be monitored more frequently throughout treatment.

- The IRB has reviewed the protocol for protection of patient's rights as well as for scientific soundness.

- Review boards of scientists oversee the operation of clinical trials.

- Participating in a clinical trial often makes parents feel that they did everything medically possible for their child.

- Some clinical trials provide all treatment and follow-up care at no cost to the family.

Cons to consider are:

- The experimental arm may not provide treatment as effective as the standard, or it may generate unexpected side effects or risks.

- Not all patients in a study receive the new treatment.

- Some clinical trials require more hospitalizations, treatments, tests that may be costly or painful, or clinic visits than the standard treatment.

- Some families feel additional stress over which arm is the best treatment for their individual child.

- Participation may generate parental guilt if the child has unacceptable toxicity from the more aggressive experimental arm.

- Insurance may not cover investigational studies. Parents need to carefully explore this issue prior to signing the consent form.

When we were struggling with the decision of whether to join the study, I asked the oncologist how would we ever know if we made the right decision. He said something very wise. "You will never know and you should never second guess yourself, no matter how the study turns out. Statistics are about large groups of kids, not your child. Your child might relapse no matter which arm she is on and she might be cured on an arm where most of the other kids relapse. Statistics for you will be either 100 percent or 0 because your child will either live or die. I can't tell you which will be the better treatment, that is why we are conducting the study. But no matter what, we will be doing absolutely the best we can."

Catheters

Do what you can, with what you have,
where you are.

—Theodore Roosevelt

MANY CHILDREN WITH CANCER require chemotherapy, intravenous (IV) fluids, IV antibiotics, blood and platelet transfusions, frequent blood sampling, and sometimes IV nutrition. The intensity of therapy is based on the type and stage of disease. Indwelling catheters have proved to be a very effective method for allowing entry into the large veins for intensive therapy. They eliminate the difficulty of finding veins for IVs and allow drugs to be put directly into a large vessel of the heart where they are rapidly diluted and spread throughout the body.

Other names for indwelling catheters are: venous access device, right atrial catheter, implanted catheter, central venous catheter, central line, Hickman, Broviac, Port-a-cath, Medi-port, or PICC lines.

The two types of indwelling catheters most commonly used in children are the external catheter and the subcutaneous port. PICC lines, or peripherally inserted central catheters, are used less frequently.

External catheter

The external catheter is a long, flexible tube with one end in the right atrium of the heart and the other end outside the skin of the chest. The tube tunnels under the skin of the chest, enters a large vein near the collarbone, and threads inside a big vein leading to the heart (see Figure 6-1). Because chemotherapy drugs, transfusions, and IV fluids are put in the end of the tube hanging outside the body, the child feels no pain. Blood for complete blood counts (CBC) or other tests can also be drawn from the end of the catheter.

The commonly used external catheters are the Hickman or Broviac. With meticulous care, the external catheter can often be left in place for years.

How it's put in

External catheters are usually put in under general anesthesia. Once the child is anesthetized, the surgeon makes two small incisions. One incision is near the collarbone over the spot where the catheter enters the vein, the other is the area on the chest where the catheter exits the body. To prevent the catheter from slipping out, it is stitched to the skin where it comes out of the chest (see Figure 6-1). There is a Dacron cuff around the catheter right above the exit site (under the skin) into which body tissue grows. This further anchors the catheter and helps prevent infection.

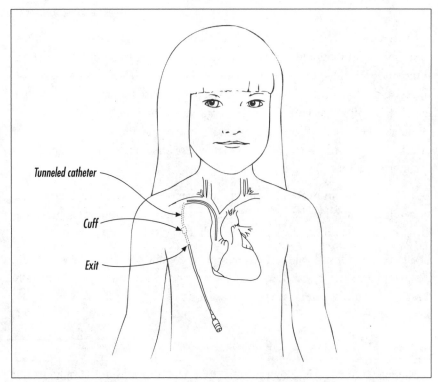

Tunneled catheter

Cuff

Exit

Figure 6-1. External catheter

Daily care

The external catheter requires careful maintenance to try to prevent infection or the formation of clots. The site where the catheter exits the body must be cleaned frequently (schedules range from every other day to weekly) and a fresh, sterile dressing needs to be applied and taped in place. The site should be checked for redness, swelling, or drainage. To prevent clots, parents or older patients are taught to flush the line with a heparin solution. Different institutions use different schedules for how often the line should be flushed. Nurses at the hospital instruct parents in catheter care, and plenty of practice should be provided until both parent and child are comfortable with the entire procedure.

> *We were very grateful for Matthew's Hickman line. Like a lot of children, he was terribly afraid of needles. The maintenance that was necessary to keep his line working properly became second nature to me. After his diagnosis, and again after his relapse, he had a Hickman implanted. In total, he had his external catheter for more than four years.*

Risks

The major complications of using the external catheter are infections—either in the blood or at the insertion site—and the formation of clots in the line. Clots can also form in the blood vessel where the catheter is placed. Rare complications are kinking of the catheter or the catheter becoming dislodged from its proper position.

Infections

Even with the best care, infections are common in children with external lines. Children who are immunosuppressed (have low blood counts) for long periods of time are at risk for developing infections. The need for frequent flushing of the external line also increases the chance for bacteria to enter the catheter. Most infections are caused by a bacterium called staphylococcus epidermidis, although a host of other organisms may also cause infections.

If the child develops a fever over 101°F (38.5°C), redness or swelling at the insertion site, or pain in the catheter area, infection is suspected. To determine if bacteria are present, blood will be drawn from the catheter to culture (grow in a laboratory for 24 to 48 hours). Treatment with antibiotics is usually effective. Treatment will start whenever there is a suspected infection and will end if the culture comes back negative. If the culture is positive, treatment usually continues for ten to fourteen days.

> *In July 1997, my son Trevor (four years old) was diagnosed with Wilms tumor. He had a nephrectomy (kidney removal) and an eighteen-*

week course of chemotherapy. During the nephrectomy, the surgeons also inserted a tube—called a Broviac—into Trevor's chest. This enabled Trevor to receive his chemotherapy treatment without getting a new IV put in each week. My husband and I were responsible for cleaning and flushing the Broviac tube daily.

Throughout the whole thing, Trevor was so strong and brave. By November he had completed all his treatments, but the catheter needed to stay in for a few more weeks. However, in December, Trevor was admitted back to the hospital when his catheter became infected. The doctors treated him with antibiotics and decided to remove the Broviac a little early. He was evaluated, and four days before Christmas we got the news: Trevor was cancer-free. The Broviac prevented a lot of unnecessary pain, and we were grateful that he had it.

Some physicians require that the child be hospitalized for antibiotic treatment, while others allow the child to go home. If the infection does not respond to treatment, the catheter may have to be removed.

When my daughter had a line infection, I wanted to use the antibiotic pump at home. It was hard, though. It took two hours per dose, three doses per day, for fourteen days. I would get up at 5 a.m. to hook her up, so that she would sleep through the first dose. The second dose I would give while she watched a tape in the early afternoon. Then I would hook her up at bedtime so she would sleep through it. I had to wait up to flush and disconnect, so I was very tired by the end of the two weeks.

Clots

Even with excellent daily care, some external lines develop blockages and/or clots. If the catheter becomes blocked, it will be flushed with streptokinase to dissolve the clot. If the line is blocked by a drug precipitate (usually only seen with the drug VM-26), diluted hydrochloric acid may be used to dissolve the blockage.

Two months before the end of Kristin's treatment, her line plugged up. We tried several maneuvers at home unsuccessfully. We had to bring her in for the IV team to work on it. I think the bumpy ride to the hospital loosened it because they were able to dislodge the clot just by flushing it with saline.

Kinks

Rarely, a kink develops in the catheter due to a sharp angle where the catheter enters the neck vein. Some parents and nurses are able to work around this problem by experimenting with different positions for the child when the blood is drawn. Another method is to teach the child a Valsalva maneuver such as bearing down as if to have a bowel movement.

Breaks in the line do happen, but they are very rare. If the break or rupture of the line occurs when it is not in use, only heparin will leak into surrounding tissues. If the break occurs when corrosive chemotherapy drugs are flowing through the catheter, they may leak and cause damage to surrounding tissue. The risk of an internal line leaking is far lower than the chance of leakage from an IV in a vein of the hand or arm.

Other factors to consider

To use an external catheter successfully it takes a well-organized and motivated family. The site needs to be cleaned and dressed frequently, and heparin must be injected using sterile technique. Because the dressing must be secured to the skin with a very sticky large tape, if your child is very tape sensitive (cries whenever tape is removed or skin reddens and breaks out), the external line may not be a good choice. An external catheter requires restrictions on showering, bathing, and swimming, since it is important to keep the exit site and catheter dry.

The external line is a constant reminder of cancer treatment and causes changes in body image. Both parent and child need to be comfortable with the idea of seeing and handling a tube that emerges from the chest. It is noticeable under lightweight clothing and bathing suits. If there is a younger sibling who might pull or yank on the catheter, the Hickman or Broviac might not be the appropriate choice.

On the other hand, the reason external lines are chosen so frequently is that there are no needles and no pain. This is a very important consideration for young children or any person who is frightened of needles and/or pain. In addition, some protocols require double lumen access and the external catheter is the only appropriate option.

Subcutaneous port

Several different types of subcutaneous (under the skin) ports are used; the Port-a-cath is the most common. The subcutaneous port differs from the external catheter in that it is completely under the skin. A small metal chamber (1×1×1/2 inches) with a rubber top, is implanted under the skin of the right chest. A catheter threads from the metal chamber (portal) under the skin to a large vein near the collarbone, then inside the vein to the right atrium of the heart (see Figure 6-2). Whenever the catheter is needed for a blood draw or infusion of drugs or fluid, a needle is inserted by a nurse through the skin and into the rubber top of the portal.

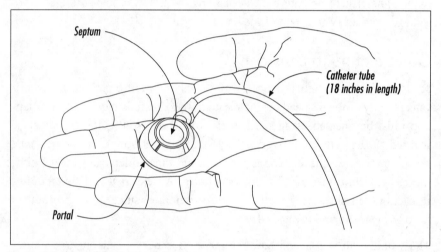

Figure 6-2. Parts of the Port-a-cath

How it's put in

The subcutaneous port is implanted under general anesthesia in the operating room in a procedure that generally takes less than an hour. Sometimes local anesthesia is used for older children or teens. The surgeon makes two small incisions: one in the chest where the portal will be placed, and the other near the collarbone where the catheter will enter a vein in the lower part of the neck (see Figure 6-3). First, one end of the catheter is placed in the large blood vessel of the neck and threaded into the right atrium of the heart. The other end of the catheter is tunneled under the skin where it is attached to the portal. Fluid is injected into the portal to ensure that the device works properly. The portal is then placed under the skin in the right chest, and stitched to the underlying muscle. Both incisions are then closed. The only evidence that a catheter has been implanted are two small scars and a bump under the skin where the portal rests.

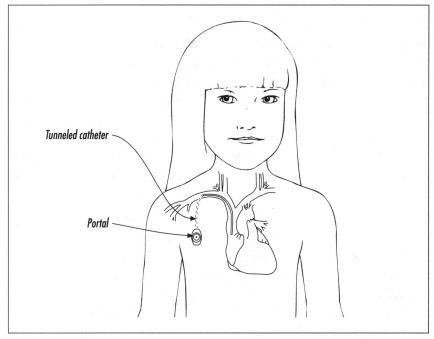

Figure 6-3. Subcutaneous port

Before my child's surgery to have a port implanted, I saw other children being wheeled into the operating room screaming and trying to climb off the gurney to return to the parents. It broke my heart. When it was Jennifer's turn, I asked them to give her enough premedication so that she was relaxed and happy to go. I also insisted that I be in the recovery room when she awoke.

· · · · ·

Christine had her port surgery late at night. The resident gave her some premedication, then the chief resident ordered him to give her more. She felt so silly that she looked at me, giggled, and said, "Mommy has a nose as long as an elephant's." I asked the surgeon if I could be in the recovery room before she awoke, and he said, "Sure." When I told the nurse that I had permission to go in recovery, she refused. When I persisted, she became angry. I told her that my child was expecting to wake up seeing my face, and I intended to be there. I added that she should go in and ask the surgeon to resolve the impasse. When she came out, she let me in the recovery room.

How it works

Because the entire Port-a-cath is under the skin, the device must be accessed in order to use it. To access the catheter, the skin is thoroughly cleansed with antiseptic, then a special needle is inserted through the skin and the rubber top of the portal. The needle is attached to a short length of tubing which hangs down the front of the chest. EMLA cream can be applied one hour prior to the needle poke to anesthetize the skin or ethyl chloride can be sprayed on right before the poke. Subcutaneous ports have a septum that is self-sealing after needle removal, and are designed to withstand years of needle insertions.

If the child is in a part of treatment where the line must be used every day, the nurse will attach the tubing to IV fluids or will close the end off with a sterile cap after flushing with saline solution. A transparent dressing will be put over the site where the needle enters the port. The port can remain accessed in this way for up to seven days. After that time, to avoid the risk of infection, the needle should be removed and the port reaccessed when necessary. If the needle and tubing are to be left in place, it is important to tape them securely to the chest to avoid accidents.

> At the end of treatment while getting cytoxan, Meagan (three years old) got a line infection. Because she hated tape removal, we did not secure the IV tubing to her stomach or chest. On one of her many trips to the potty, we accidentally tugged on the tubing and caused a very small tear in the skin around the needle. It became infected. We did home antibiotics on the pump and felt very fortunate that we were able to clear the line with vancomycin and rifampin (two strong antibiotics). We were glad our doctor was not too quick to remove the line, but it did require two weeks off chemotherapy.

If the port is needed only infrequently, this will be the sequence of events: the site will be cleaned, needle put in, line rinsed with saline, drug given or blood drawn, line rinsed with saline, heparin added to line, needle withdrawn, and a Band-Aid placed over the site.

Care of the subcutaneous port

The entire port and catheter are under the skin and therefore require no daily care. The skin over the port can be washed just like the rest of the body. Frequent visual inspections are needed to check for swelling, redness, or drainage.

The subcutaneous port must be accessed and flushed with saline and heparin at least once every 30 days, which usually coincides with the monthly clinic visit and blood checks. This procedure is done by a nurse or technician. The port system requires no maintenance by the parent or patient.

Risks

The risks for a subcutaneous port are similar to those for the external catheter: infection, clots, and rarely, kinks or rupture. If the needle is not properly inserted through the rubber septum, fluids can leak into the tissue around the portal.

> *Brent (eight years old) has had a Port-a-cath for 33 months with absolutely no problems. He uses EMLA to anesthetize it prior to accessing. He hates finger pokes so much that he has his port accessed every time he needs blood drawn.*

Infection

Most studies show that the infection rate of subcutaneous ports is lower than that of external catheters. If the subcutaneous port does become infected, it is treated exactly the same as those in external catheters.

> *Katy had two infections in her Port-a-cath during treatment. One occurred when the tape loosened during a blood transfusion. She developed a fever the next day and required fourteen days of vancomycin. On another occasion, she became ill in the car on the way home from the clinic. Her skin became white and clammy, and she felt faint and nauseated. She spiked a 102°F temperature which only lasted for two hours. The blood culture both times grew staphylococcus epi.*

Kinks, clots, ruptures

These events rarely occur with the subcutaneous port or the external catheter. If they do occur, they are treated as described earlier in "External catheter."

Peripherally inserted central catheters

A peripherally inserted central catheter is also referred to as a PICC line. This type of catheter is placed in the large antecubital vein (a large vein in the inner elbow area) and threaded into a large vein above the right atrium of the heart (see Figure 6-4). Unlike other catheters, a PICC line can be inserted by an IV nurse, rather than a surgeon.

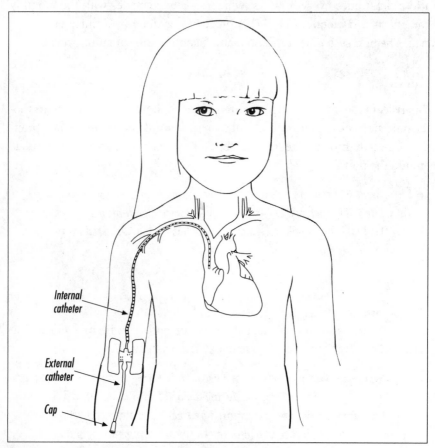

Figure 6-4. Peripherally inserted central catheter

The PICC line can remain in place for many weeks or months, avoiding the need for a new IV every few days. PICC lines can be used to deliver chemotherapy, antibiotics, blood products, other medications, and intravenous nutrition. When the PICC line needs to be accessed, an IV line is connected to the end of the catheter. When it is not in use, the IV is disconnected and the catheter is flushed and capped.

How it's put in

The peripherally inserted central catheter can be inserted in your child's hospital room by an IV nurse or physician. Your child will be positioned on a flat surface, and she will need to keep her arm straight and motionless during the procedure. An injection to numb the area is given to decrease discomfort during insertion. A special needle is used to place the PICC line into the arm vein. The catheter is then threaded through the needle. Once the line is in place, a chest x-ray is taken to ensure that it is positioned properly.

> Brian had his Hickman pulled in February 1997, but two weeks later he developed pancreatitis and needed total parenteral nutrition. Since he was still on active treatment, he was given the choice of another Hickman or a PICC, which he decided to try. It was inserted right in our room with no anesthetic other than the morphine pump he was already on for the pancreatitis pain. He pushed his PCA button moments before it was inserted, because he was not sure what to expect. The procedure was uncomfortable, but not terribly painful. They did an x-ray to make sure it was in the right place. It wasn't, but after some aerobics (moving him into different positions) and lots of flushing, they checked again, and it was.

Care of the peripherally inserted central catheter

The PICC line, like the Hickman catheter, requires meticulous care to prevent problems. You will be taught by the nurses to change the dressing, flush the line, change the injection cap, and inspect the site for possible signs of infection. The dressing covering the exit site is changed on a weekly basis, unless it becomes wet or exposed to the air. The line must be flushed after every use or every day. You should get plenty of practice under the supervision of a nurse until both you and your child are comfortable with caring for the line. The care required for your child's PICC line may be slightly different from what has been described in this section since institutional preferences vary.

> Kelsey had a PICC line in her right arm, and she would not straighten it out, but kept it a little bent. I definitely think she was protecting it, and also I think when she tried to straighten it, it pulled on the suture and on the dressing in an uncomfortable way that could have been painful, so she just wouldn't try. I had to do a heparin flush every day, and change the dressing twice a week. She could not tolerate Tegaderm so

we used another kind of adhesive bandage, and doused it with Detachol,
which dissolved the adhesive within a few minutes, allowing us to get the
bandage off quite easily. The Detachol was a godsend for her, as remov-
ing the adhesive was like pulling teeth and a source of unnecessary pain.

Risks

The problems associated with a PICC line are similar to those of any external catheter. Veins may become irritated, infection can occur, or the line can
be accidentally torn or moved.

Irritated veins

The vein where the catheter is located may become irritated. This is most
likely to occur during the first few days after it has been inserted. Signs of
irritation include swelling or pain in the area, or the development of small
veins near the site. Often, a warm moist cloth placed on the vein will help
alleviate discomfort. Raising the arm is also sometimes helpful.

Infection

Meticulous care using sterile techniques is very important to reduce the risk
of infection. The dressing exit site should be changed every week, or if it
becomes wet or exposed to the air. Injection caps must also be regularly
changed using sterile techniques when the line is not in use, and the line
must be flushed on a regular basis. Signs of infection include redness, swelling, pain, drainage, or warmth around the exit site. Fever, chills, tiredness,
and dizziness may also indicate that the line has become infected. You
should notify the doctor if any of these signs are present or if your child has
a fever above 101°F (38.5°C).

Torn catheter

Accidents sometimes happen, and it is possible that a hole or tear in the line
can occur. The only prevention for this is ensuring that care is taken when
handling the catheter. You should suspect a torn catheter if fluid leaks out of
the line, especially during an injection. If a tear is found, you should find the
hole, fold the line above the tear, tape it together and cover it with sterile
gauze. You should immediately notify your child's doctor of the problem.

Displacement of the catheter

Like the external catheters discussed earlier in this chapter, it is important that the PICC line is securely taped to the exit site to prevent movement. Signs of a displaced catheter include chest pain, burning or swelling in the arm above the exit site or in the chest, fluid leaking around the catheter, or pain when fluid is injected into the line. If you suspect that the line has been moved, you should tape the catheter in place and immediately notify your child's doctor.

Choosing not to use a catheter

Some physicians do not recommend using implanted catheters in their pediatric patients with specific types of childhood cancer. Ask the physician the reason for her recommendation, and request a second opinion if you think a catheter might be helpful to your child.

> Stephan (six years old) has no catheter. Sometimes I wish he had one. It seems like it would be easier. We were told he didn't need it. He is running out of usable veins and it is getting harder and harder.

· · · · ·

> Our physician gave us the option of using a catheter for our six-year-old daughter, but he recommended against it. He said if she could stand the pokes it was better not to use it due to the chance of infections. She had several sessions with the staff psychologist to teach her visualization and imagery which she used successfully to deal with the two years of IVs.

To help you make the best decision for your particular situation, the table "Comparison of Catheters," outlines the pros and cons for each catheter. There is no right or wrong choice; different options are available because each child, each parent, each family, is unique.

Comparison of Catheters

	External Catheter	Subcutaneous Port	Peripherally Inserted Central Catheter
Infection Rate	Higher	Lower	Higher
Maintenance	Daily	Monthly	Daily
Body Image	Tube outside body	Lump under skin	Tube outside body

	External Catheter	Subcutaneous Port	Peripherally Inserted Central Catheter
Pain	Dressing changes	Needle poke to access (use EMLA)	Needle poke to insert the line, dressing changes
Anxiety	Low to high	Low to high	Low to high
Cost	More due to daily maintenance	Less—monthly maintenance	More due to daily maintenance
Risk of drugs leaking into tissues	Lowest	Low	Low

The decision: Which catheter for your child?

After reviewing the information presented and the comparison chart, discuss with your doctor his opinion of the merits of each catheter. Talk over the pros and cons with your child if she is old enough. Then make the rounds of the cancer ward, asking both parents and children which type of catheter they chose and why. You will probably hear many strong opinions on the benefits and drawbacks for each catheter.

> *When we asked one of the young children on the ward which catheter she had, she pulled up her shirt with a big grin to show us her Hickman. She had a coil of white tubing neatly taped to her chest. My husband's face turned as white as her tubing.*

. . . . .

> *My four-year-old daughter loved ballet and was extremely interested in her appearance. Her younger sister was very physical, and we were worried that if we chose the Hickman she would grab and pull on the tubing. We chose the port so that she could wear her tutus without reminders of cancer and so that the children could play together without mishap.*

The nurses in the clinic and on the ward are another source of valuable information. They will have seen dozens (or hundreds) of children with catheters, and will be able to give excellent advice, given your family situation. There is no right or wrong choice, just different options for each unique child.

Removal of indwelling catheters is explained in Chapter 25, *End of Treatment and Beyond*.

When Scott (age three) was diagnosed with stage IV neuroblastoma, his doctor gave us a choice of which central line we could use. He showed us a mannequin with a Broviac and a Port-a-cath. He also told us the pros and cons of each type, then asked us to decide. We chose the Broviac, and feel it was the best decision for Scott. The day it was installed was the end of a lot of unnecessary pain (from needle sticks) for Scott.

Scott finished all his treatments three months ago, and yesterday he had his Broviac removed. It went extremely smoothly. He had only one cuff and it was halfway out already. And to think, I fretted and worried about the removal all week!

He has lots and lots of energy. His hair is coming back in and he actually has color in his face. He looks so healthy! I love it!

CHAPTER 7

Surviving Your Child's Hospitalization

Every day is a journey,
and the journey itself is home.

—Matsuo Basho

THERE ARE FEW THINGS in life worse than arising from a lumpy, pullout couch to face another day of your child's hospitalization for cancer. Hospitals are huge, noisy bureaucracies on a time schedule all their own. For a child, being hospitalized means being separated from parents, brothers, sisters, friends, pets, and the comfort and familiarity of home. A child's hospitalization can rob both the parent and child of a sense of control, leaving them feeling helpless. There are ways, however, to wrest back some power, while adding a great deal of cheerfulness to the proceedings.

The room

Hospital rooms are often painted an institutional shade of gray or green, and somehow, most windows seem to look out over the power plant. Covering the walls with big, bright posters (Disney characters, sports figures, rock groups) can liven up the room immensely.

> *The first thing we put up in Meagan's room was a huge poster of the Little Engine That Could saying, "I think I can, I think I can."*

Display cards on the walls, hanging from strings like a mobile, or taped around the window sills. Put up pictures of the child engaged in her favorite activity, and add photos of friends, too. Most hospitals don't allow flowers on oncology floors since they can grow a fungus which can make the child sick, but it's fun to have bouquets of balloons bobbing in the corners. Younger children derive great comfort from having a favorite stuffed animal, blanket, or quilt on their bed. If it doesn't bother your child, make the room smell good with potpourri or aromatherapy oils.

To personalize the visit of each member of the medical staff, some parents bring a guestbook to sign. Others put up a visitor sign-in poster, which must be signed before examinations begin or vital signs are taken. Another variation of the sign-in poster is to have each staff member outline her hand and write within the print.

> In my position as a parent consultant, I suggest that a journal be kept in the child's room for any visitor, family member, or medical care giver to write in at any time. Leaving a message if the child is sleeping or out of the room for procedures can be a nice surprise. Later, a surviving child and her family, or the family of a child who has died, have a memory book of those who have touched their lives.

Bringing music will help block out some of the hospital noise as well as help everyone relax. A small cassette player, Walkman with earphones, or a CD boom box is portable and useful.

> My daughter's preschool teacher sent a care package. She made a felt board with dozens of cutout characters and designs that provided hours of quiet entertainment. She also included games, drawings from each classmate, coloring books, markers, get well cards, and a child's tape player with ear phones. Because we had run out of our house with just the clothes on our backs, all of these toys were very, very welcome.

Although many hospitals provide brightly colored smocks for the patients, most children and teens prefer to wear their own clothing if at all possible. This can pose a laundry problem, so check to see if the floor has washers available for families to use.

As soon as possible after admission, ask for a "floor tour." Find out if a microwave and refrigerator are available, learn what the approved parent sleeping arrangements are, and ask about showers and bathtubs for both patients and parents. Obtain a hospital handbook if one is available. These booklets often include information on billing, parking, discounts, and other helpful items.

Many children's hospitals have VCRs available. Sign up for a convenient time and bring in or rent a favorite funny video. Humor helps. Bring in age appropriate games, puzzles, and books.

> *A friend brought in a bag full of fun stuff from the local dime store. He included a water pistol (good for unwelcome visitors or unfriendly interns), play dough, Slinky, checkers, dominos, bubbles, a book of corny jokes, and puzzles.*

Food

Buying meals day after day in the hospital cafeteria is expensive. In addition, many of the food items available in the cafeteria deserve the notorious reputation of "hospital food." Check to see if the floor has a refrigerator for parent's food and stock it from home. Remember to put your name in a prominent place on your containers. Many hospitals have cooking facilities for families where they can cook or microwave favorite meals. Ask family and friends to bring food in when they visit, and consider ordering extra items to come up on your child's tray. Ordering out for dinner can also be a nice change of pace for you and your child. As long as there are no medical restrictions, there's no reason why pizza can't be delivered to the hospital. Ask the nurses if they have menus from local restaurants.

> *Just the smell of food nauseated my daughter. I'll never forget taking the tray out in the hall, and gobbling it down myself. I always felt so guilty, and thought that staff viewed me as that parent who ate her kid's food. But it saved money and prevented her meals from going to waste. I also did not want to leave her side for the few minutes it took to go to the cafeteria, although in hindsight, the walk would have done me some good.*

Parking

Most parents of children with cancer have unpleasant memories of driving around in endless loops looking for a parking space while their child is throwing up in a bucket in the back seat (or even worse when the bucket was left at home). Learn about both long- and short-term parking arrangements. Ask other parents if parking passes are available or where the cheapest parking is located.

> *I had no idea that the hospital gave out free parking passes to their frequent customers. Now I tell every new parent to check as soon as possible to see if they can get a parking pass. It will save them lots of money*

that they would have spent on meters and parking tickets, and time they would have spent running out to move the car out of the emergency parking spot.

The endless waiting

Parents need to become experts in learning how to wait without losing their minds. They need to expect long waits for everything from blood draws to procedures. Many parents find themselves getting nervous or angry while waiting for the doctors to appear during "rounds" each morning (when the attendings, residents, and interns move from room to room in a large group), then feel let down when the visit lasts only a few moments. If you have questions to ask the doctors, write them down and tell the doctors when they come in that you would like a few moments to discuss concerns or ask questions.

It helps to come prepared for long waits each time that you go to the hospital. Some progressive (and well funded) institutions have VCRs and games available, but usually you need to bring your own things. Have your child pick out favorite card games, board games, computer games, drawing materials, and books. Remember to bring food and drinks. Some children will take comfort from taking a favorite blanket or pillow along with them for a day in the clinic or a lengthy hospitalization.

Befriending the staff

Hospitals are staffed by many wonderful and some not so wonderful people. Many parents find that their heightened stress makes them less tolerant of inefficiency or confusion. As discussed in Chapter 4, *Forming a Partnership with the Medical Team*, working together, rather than becoming adversaries, will provide your child with a sense of security. Doing things like helping change soiled bedding, taking out food trays, and giving baths frees up overworked nurses to take care of medicines and IVs. Nurses really appreciate the help, and usually reciprocate by answering questions or negotiating with the doctors for you.

As soon as possible, learn about the shift changes on the oncology floor. If you need to leave, don't leave a request with one nurse if another will be coming on duty soon. If you have a request or reminder, you can post it on the child's door, the wall above the bed, or on the chart.

Being an advocate for your child

Hospitals can be frightening places for children. Parents need to provide comfort, protection, and advocacy for their vulnerable child. To fulfill these roles, parents need to be present.

Most pediatric hospitals are quite aware of how much better children do if a parent is allowed to sleep in the room. Sometimes small couches convert into beds, or parents can use a cot provided by the hospital.

> Whenever my husband couldn't be at the hospital at bedtime, he would bring in homemade tapes of him reading bedtime stories. Our son would drift off to sleep hearing his daddy's voice.

If hospital policy requires the parent to leave, insist on staying. Geralyn Gaes tells a story in *You Don't Have to Die* about a confrontation at her local community hospital:

> One night a nurse came into Jason's room and curtly informed me that I would have to leave, since it was past visiting hours. With my son pale and retching from chemotherapy, I was not about to go anywhere. Looking her in the eye, I said "You can send security after me if you like, but I'm not leaving here." No one disturbed me again.

Of course, sometimes it isn't possible to stay with your child if you are a single parent or if both parents work full time. Many families have grandparents or close friends who stay with the hospitalized child when the parents cannot be present. Older children and teenagers may not want a parent in the room at night, but they need an advocate there during the day just as much as the preschoolers.

Whenever a family member cannot be present, children who are old enough should be taught to use the telephone. Tape a phone number nearby where a parent can be reached and have the child call if anyone tries to do procedures that are unexpected. The hospital staff should be informed that any changes in treatment (except emergencies) need to be authorized by a parent.

Having cancer strips children of control over their bodies. To help reverse this process, parents can take over most nursing care. Children may prefer parents to help them to the bathroom or to clean up diarrhea or vomit.

I was embarrassed to have the nurse change the sheets when I had an accident in the bed. I couldn't help it when I was taking the cytoxan, but I was still embarrassed.

Making the bed, keeping the room tidy, changing dressings, and giving back-rubs help your child feel more comfortable and lighten the burden of the over-worked nurses. However, some children may do better with the nurses. Parents should allow the child to express his needs, even if it feels like rejection.

Parents can help their child regain some control by encouraging choices whenever possible. Older children should be actively involved in discussions about their treatment, while younger children can decide when to take a bath, which arm to use for an IV, what to order for meals, what position for procedures, what clothes to wear, and how to decorate the room. Some children request a hug or a handshake after all treatments or procedures.

Where do the kids play?

Children need to play and teens need to socialize, especially when hospitalized. Ask whether the hospital has a recreation therapy department (play therapy is discussed in Chapter 2, *Coping with Procedures*). Often, a large room is devoted to toys, books, dolls, and crafts, and is staffed by specialists who really know how to play with children. These rooms provide many therapeutic activities such as medical play with dolls, which help children to express fears or concerns about what is happening to them. By encouraging contact with other children in similar circumstances, recreation therapy helps children feel less alone, less different from other children. The rooms are a cheerful change from lying in a hospital bed and are full of fun-filled activities and smiling staff people. If the child is too ill or her counts are too low to go to the play area, arrangements can be made for a recreational therapist to bring a bundle of toys, games, and books to the room. This can give the parent time to go out to eat or take a walk.

When I wanted to have a conference with the oncologist about Katy's protocol, I called recreation therapy and they sent two wonderful ladies to the clinic. The doctor and I were able to talk privately for an hour, and Katy had a great time making herself a gold crown and decorating her wheelchair with streamers and jewels.

Find out if there are support groups for teens. You might also try to bend the rules a bit to allow your teen to have friends in visiting as much as possible.

Exercise is important, too. For kids strong enough to walk, exploring the hospital can be fun. Plan a daily excursion to the gift shop or the cafeteria. Go outside and walk the entire perimeter of the hospital if weather and the neighborhood permit. Don't feel limited by an IV pole; it can be pushed or pulled and will feel normal after a while. Many children have been seen standing on the base of the IV pole—hanging on for dear life—with a parent wildly pushing them down the hall at breakneck speed. Check to see if the hospital has a swimming pool (for you to swim in; your child probably can't use it).

Many neutropenic (low white count) children or teens feel refreshed by going up on the roof just to feel the wind on their face and have the sun warm their skin. Some hospitals even grant "passes" to young patients whose white counts are high enough.

Any action that parents, family members, and friends take to support and advocate for the youngster with cancer buoys up the spirit. Remember: courage is contagious.

Sometimes you can create your own fun with just a little imagination. On one particular occasion, Matthew was feeling especially bored. With a little ingenuity, we soon discovered that four unused IV poles and as many blankets as we could "steal" from the linen cart made for one pretty cool tent. We then used the mattress from a roll-away cot, and spent the night "camping" in his hospital room. He had a wonderful time.

CHAPTER 8

Neuroblastoma

The world breaks everyone and afterward
many are strong at the broken places.

—Ernest Hemingway
A Farewell to Arms

NEUROBLASTOMA IS A CANCER of the sympathetic nervous system. The average age at diagnosis is two years, with the majority of cases presenting before the age of five years. While neuroblastoma can arise at any place along the sympathetic nervous system from the neck to the pelvis, more than half originate at the adrenal gland in the abdomen. Symptoms of this disease vary depending on the location of the primary tumor.

This chapter first looks at the structure and function of the sympathetic nervous system. Then it examines who gets neuroblastoma, what the signs and symptoms are, how it is diagnosed, and how doctors determine the prognosis. The chapter ends with a discussion of the current treatments and looks ahead to future and experimental treatments.

The sympathetic nervous system

The human body is equipped with the most impressive information system known to man. Chemical messengers, called neurotransmitters, relay information throughout the body using the two networks which comprise the nervous system. The central nervous system (CNS) includes the brain and spinal cord. The brain acts as the central control room, while the spinal cord operates as a link to other important elements of the nervous system. The peripheral nervous system (PNS) connects the CNS to other organs and systems. The network of nerves that make up the sympathetic nervous system is part of the PNS.

The sympathetic nervous system performs automatically in response to the environment and emotions. For example, if a person is surprised or angered, the sympathetic nervous system leaps into action by accelerating the heart-beat, increasing blood sugar, and cooling the body through perspiration.

The adrenal glands are relatively small glands that sit on top of each kidney, and are responsible for producing many different hormones. The adrenal gland has two parts. The outer portion, called the cortex, secretes hormones such as cortisone and aldosterone that are used by the body for fluid and electrolyte balance. The central portion, called the medulla, produces the hormones adrenaline and noradrenaline, which help the body respond to stress.

Who gets neuroblastoma?

Neuroblastoma accounts for approximately 8 to 10 percent of all childhood cancers. Each year more than 600 new cases are diagnosed in the United States and an additional 65 are diagnosed in Canada. Males are diagnosed more often than females, and there is a slightly higher incidence among white than black children. About half of all neuroblastomas are diagnosed by two years of age and about 75 percent are diagnosed before five years of age. Neuroblastoma is also diagnosed in newborns.

> My son was only two years old when his first symptoms began. It was on the day of his third birthday that we received the diagnosis of neuroblastoma. A tumor was found attached to his left adrenal gland, and cancer cells were also discovered in his bones and bone marrow. I remember thinking that I had never heard such a strange and ugly sounding word as neuroblastoma before in my life.

Genetic factors

There is no known genetic cause of neuroblastoma. Children with some disorders, however, have a higher risk of developing neuroblastoma. Two examples of these associated disorders are Hirschsprung disease (a developmental abnormality which involves the colon) and von Recklinghausen neurofibromatosis.

Environmental factors

Although certain types of cancer have been linked to environmental factors, this is not true for neuroblastoma. Many research studies have been conducted to evaluate possible environmental causes, but no conclusive answers have yet been found.

Signs and symptoms

Children with neuroblastoma may exhibit a number of different symptoms. The signs and symptoms of disease depend largely on the location of the primary tumor and whether the disease has spread (metastasized) to other distant locations in the body.

> *Mikey (four years old) was always a sickly child and he was constantly on antibiotics for one ailment or another. The night before we took him to the emergency room, he had fallen into his toy box and hurt his abdomen. He wasn't in any pain, but overnight a huge mass began to appear. He was asleep on my bed laying on his side and we could see a mass protruding from his upper left abdomen area. We never imagined it could be a tumor.*

· · · · ·

> *My son was fourteen years old when he was diagnosed. Greggory could run a mile in 5 minutes and 4 seconds. Who would have thought that he had a 5×6 inch tumor attached to his kidney? He complained off and on about back pain, but it was usually after shoveling snow or sledding or whatever else boys his age do. There was always a reason.*

In many cases, parents find a lump or mass in the abdomen while dressing or bathing their child. The abdomen may appear enlarged. The child may stop eating, lose weight, and experience diarrhea and vomiting. If disease has spread to the skeleton, the child may begin to limp, refuse to stand, or complain of pain in the bones. Children with neuroblastoma may have fever and they may be unusually tired and irritable. In addition, children whose disease has spread to the bones around the eye socket may have dark circles around the eyes. This is often referred to as "raccoon eyes."

> *Initially, when our son began limping, we attributed it to normal growing pains. There were no other signs that it could be a more serious situation. We took him to a doctor a few days after the limping started, and he didn't seem to feel it was a cause for great concern, either. Shortly after that, our son began to complain of leg pains and he was unable to walk at all.*

If the tumor involves the spinal cord, the child may complain of back pain and have difficulty passing urine or stool. Tumors located in this area sometimes cause spinal cord compression which can result in paralysis. Children whose disease has spread to the bone marrow may have pale skin and sometimes tiny red dots under the skin (petechiae). Tumors growing in the chest may cause a chronic cough or difficulty breathing.

Horner syndrome is a rare disorder that is sometimes associated with a mediastinal (in the chest) or cervical (in the neck) neuroblastoma. This syndrome occurs when the sympathetic nerve to the eye is damaged or disrupted. The eyelid droops, the pupil looks small, and the child may not sweat on the side of the face of the affected eye.

> My son had a strange reaction after his surgery in which he developed a red flush on exactly one side of his face and neck. The anesthesiologist called it Horner syndrome, and was interested in it enough to take a photograph of it for research purposes.

· · · · ·

> Scott has a minor complication from surgery called Horner syndrome. His left eyelid droops, and the pupil is smaller than that of the right eye. It doesn't impact his vision, but it is clearly noticeable when you look at him.

Opsoclonus-myoclonus is another rare and unusual sign that can accompany neuroblastoma. It is sometimes referred to as "dancing eyes-dancing feet syndrome" because of its symptoms—rapid, uncontrollable movement of the eyes, and sudden, jerky movements of the feet and legs.

> At the age of nineteen months, Justina lost all her motor skills. At first she was clumsy and staggering, but it progressed very rapidly (over a period of four days) to a point where she was not able to pull herself up or even sit. Her eyes would bounce, roll back, and circle. She was scared, since she had no concept of where her body was in space. She always felt as if she was falling. Justina was misdiagnosed for four months until we finally learned what was wrong. She had neuroblastoma along with opsoclonus-myoclonus.

Diagnosis

Many tests are necessary to confirm a diagnosis of neuroblastoma because symptoms of this disease can mimic other illnesses, including other cancers. The oncologist will perform a thorough physical examination and order a complete blood count (CBC). Computed tomography (CT) or magnetic resonance imaging (MRI) scans are obtained. Chest x-rays and ultrasonography of the abdomen help determine if a mass is present. A bone scan is usually ordered to check the presence or extent of skeletal involvement. An MIBG scan, performed in the nuclear medicine department, is frequently ordered since it is very specific in detecting the presence of neuroblastoma. However, the radiopharmaceutical used for this scan can be difficult to get, so it is not available at all pediatric facilities. For further information on each of these procedures, see Chapter 2, *Coping with Procedures*.

> *Little alarm bells started going off when the radiologist had the technician scan Cam's abdomen twice. She wanted to get a good look at his liver and all the way to the bottom of his kidneys. A few hours later, the oncologist, psychologist, and nurse clinician all showed up and my stomach sank.*

Hormone tests, biopsies, and evaluation of a host of biologic factors also help the oncologist diagnose neuroblastoma. Approximately 95 percent of all neuroblastomas secrete hormones called catecholamines, which are usually produced by the adrenal medulla. Catecholamines, and their metabolic end products vanillylmandelic acid (VMA) and homovanillic acid (HVA), are found in the urine. A 24-hour or "spot" urine sample (urine collected one time, rather than all urine collected for a 24-hour period) is collected and tested for catecholamine levels. This test is valuable for making the initial diagnosis and for following the child's response to treatment.

> *Rachel was three years old when she first developed symptoms. One of her eyes started turning in and she lost most of her vision in that eye (she regained it after treatment). The doctor did some scans and a biopsy, and diagnosed her neuroblastoma. She had a primary tumor on her right adrenal gland, but there was a much larger tumor in her sinus cavity, behind her right eye. Her urine catecholamine levels were never elevated.*

In order to make a diagnosis, the oncologist needs actual tumor tissue obtained from a biopsy or operation. Every child with suspected neuroblastoma will also have a bone marrow aspiration. The tumor sample and bone marrow aspirate are studied under a microscope by a pathologist. These samples are then tested for a variety of biologic factors.

Staging

Once a diagnosis of neuroblastoma has been made, the oncologist will order further tests and scans to determine the extent (stage) of the disease. There are three systems currently in use to stage neuroblastoma: the Children's Cancer Group (CCG) system, the Pediatric Oncology Group (POG) system, and the International Neuroblastoma Staging System (INSS). The INSS was developed to provide researchers with a system to compare data and facilitate the international exchange of information.

Using the INSS, neuroblastoma is categorized into five distinct stages:

- Stage 1. The tumor is limited to the site of origin and can be completely removed (resected), with or without microscopic residual disease (extremely small amounts that are visible only with the aid of a microscope); lymph nodes on both sides of the abdomen are negative (no cancer found when viewed under a microscope).

- Stage 2A. The tumor affects only one side of the body and is limited to the site of origin; the cancer cannot be completely resected (microscopic disease remains); lymph nodes on both sides of the body are negative microscopically.

- Stage 2B. The tumor affects only one side of the body and is limited to the site of origin; complete resection may or may not be possible; lymph nodes on the same side of the body near the tumor are positive (contain neuroblastoma cells); lymph nodes on the opposite side of the body are negative microscopically.

- Stage 3. The tumor has moved across the midline and is unresectable; regional lymph nodes may or may not be positive; or the tumor affects only one side of the body with related lymph node involvement of the opposite side of the body; or the tumor begins in the midline with lymph node involvement on both sides of the body.

- Stage 4. The tumor has spread from the site of origin to distant lymph nodes beyond the cavity, bone, bone marrow, liver, and/or other organs in which the tumor began (except as defined for stage 4S).

- Stage 4S. This stage includes only infants under one year of age. The tumor is confined to the site of origin as described in stage 1 or 2, with spread limited to liver, skin, and/or, to a limited extent, bone marrow.

Prognosis

Treatment for childhood neuroblastoma has steadily improved in the last two decades. In the 1960s, virtually all children with neurobalstoma died.

Now, the success rate of treatment varies with the stage at diagnosis. The majority of children with stage 1, 2, 4S, or 4 (if the child is less than one year old at diagnosis) are cured.

Doctors determine the appropriate treatment for each child by considering the child's age, the stage of the tumor, and a variety of biologic factors. Children with neuroblastoma are grouped into low, intermediate, and high risk subgroups in order to give the child the best possible treatment for her disease.

To determine these risk levels, several prognostic factors are used, including the following:

- N-myc amplification. N-*myc* (also known as MYCN) is a gene that under certain conditions helps to change a normal cell into a cancerous cell. Amplification means that the cell makes multiple copies of the gene.

- Tumor pathology. The Shimada index is a method to grade the tumor based on how it looks under a microscope (histopathologic classification). This index, developed by Dr. H. Shimada, is widely used to evaluate neuroblastoma tumors.

- DNA index. This is a measurement of the amount of DNA material in neuroblastoma cells. An increase in the number of chromosomes is called hyperdiploid DNA.

- Abnormalities of chromosome 1.

> When Adam was three weeks old we took him to the pediatrician because his abdomen was swollen. We were shocked to learn that it was cancer—stage 4S neuroblastoma. He didn't receive any treatment for his disease at that time, because his doctor felt he didn't need it. Instead, we just watched him very closely. His tumors eventually calcified, and he was fine until five years later when he suffered a relapse and required chemotherapy. He has done very well, and recently we celebrated his twelfth birthday.

Treatment

At diagnosis, many parents are confused about how to find the best doctors and treatments for their child. State-of-the-art care is available from physicians who participate in the Children's Cancer Group (CCG) and/or the

Pediatric Oncology Group (POG). These study groups, composed of pediatric surgeons and oncologists, urologists, radiation oncologists, researchers, and nurses, establish the standard of care for patients worldwide, conduct new studies to discover better therapies, and establish follow-up for survivors. They are in the process of merging into one entity called the Children's Oncology Group (COG). If the treatment center you are referred to is a member of one of these groups, you can rest assured that your child will have access to the best thinking on the treatment of pediatric cancers.

The oncologist chooses the best treatment or clinical trial (see Chapter 5, *Clinical Trials*) based on these risk categories:

- **Low risk.** Children with early stage disease and infants with stage 4S do not require aggressive treatment. They usually have surgery and in some cases, mild chemotherapy.

- **Intermediate risk.** Children with intermediate risk disease generally require chemotherapy and surgery. Occasionally radiation is necessary.

- **High risk.** Children at high risk of relapse need aggressive treatment, including chemotherapy, surgery, radiation, and sometimes bone marrow or peripheral stem cell transplantation.

The goal is to achieve a complete remission by obliterating all cancer cells as quickly as possible. Complete remission occurs when all signs and symptoms of neuroblastoma disappear and abnormal cells are no longer found by any standard evaluation (CT, bone scan, routine bone marrow aspirate, and biopsy).

Surgery

Surgery is used to treat virtually all neuroblastomas and has many important roles (see Chapter 18, *Surgery*). It is used to establish the diagnosis, to obtain tumor tissue for examination, to stage the disease, and for second-look procedures. If the tumor is localized and appears resectable, surgery is performed soon after diagnosis before further therapy is begun. Most often, however, this is not possible and chemotherapy is used to shrink the tumor prior to surgery. Even after chemotherapy, surgical removal is often incomplete, and radiation is required to ensure that all tumor cells are destroyed, notably for stage 3 and 4 disease.

The surgery to remove the tumor took about four hours, and there were no major complications. Scott spent three hours in the recovery room before being ready to go to the ward. His first words after waking were, "I love you, mom," which obviously touched Karen. While in the recovery room, we realized that Scott's stuffed Yoshi toy, who also went to the operating room, returned with a neck bandage identical to Scott's. Someone had a sense of humor!

· · · · ·

Kirsten's tumor had shrunk enough after four cycles of chemotherapy for a near total resection. However, the tumor was still considered active, and she went on to receive three further cycles.

Complications can occur in 5 to 10 percent of aggressive surgical procedures. The goals of initial surgeries should be developed on an individual basis because each child is unique. Factors considered include tumor location, resectability, relationship to major blood vessels, and the child's prognosis. Lymph nodes near the tumor are usually sampled to determine if the disease has spread. Sometimes a liver biopsy is taken during the initial surgery, although the value of this practice is unclear if the liver appears normal on the scans and during surgery.

Spinal cord compression, often called "dumbbell" extension, occurs when a tumor invades the spinal canal. In this situation, a surgical procedure called laminectomy is sometimes performed. A laminectomy removes part of the bone covering the spinal canal, relieving symptoms caused by compression of the cord and nerve roots. Most often, spinal cord compression from neuroblastoma is treated with chemotherapy, avoiding the need for laminectomy.

Chemotherapy

Chemotherapy is used to treat almost all children with neuroblastoma. Response rates have improved considerably through the use of multidrug regimens (treatments using more than one chemotherapeutic agent). The most commonly used chemotherapy agents include cyclophosphamide, cisplatin, doxorubicin, vincristine, teniposide, and etoposide. Some studies use only one drug at the beginning of therapy in a "window" study. This kind of study attempts to find out if the drug being studied has an effect on neuroblastoma on its own. These drugs include carboplatin and ifosfamide. Other chemotherapy drugs that are used to treat neuroblastoma include topotecan, irinotecan, and melphalan.

> *After seven months of ups and downs, ins and outs, chemotherapy, fungal infections, bone marrow biopsies, and surgeries, Michael finally reached remission.*

· · · · ·

> *Luke (two years old) had side effects from his chemo protocol that were relatively minor compared to what other children experience. He did have nausea, but it usually consisted of one to three vomiting episodes over one or two days and were over quickly. Over the entire eight course cycle he did have numerous neutropenic bouts, with several visits to the emergency room for night-onset fevers resulting in short-term hospitalizations to get IV antibiotics. He did get two or three infections in his broviac which also required hospitalizations for antibiotics. However, he only needed one blood and one platelet transfusion during the entire protocol. He ate incredibly well all during his protocol and even gained steadily in weight and height.*

Generally, therapy will be mapped out in a protocol, which is an outline of the drugs to be used, the maximum dose to be given, as well as the preferred schedule and routes of administration. For more information, see Chapter 15, *Chemotherapy*.

Radiation

Neuroblastoma is very sensitive to radiation. The primary role of radiation is to locally control tumors that cannot be resected even after several courses of chemotherapy. It is also a component of some bone marrow transplant programs (total body radiation). Finally, it can be used for symptomatic relief of painful bony lesions at any time. Children with INSS stages 2B and 3 often are given radiation therapy in combination with chemotherapy. Radiation in doses of 1500 cGy (centigrays—measured units of radiation) to 2500 cGy are given in 150 cGy fractions over ten to twenty days. For more information, see Chapter 17, *Radiation*.

> *Matthew received palliative doses of radiation to bony areas that were causing him great pain. It worked very well, and generally he had considerable relief within 24 hours.*

My son experienced very few side effects from the local radiation he received to his abdomen and chest. He was premedicated each time with Zofran and only had a few bouts of vomiting over a two-week course. Other than diarrhea, he tolerated it great and wasn't even very fatigued.

In infants with stage 4S disease, 300 cGy to 600 cGy given to the liver is sometimes used in single or multiple fractions if there is respiratory distress because of a markedly enlarged liver.

Bone marrow transplantation

In the last decade, autologous bone marrow transplants and peripheral blood stem cell transplants have been used with increasing frequency to treat children with high-risk or relapsed neuroblastoma. Various regimens are used to prepare the child for transplant. These include chemotherapy drugs such as melphalan, cisplatin, teniposide, and doxorubicin with or without total body irradiation (TBI). For more information, see Chapter 19, *Bone Marrow and Stem Cell Transplantation*.

Rachel was three years old when she received an autologous bone marrow transplant as part of her protocol for high-risk neuroblastoma. It was a difficult experience for her and she was incredibly sick. During transplant, her personality changed and for weeks she just didn't seem like Rachel. She had awful sores on her mouth and bottom. She developed a severe case of mucositis and was placed in an oxygen tent to maintain her oxygen levels. Morphine was given to control pain, and we were in the hospital for a month. She's seven years old now, and has done well since she finished treatment in 1996.

• • • • •

The transplant was part of Zach's (age seven) upfront treatment protocol for stage IV neuroblastoma. We were scared, but it went so much easier than we expected. Zach breezed through, according to his doctor, and he was in and out of the hospital in three weeks. He had constant vomiting for three days because of the high dose chemotherapy, though. The stem cell infusion and the wait for his counts to recover were uneventful with just some boredom and fatigue. Currently, he's doing great. He is receiving 13-cis-retinoic acid now to finish up his protocol.

Biologic modifiers and more

Many brilliant researchers have devoted their lives to unlocking the neuro-blastoma mystery, resulting in vastly improved prognoses for many children. Some exciting new treatments are currently under investigation:

- Promising results have been achieved using a derivative of vitamin A, called 13-cis-retinoic acid, following autologous bone marrow transplants. 13-cis-retinoic acid has minimal toxicity and can cause neuroblastoma cells to stop growing. Confirmation of its efficacy is underway.

- GD2 is a substance found in large amounts in some neuroblastoma cells. Some institutions are researching using antibodies that attack the GD2 in neuroblastoma cells while limiting damage to healthy cells.

- Cytokine gene therapy (also called vaccine therapy) uses agents such as IL-2 to help the child's immune system destroy cancerous cells. Neuroblastoma cells are removed from the child, modified in a lab, then injected back into the child.

- Some institutions are getting good results with a new radiotherapy technique using ^{131}I-MIBG and ^{125}I-MIBG. For more information, see Chapter 17.

Newest treatment options

To learn of the newest treatments available, call (800) 4-CANCER and ask for the PDQ (physicians data query) for neuroblastoma. These free statements, also available on the Internet at *http://cancernet.nci.nih.gov/*, explain the disease, state-of-the-art treatments, and ongoing clinical trials. There are two versions available: one for patients, which uses simple language and contains no statistics, and one for professionals, which is technical, thorough, and includes citations to scientific literature.

> *Paige was four years old when she was diagnosed with stage 4 neuro-blastoma. She hadn't been sick at all, and the disease was found during a well child visit with the pediatrician. I remember feeling completely shocked and terrified. It happened so fast, and within 24 hours she had already had her catheter installed for her chemotherapy. Things were very difficult, but they got much worse when Paige relapsed while she was*

still receiving treatment. Her doctors decided that her only chance of survival would be a stem cell transplant. The experience was grueling, and it felt like we were living in another, weird world.

Paige is now a happy eight-year-old. Her diagnosis was the worst thing that has ever happened in our lives, but we have survived.

CHAPTER 9

Wilms Tumor

To keep a lamp burning we have to keep
putting oil in it.

—Mother Teresa

WILMS TUMOR, ALSO CALLED NEPHROBLASTOMA, is a cancer that originates in the kidney. The disease gets its name from a German doctor, Max Wilms, who wrote one of the first medical articles about it in 1899.

Ninety percent of all kidney cancers in children are Wilms tumor. The remaining ten percent are rare forms of childhood kidney cancers: clear cell sarcoma of the kidney, malignant rhabdoid tumor of the kidney, and occasionally renal cell carcinoma.

This chapter first looks at the structure and function of the kidney. Then it examines who gets kidney cancer, what the signs and symptoms are, how it is diagnosed, and how doctors determine the prognosis. The chapter ends with a discussion of current and future treatments.

The kidneys

The kidneys, located near the middle of the back, are responsible for filtering the blood and removing harmful waste products. These two bean-shaped organs are each about the size of a fist.

The kidney operates as a recycling depot complete with high-tech sanitation engineers. Its main job is to filter harmful waste products from the blood and to regulate the return of reusable chemicals—sodium, phosphorus, and potassium—back to the body.

Inside each kidney are millions of microscopic structures which filter out large particles, such as white and red blood cells, as well as most proteins, allowing them to return to the bloodstream. What remains in the kidney after this process is called urine. The urine flows from the kidney through a long tube (ureter) into the bladder, where it is stored until it is eliminated from the body by urination (see Figure 9-1).

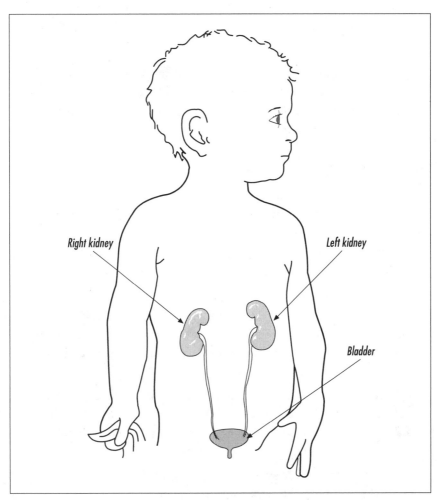

Figure 9-1. The kidneys

Who gets Wilms tumor?

Wilms tumor is the second most common type of all childhood solid tumors, not including brain tumors. It accounts for approximately 6 percent of all childhood cancers. The average age at diagnosis is between two and three years when the disease is unilateral (affecting only one kidney), but it is generally diagnosed at a younger age in children when the disease is bilateral (affecting both kidneys). Seventy-five to eighty percent are diagnosed before the age of five. Approximately 450 new cases are seen annually in North America. There is a higher incidence in black children than in white children. Conversely, there is a lower incidence among Asian compared to white children. Girls are only slightly more at risk of developing Wilms tumor than boys.

> Matthew was one year old when he was diagnosed with Wilms tumor. Everyone used to tell me how lucky I was because he was so young and he probably wouldn't remember anything. Funny, because lucky was not a word I would use to describe the scenario.

Genetic factors

Wilms tumor is believed to result from mutations or changes in certain genes. The involved genes and other genes located nearby are not only associated with Wilms tumor, but several other rare conditions. Approximately 15 percent of children diagnosed with this cancer also have one of the following birth defects or syndromes:

- **Aniridia.** A rare condition in which there is incomplete formation of the iris of the eye. It is a congenital defect that can cause blindness. Because of its association with Wilms tumor, children with this rare syndrome should be screened periodically for Wilms tumor. There is no specific genetic testing available for aniridia.

- **WAGR syndrome.** A rare genetic condition associated with Wilms tumor. WAGR is an abbreviation for Wilms tumor, aniridia, genitourinary tract abnormalities, and mental retardation. A child with this syndrome has a greater than 30 percent chance of developing Wilms tumor.

- **Beckwith-Wiedemann syndrome.** A congenital disorder characterized by larger-than-normal internal organs and hypoglycemia at birth.

- **Hemihypertrophy.** A condition in which one side of the body may grow larger than the other. Because of its association with Wilms tumor, children with this syndrome should be screened periodically for the disease.

- **Denys-Drash syndrome.** Characterized by abnormal kidney function and genital abnormalities called pseudohermaphroditism (a condition in which genitalia are ambiguous, making it difficult to determine if the child is male or female). This syndrome occurs mostly in boys.

- Nephroblastomatosis. The presence of small pockets of embryonal kidney tissue under the capsule of the kidney that is usually bilateral. If present, there is a high risk of developing a tumor in the kidney and ultrasound is usually recommended for up to ten years.

- Hereditary Wilms tumor. Characterized by tumors in both kidneys and a family history of the disease. It is uncommon; 4 to 5 percent of all patients diagnosed have bilateral tumors and 1 to 2 percent have a family history of Wilms.

Environmental factors

There has been no consistent link between development of Wilms tumor and any environmental factors.

Signs and symptoms

Wilms tumor is often a difficult disease to diagnose. Usually, a parent notices a lump or mass in the abdominal area while dressing or bathing her child who has no other symptoms. By this time, the tumor is generally very large. Sometimes the tumor is found during routine visits when the pediatrician palpates the toddler's abdomen. Wilms tumor is occasionally diagnosed when the child is evaluated for other unrelated reasons, such as accidental trauma to the abdominal area.

> We thought she had the flu. After she had been throwing up for a few hours and was too weak to stand on her own, I was holding her up in the bathroom. As she leaned over my hands, I could feel a lump in her abdomen. The doctor knew what it was the second he felt it. We had tests at the local hospital that confirmed the diagnosis of Wilms tumor.

Some children with Wilms tumor have abdominal pain and up to 25 percent will have hematuria (blood in the urine). Blood may be visible to the naked eye or it may only be seen with microscopic evaluations. In addition, up to 25 percent of children have high blood pressure at diagnosis.

Other symptoms that may be present include fever, diarrhea, weight loss, shortness of breath, urogenital infections, and anemia (low number of red cells). The child may feel generally tired and unwell. Nausea and vomiting are infrequent symptoms of a Wilms tumor.

The vomiting and the lump were the only symptoms that Elizabeth had. I have seen the list of symptoms for Wilms tumor and I'm always startled by them. She never had signs of any of those things. I feel very fortunate that we caught her cancer so soon and with so little indication of anything being wrong. This is especially true since I know Wilms tumor is a fast growing cancer and we were fighting against time.

Diagnosis

Several tests and procedures are necessary to diagnose Wilms tumor. The doctor will first perform a physical examination and obtain the child's medical history. This is usually followed by an abdominal ultrasound and/or a CT scan. Occasionally, a scan called magnetic resonance imaging (MRI) is done. Because some children with Wilms tumor have bilateral involvement, both kidneys need to be examined. A complete blood count (CBC) is ordered, as well as urinalysis to check for signs of hematuria (blood in the urine). Kidney function tests are also taken.

I have to say that on diagnosis day our pediatrician was wonderful. When I called the doctor's office and told them about the lump that I had found in her abdomen and the vomiting, no one even hinted at what might be wrong. I was simply told to bring her in as soon as possible. The doctor was examining her less than two hours after my call to his office. He didn't tell me initially what he suspected. Later, he told me that he wanted to be sure before he even mentioned the word to me. He sent us to the local hospital where she underwent her first CT scan. The doctor was waiting for us with the news when we returned to his office.

X-rays and CT scans of the chest should be ordered to determine if the disease has spread to the lungs. Approximately 10 percent of children with Wilms tumor have lung metastases at diagnosis.

A chemical survey of the blood (called blood chemistries) is done to establish baseline kidney function, since one kidney is usually removed as part of the treatment protocol. Chemical surveys also check for liver disease and elevated levels of urates and phosphate. For more information on these tests, see Chapter 2, *Coping with Procedures*.

Staging

Once Wilms tumor has been diagnosed, surgery and/or more tests are done to determine if the cancer has spread to other parts of the body. This process is called staging and it helps the doctor choose the most appropriate treatment for the child.

> *Elizabeth's cancer was found by CT scan. That probably gave the doctors up front a good indication of what they were facing (how large the tumor is, how far it has spread). I was not told an estimate of what stage we might be at (those first days I wouldn't have understood anyway, and we all know that surgery can show something entirely different from what they expect). They said that she had a cancerous tumor called Wilms, and we were sent to the children's hospital.*

> *Surgery was immediately scheduled. I was told that what happened following the surgery would depend on what they found in surgery. I was also told at the very beginning that she would lose her kidney. If it was discovered that the cancer had progressed beyond the kidney (to the lung, etc.), it was possible that further surgery would be done.*

> *Following the surgery, tissues were typed and staged. A few days after the surgery, the doctors and I sat down in the conference room. It was then that I was given the staging information and the list of all of the stages so that I could see how we fit into the big scheme of things.*

Wilms tumor is staged by the following system, devised by the National Wilms Tumor Study Group (NWTSG):

- **Stage I.** The tumor is limited to the kidney and is able to be completely removed surgically.

- **Stage II.** The tumor extends beyond the kidney, but it is able to be completely removed surgically.

- **Stage III.** The tumor is not able to be completely removed surgically or is spilled at surgery, but disease is still limited to the abdomen.

- **Stage IV.** The disease has spread from the abdomen through the bloodstream and may be found in the lung, liver, bone, or brain, as well as distant lymph nodes.

- **Stage V.** The tumor is found on both kidneys at the time of diagnosis.

Prognosis

Treatment of Wilms tumor in children is one of medicine's success stories. Due to improvements in surgical techniques, drug therapies, and radiation, 85 to 90 percent of children with Wilms tumor who receive state-of-the-art treatment are cured. The best treatment for each child with Wilms is determined by analysis of several clinical and biologic features.

After a biopsy or surgery, the pathologist examines the nucleus of the cancerous cells under a microscope. If the nuclei of some of the cells appear larger than normal or irregular in shape, it is called anaplasia. Local anaplasia does not appear to affect prognosis. If there is a large proportion of anasplasia scattered throughout the tumor, it is called diffuse anasplasia and has a poorer prognosis.

Tumor cells that are not anaplastic are said to be Wilms tumor of favorable histology. The vast majority, approximately 95 percent, of children diagnosed with Wilms have cells with a favorable histology.

The oncologist will determine the prognosis using many criteria, including stage of disease, histology of the tumor cells, age of the child, and size of the tumor. These factors affect the aggressiveness of treatment needed. For example, a child diagnosed with stage II, favorable histology receives less intensive therapy than does a child with stage IV, unfavorable histology.

> *Elizabeth was diagnosed with stage II nephroblastoma (Wilms tumor), non-aggressive, favorable histology. That is only one notch away from as good as it gets. She was given a prognosis of 90 percent chance of five-year survival. We are currently only fourteen months and two weeks away from achieving that (but who's counting?).*

Treatment

The vast majority of children with Wilms who receive optimal treatment are cured of the disease. At diagnosis, many parents are confused about how to find the best doctors and treatments for their child. State-of-the-art care is available from physicians who participate in the National Wilms Tumor Study Group, the Children's Cancer Group (CCG), and the Pediatric Oncology Group (POG). These study groups, composed of pediatric surgeons and oncologists, urologists, radiation oncologists, researchers and nurses, establish the standard of care for patients worldwide, conduct new studies to discover better therapies or fine tune old ones, and establish follow-up for survivors. They are in the process of merging into one entity called the Children's Oncology Group (COG). If the treatment center you are referred to is a member of one of these groups, you can rest assured that your child will have access to the best thinking on the treatment of pediatric cancers.

The doctor will choose the best treatment or clinical trial (see Chapter 5, *Clinical Trials*) based on many factors, including your child's age, stage of disease, and size and histology of the tumor. For most patients, treatment is surgery followed by chemotherapy. Some children also require radiation.

Surgery

Children diagnosed with Wilms tumor usually have a surgical procedure, called a nephrectomy, performed before any other therapy is initiated (see Chapter 18, *Surgery*). Occasionally, if the diagnosis is questionable, a biopsy will be performed prior to nephrectomy. In North America, only children with bilateral Wilms tumor receive chemotherapy prior to surgery.

There are three different types of nephrectomies:

- **Simple nephrectomy.** Removal of the tumor as well as the entire kidney and ureter. The remaining kidney is able to compensate for the loss.

- **Partial nephrectomy.** Removal of the tumor and a portion of the affected kidney. It is done usually if the other kidney has already been removed or is damaged.

- **Radical nephrectomy.** Removal of the tumor, kidney, and some surrounding tissue.

During surgery, the surgeon evaluates the remaining kidney for disease and takes samples from lymph nodes in the area. The surgeon may also biopsy areas of the liver if she suspects that disease may be present.

> I was told that the surgery would take between two and three hours. It was just over four hours, which drove me insane in the waiting room. I hadn't been told anything about what Elizabeth would look like after the surgery. My cousin is a surgical nurse at a nearby hospital. She stopped by during my wait and prepared me. If she hadn't told me what to expect, I think I would have broken down from the shock. I wasn't prepared for all of the tubes and wires and the puffy face and anesthesia reactions. And no one told me about the central line. I had to ask one of the nurses after the fact what it was.

Elizabeth was expected to be out of bed and moving around on the second day. By the end of day three she was beginning to move around more like her old self, and by day four there was no slowing her down.

Her scar is her big smile, from her viewpoint. It was a long frown, from my viewpoint, that ran from one hip to the other. As she has grown, it has grown smaller and no longer extends all the way out to her hips.

Chemotherapy

All children diagnosed with Wilms tumor receive chemotherapy (drugs that kill cancer cells) as part of their treatment protocol.

There are several chemotherapy drugs that are effective against this type of cancer. The use of dactinomycin and vincristine has dramatically increased survival rates. Children with early stage disease often are treated with just these two drugs. For those who are diagnosed at more advanced stages, doxorubicin, cyclophosphamide, etoposide, ifosfamide, and carboplatin may be added. For information about these drugs, see Chapter 15, *Chemotherapy*.

Matthew received Adriamycin, dactinomycin, and vincristine for six months on an outpatient basis. His blood counts would drop between courses, but the lowest his ANC (absolute neutrophil count) ever got was 321. On one occasion his hematocrit dropped to 21, though he didn't need a blood transfusion.

Most children with Wilms tumor enter a clinical trial tailored to the stage and histology of their disease. The clinical trial protocol outlines the chemotherapy drugs and dosages that are used. Since chemotherapy can damage healthy, normal cells, the oncologist may need to adjust the actual dose that is administered. The goal is to minimize potential side effects (see Chapter 16, *Common Side Effects of Chemotherapy*), while providing adequate treatment for the disease.

My daughter's main side effects from the dactinomycin and vincristine were constipation and nausea. She was given a standard dose of Senecot every day for the constipation, and we were given a standing prescription for Zofran to control the nausea. Both of these drugs worked wonders for her. She really suffered very little discomfort during chemotherapy.

Radiation

The decision to use radiation therapy to treat a child with Wilms is based largely on the stage and histology of the tumor. Children with stage I and stage II favorable histology disease do not require radiation. For children with more advanced stages of disease, external beam radiation therapy is given (see Chapter 17, *Radiation*). This type of treatment uses high energy rays, delivered from outside the body, to kill cancer cells. The amount of disease present will determine the size of the area to be radiated. Usually, 1000 cGy, with an optional 1000 cGy boost to the tumor, is the recommended dose of radiation given to children with advanced stage diseases or tumors with unfavorable histology.

> *My one-year-old son had a huge tumor that went from his diaphragm to his bladder and crossed the midline. He had a simulation that lasted one and a half hours, then radiation to the spinal cord and abdomen, once a day for five days. He tolerated it very well. The only side effect he had was red peeling skin. He did have doxorubicin for the following six months, and had radiation recall several times. His peeling skin would return for a couple of days, then disappear.*

Newest treatment options

To learn about the newest treatments available, call (800) 4-CANCER and ask for the PDQ (physicians data query) for Wilms tumor. These free statements, also available on the Internet at *http://cancernet.nci.nih.gov/*, explain the disease, state-of-the-art treatments, and ongoing clinical trials. There are two versions available: one for patients, which uses simple language and contains no statistics, and one for professionals, which is technical, thorough, and includes citations to scientific literature. The PDQs for Wilms also cover clear cell sarcoma of the kidney and malignant rhabdoid tumor of the kidney.

Other types of childhood kidney cancers

While 90 percent of all kidney cancers in children are Wilms tumor, the remaining 10 percent are clear cell sarcoma of the kidney, rhabdoid tumor of the kidney, or renal cell carcinoma. Treatment for these aggressive malignancies is more intensive than that used for Wilms tumor. A combination of nephrectomy, radiation, and chemotherapy are used.

I had Wilms tumor in 1962 when I was two years old. I had one kidney removed, then radiation and chemotherapy. I recovered and had a perfectly normal childhood. Other than not wearing bikinis because of the big scar right around my waist, it didn't affect me much. I played hockey, basketball, and other contact sports without problems. I have no late effects from the treatment other than slight curvature of the spine and a few less pockets of fat on the side they irradiated. They told me that one of my fallopian tubes was damaged, but I have had three sons, all over seven pounds. My childhood cancer experiences created a deep fascination with medicine, and I am now a nurse.

CHAPTER 10

Soft Tissue Sarcomas

When it is dark enough, you can see the stars.

—Charles A. Beard

SOFT TISSUE SARCOMAS ARE cancerous tumors that arise in various soft tissues of the body. Soft tissues connect, surround, and support other body structures and organs. They include muscles, tendons, fibrous tissues, fat, nerves, blood vessels, and synovial tissues. The most prevalent of all childhood soft tissue sarcomas is rhabdomyosarcoma. Other rare soft tissue sarcomas include fibrosarcoma, neurofibrosarcoma, leiomyosarcoma, liposarcoma, synovial sarcoma, hemangiopericytoma, alveolar soft part sarcoma, and malignant fibrous histiocytoma.

This chapter first looks at the structure and function of muscles and connective tissues. Then it examines who gets soft tissue sarcomas, what the signs and symptoms are, how they are diagnosed, and how doctors determine the prognosis. Finally, it discusses current and future treatments for rhabdomyosarcoma and other soft tissue sarcomas.

Muscles and connective tissues

The human body comes equipped with more than 650 muscles. These muscles, together with other connective tissues (tendons and cartilage), form the support system for the skeleton. It is the muscular system that enables body movement through the process of contraction and relaxation.

There are three types of muscle:

- **Skeletal muscles.** Also called striated, these muscles manipulate the skeleton to cause movement. Skeletal muscles are voluntary muscles because their actions can be controlled.

- **Smooth muscles.** These involuntary muscles are found in many internal organs, such as the bladder, arteries, veins, and the digestive tract.

- **Cardiac muscle.** This type of involuntary muscle is found only in the heart. Several layers of tough, muscular wall, called the myocardium, keep the heart pumping through a process of contraction and relaxation.

Skeletal muscles are attached to bones by tendons. These cords of tissue are flexible and very strong. Their primary purpose is to move the force of muscular action to the bone to cause movement. For example, the Achilles tendon connects the calf muscles to the bone in the heel and allows the foot to push against the ground when walking.

Another important feature of the musculoskeletal system is the joint. Its main function is to connect bone to other bone and to allow movement where it is needed. Joints and tendons are surrounded by synovial tissue—a sheath which secretes a clear, thick lubricating fluid.

There are three types of joints and each serves a different purpose. Some, such as those found in the skull, do not move at all, while others, such as those found in the spine, have restricted movement. Joints in the arms, legs, and shoulders permit a great deal of movement.

Ligaments cross over joints and help join bone to bone. The ligaments strengthen joints and provide support to prevent dislocation.

The muscular system is a network of complex tissues working together, much like levers and fulcrums, which enables the body to move. Soft tissue sarcomas can arise at any point within this system.

Rhabdomyosarcoma

Childhood rhabdomyosarcoma is a soft tissue cancer that arises in the muscles. It accounts for approximately 4 percent of all cases of childhood cancer.

Rhabdomyosarcoma can start anywhere in the body; however, the point of tumor origin is often associated with age at diagnosis. Most head and neck tumors occur in children under the age of eight, whereas extremity tumors are most commonly found in adolescents. Less common primary sites for this cancer are the genitourinary tract, including the bladder and prostate in the male and the vagina in the female.

There are distinct histologic types (referring to how the cells look under a microscope) of rhabdomyosarcoma:

- **Embryonal.** This type accounts for approximately 60 to 70 percent of all childhood rhabdomyosarcomas. Tumors with this histology usually arise in the head, neck, and genitourinary areas.

- **Botryoid.** Botryoid tumors are a variant of the embryonal type and account for 10 percent of rhabdomyosarcoma cases. They are most commonly found in the genitourinary region and occur most often in infants.

- **Alveolar.** These tumors are usually found in the trunk or limbs. They are a more aggressive form of rhabdomyosarcoma and occur most often in adolescents.

- **Rare forms.** Pleomorphic and undifferentiated tumors are rarely found in childhood rhabdomyosarcomas.

Who gets rhabdomyosarcoma?

Rhabdomyosarcoma is the most common childhood soft tissue sarcoma. Approximately 250 children are diagnosed with rhabdomyosarcoma in the United States each year. Two-thirds of these cases are diagnosed in children under the age of six. The disease has a slightly higher incidence in males than in females. The occurrence of disease found in white and black males is very similar; however, the incidence in black females is only half of that in white females. The disease is more common in industrialized Western nations than in Asia.

> In December 1996, my two-year-old son Kenny was diagnosed with stage IV rhabdomyosarcoma. Needless to say, our lives have changed. We were told a year earlier that Kenny had a cytoma and that it would get bigger and bigger, then eventually go away. Over the course of the year, the mass did grow larger. Little did I know that the "boo boo" I touched every day was in actuality trying to kill my son.

Genetic factors

Most rhabdomyosarcomas occur sporadically; however, certain familial syndromes are associated with this form of childhood cancer. Children with Li-Fraumeni syndrome, neurofibromatosis, or Beckwith-Wiedemann syndrome have a higher chance of developing rhabdomyosarcoma than do children who do not have these congenital disorders.

Environmental factors

No known environmental factors cause rhabdomyosarcoma in children.

Rhabdomyosarcoma signs and symptoms

The signs and symptoms of rhabdomyosarcoma depend very much on the location of the primary tumor and whether or not the disease has metastasized (spread) to other areas. Generally, the child will develop a lump or mass that is not related to trauma to the area. Sometimes a normal body function is disrupted by a growing tumor. For example, large masses in the genitourinary system can cause difficulty with urination.

> Cassandra had been complaining of pain in her left knee while sleeping at night for one month previous to her diagnosis. I brought this to the attention of her pediatrician at a well child visit. The doctor looked her over and said that it was probably growing pains, and to elevate her leg in the evening and see if that might help. Following his advice, I began to elevate her leg at night with a pillow—a practice that my mother used when I had similar pains in my legs as a child. This didn't help alleviate the pain, though, and in fact, it seemed to intensify as days went by.

> One week later we were at a local Starbucks and Cassandra had to go to the bathroom. I went in with her, and while I was helping her with her tights I noticed a large lump on her left buttock.

Primary tumors located in the head or neck region can cause many different signs and symptoms. Orbit tumors can cause eyelid swelling or drooping, called ptosis. The eye may appear to protrude or bulge, and the muscles surrounding the eye may be weakened. The child may also complain of double vision.

> I called a dear friend who had graduated from being our babysitter during her four years of college to her current status as second year medical student. I told her I needed to do some research, listed Joseph's symptoms, told her what the ophthalmologist said, then asked about tumors in the eye area. She opened her cancer book and under orbital tumors found a word—a cancer—I'd never heard of before.

> *"Okay," she said, "this is the most common orbital tumor in children, it causes ptosis and proptosis (which she kindly stopped to define for me), hits kids most commonly between the ages of two and six, is more common in boys than in girls, and is highly malignant."*
>
> *As she described its symptoms, she was literally describing Joseph's face. She spelled the word out for me, and I still have the piece of paper on which I took those notes, on which I first wrote the word "rhabdomyosarcoma."*

Tumors that arise in the sinus area or the middle ear can cause nasal obstruction, sometimes with discharge and intermittent bleeding. The child may have a nasal voice.

Rhabdomyosarcomas are often found in the bladder and prostate. Symptoms include blood in the urine, difficulty passing urine, urinary obstruction, and pain. Prostate tumors tend to be found as a large mass, sometimes accompanied by constipation.

A painless scrotal enlargement may be found in boys with tumors in the paratesticular area (the areas next to the testicles).

Vaginal tumors generally present with a mass that looks like a bunch of grapes at the vaginal opening, often accompanied by a vaginal discharge. Tumors originating in the cervix or uterus are diagnosed more frequently in older girls, and may present with a mass and sometimes discharge.

Tumors that occur in the extremities and trunk most often will cause swelling, pain, tenderness, and redness in the affected area.

> *The pediatrician looked concerned as she examined Cassandra and told me that it was some type of "mass." I didn't think the word "cancer" at all. She made an appointment for me to see a surgeon at Children's Hospital in Seattle for later that afternoon.*
>
> *I knew that this was something serious, but had no idea just how bad until later that evening when the surgeon gave me the results of the CT scan: cancer in her left buttock, with metastatic lesions in her lungs. When I heard this news, I was reeling. My sister had died just two years before of breast cancer, and my younger brother had just finished treatment for testicular cancer. I thought, "This can't be happening again!"*

Diagnosis of rhabdomyosarcoma

Many tests are performed to diagnose rhabdomyosarcoma as well as to distinguish it from several other childhood cancers that can appear very similar.

First, the doctor obtains the child's medical history and performs a physical examination. Usually, he orders a complete blood count (CBC). A computed tomography (CT) scan or magnetic resonance imaging (MRI) may reveal a mass. The lump will then be sampled, either with open or needle biopsy. For further information on each of these tests and procedures, see Chapter 2, *Coping with Procedures*.

Rhabdomyosarcoma can appear very similar to other childhood cancers at the microscopic level, and extra tests may be needed to help differentiate between malignancies and establish the proper diagnosis.

> At the end of all the tests, the ophthalmologist asked me to come back into his office alone to speak with him. He told me that Joseph had some kind of growth pressing out on his eyeball from above and behind. I looked down at the notes he had in front of him and I saw the word "TUMOR." He told me that Joseph would need further testing in the form of an MRI to tell what the growth was, and gave me a list of possibilities, at the bottom of which (and "highly unlikely") was a cancerous tumor.

Staging

Once rhabdomyosarcoma has been diagnosed, more tests are done to determine if the cancer has spread to other parts of the body. Bone marrow aspiration and biopsy may be performed to see if disease has spread to the bone marrow. Ordinary x-rays are used to detect disease that has spread to the bone or lungs. More specialized imaging techniques used to evaluate the extent of the disease include CT, MRI, and bone scans. If the mass is located within the pelvic area, ultrasonography may be done along with CT. This process is called staging, and it helps the doctor choose the most appropriate treatment for the child.

> Cassandra had to undergo a myriad of tests and procedures when she was initially diagnosed. The CT scans showed that the tumor in her bottom had spread to the lungs, so we knew that first night that she was fighting a malignant cancer. The second day at the hospital she had an MRI. While she was under anesthesia for that procedure, the doctors implanted a Hickman line in her chest that would be used for administer-

ing chemo, antibiotics, fluid, food, etc. over the next eight months. They also took samples of her bone marrow to see if the cancer had spread there—it hadn't.

The next day she had a bone scan to detect any bone involvement, of which there was none. They also ran tests on her kidney function to use as a baseline to see how the treatment would affect her kidneys. An ultrasound of her heart was done as well, also to use as a baseline, since one of the chemo drugs, Adriamycin, can cause heart problems.

The Intergroup Rhabdomyosarcoma Study Group (IRSG) currently bases treatment protocols on the following staging system:

- Stage 1. The tumor is localized to the orbit and head or the genitourinary region (excluding the bladder and prostate).

- Stage II. The tumor is localized to any primary site not included in stage I. Primary tumors must be less than 5 cm in diameter, and there must be no regional lymph node involvement.

- Stage III. The tumor is localized to any primary site not included in stage I. Primary tumors are greater than 5 cm and/or there is regional lymph node involvement.

- Stage IV. The tumor has spread to distant sites.

Another system is called the TNM system. The T represents tumor, and takes into consideration its size and location. The N represents nodes, and is used to indicate the presence or absence of lymph node involvement. The M represents metastases, indicating whether the disease has spread beyond the primary site to distant areas.

The TNM system has several benefits. It is the method used for staging rhabdomyosarcoma in many other counties, and its use allows direct comparison between studies. The system has also been shown to be very predictive of long-term outcome because location of the tumor has been found to be the most important prognostic factor—regardless of whether the surgeon achieves an excision.

Prognosis

Since the 1970s, the treatment of rhabdomyosarcoma has dramatically improved. The majority of children and teens diagnosed with non-metastatic rhabdomyosarcoma now survive the disease. The prognosis and best treatment for each child is determined by analysis of several clinical and biologic features.

The histology of the tumor is important, with alveolar tumors tending to behave more aggressively. Within any given histologic type, localized tumors respond better to therapy than do those that have metastasized. Tumors that are completely resected have the best prognoses. The degree to which resection can be achieved is determined by the size of the tumor and its closeness to vital structures. The importance of these determinants is that the aggressiveness of treatment can be increased for those with adverse features to improve their prognosis.

Treatment of rhabdomyosarcoma

At diagnosis, many parents are confused about how to find the best doctors and treatments for their child. State-of-the-art care is available from physicians who participate in Intergroup Rhabdomyosarcoma Study Group (IRSG), the Children's Cancer Group (CCG) and the Pediatric Oncology Group (POG). These study groups, composed of pediatric surgeons and oncologists, urologists, radiation oncologists, researchers and nurses, establish the standard of care for patients worldwide, conduct new studies to discover better therapies, and establish follow-up for survivors. They are in the process of merging into one entity called the Children's Oncology Group (COG). If the treatment center you are referred to is a member of one of these groups, you can rest assured that your child will have access to the best thinking on the treatment of pediatric cancers.

The oncologist will choose the best treatment or clinical trial (see Chapter 5, *Clinical Trials*) based on many factors. For most patients with rhabdomyosarcoma, treatment usually includes surgery, chemotherapy, and radiation.

Cassandra was started on a pilot study put together by Children's Cancer Group (CCG), with which our hospital was affiliated. We didn't have time to look into alternatives. Our surgeon told us that this was fast growing and very dangerous, and we wanted to start fighting immediately.

The protocol involved using multiple drugs together on an aggressive treatment plan consisting of one week of treatment, then two weeks off, then another week of treatment, etc. She would have six rounds of chemo, and then surgery to remove any residual tumor in the buttocks, have two more rounds of chemo, and finally she would end with six weeks of daily radiation.

The drugs dripped into her for 24 hours a day for six days. She was hospitalized for the treatment and then released until her immune system, so weakened by the treatment, would give in, and she would get an infection. This began to happen like clockwork. She would be admitted for treatment on Tuesday, let out on Sunday and readmitted by Thursday with neutropenia and a fever. We would then spend about a week in the hospital until her blood counts recovered, go home for a few days and then start the next round of chemo. This was our life from November 1995 until May 1996.

Surgery

All children diagnosed with rhabdomyosarcoma will have surgery, either to remove all or part of the primary tumor, or to perform an incisional biopsy to reach a definitive diagnosis. Surgery is used as early as possible in the course of treatment and is the quickest method to reduce the amount of the disease. However, complete resection may not be possible, particularly if the mass is located near vital blood vessels, if it deeply invades surrounding normal tissue, or if there are functional or cosmetic reasons for preventing such a procedure.

The doctor showed us the MRIs, and we got to see the monster in Joseph's head. It was a creepy top-down view, and we could see a big white blob behind his right eyeball, pushing it much farther out and down than the left one. Still no one used the word cancer. He explained how he would do the biopsy, cutting across the width of the whole eyelid to retrieve a bit of the mass, leaving packing and stitches that would make the eye look puffy and scary for a few days, but which would retreat into invisibility within a few months.

During surgery the doctor removes as much of the tumor as he can and then samples surrounding tissues which are later examined by a pathologist. The pathologist determines whether all of the tumor has been removed, or whether some cells remain behind. If the surgeon is able to remove the entire tumor, it is referred to as a total gross resection. If there is evidence of remaining disease, it is referred to as residual disease. If it is visible to the naked eye or can be felt by the surgeon's hand, it is called gross residual disease. If it is only visible under the microscope, it is called microscopic residual disease.

Second-look surgical procedures, done after chemotherapy, remove any remaining residual disease and determine if remission has been reached. This can be especially important for choosing appropriate further treatment, such as the amount of radiotherapy to be given. Approximately 10 percent of newly diagnosed children have tumors that are able to be completely removed. In most cases, residual disease is present. For this reason, chemotherapy is used in all treatment protocols and radiation in most. For further information about surgery, see Chapter 18, *Surgery*.

> *Sean had a ten-hour surgery during which they removed a three-pound tumor from his shoulder. He was cut from the top of his ear down to his midchest area. I believe they could not find the point of origin of the tumor and cut to the top of his ear searching for it. I have been told by the MRI technicians that the surgeon must have been a magician to leave the area so incredibly clean. Two MRIs since surgery have showed the site remains tumor-free.*

Chemotherapy

All children diagnosed with rhabdomyosarcoma receive chemotherapy, with the quantity and duration dependent on risk factors. Without chemotherapy, the majority of children with rhabdomyosarcoma would die of metastases which are usually present at diagnosis, even though they are too small to appear on scans. Giving several anticancer drugs in combination has markedly improved the survival rate for this disease. The most commonly used drugs include cyclophosphamide, vincristine, ifosfamide, etoposide, dactinomycin, and doxorubicin. For further information on these drugs, see Chapter 15, *Chemotherapy*.

> *Sean's treatment included 14 rounds of chemotherapy and 30 radiation treatments. He had every side effect imaginable. Aside from very low counts, he also had raised liver counts and had jaundice a few times. He has had pneumonia and klebsiella when neutropenic. His eyes were blood red from capillaries breaking. Amazingly, with all of the side effects he experienced, he had very little nausea during and after chemotherapy. I have seen him sit and eat greasy fried chicken and fries during chemo.*

> *Kenny started off on the VACIME protocol. After each round of chemo, his counts would bottom out and we would do G-CSF, a white blood cell booster, for up to ten days. Sometimes we would be home for one day and have to go back in for fever and neutropenia.*

Clinical trials are also evaluating melphalan, topotecan, and taxol for their efficacy against rhabdomyosarcoma. The use of higher doses of chemotherapy, followed by autologous bone marrow transplantation (see Chapter 19, *Bone Marrow and Stem Cell Transplantation*) is currently under investigation.

Radiation

Radiotherapy is an important tool used to treat children with rhabdomyosarcoma. The Intergroup Rhabdomyosarcoma Study Group has designed radiation therapy guidelines for treating this disease. Generally, children with stages I and II disease do not receive radiation therapy if their tumors are able to be completely resected. However, the need for radiation also depends on the histology of the tumor. Current protocols give patients with residual disease external beam radiation in fractions of 180 cGy a day, for up to six weeks. Total radiation may reach 4000 to 5500 cGy.

Most often, radiation is given approximately nine weeks after chemotherapy has begun. However, children with tumors in the skull, meninges (lining of the brain), or spinal cord may start radiation therapy soon after diagnosis.

> *Our son Joseph had roughly 5000 Gy delivered to his right orbit. His radiation was "hyperfractionated"—a method of giving smaller doses more often in the hopes that the patient can receive a larger total amount with fewer long-term side effects. In Joseph's case, this meant two treatments per day over six weeks. His treatments began three weeks before his fifth birthday. The radiotherapy staff handled him with patience, affection, and respect from the first day they met him, and gave us a lot of support as a family. They invited him in for a couple of trips to their treatment rooms to get used to the equipment and meet all the people before they did any of the preliminary measurements or scans. He got all the time he wanted to ride up and down on the tables and ask questions about the machines. Using me as a sample patient, they made a mold of the type of plastic mesh mask Joseph would need for his treatments so he could see what it would be like. Having my head screwed down to that*

table was NOT FUN! I'm glad I did it, though, because just as I tasted all his medicines, this gave me a chance to try a physical experience from his perspective, too.

Other soft tissue sarcomas

Childhood soft tissue sarcoma is a disease in which cancer arises in soft tissue somewhere in the body. Soft tissues include muscles, tendons, fat, blood vessels, nerves, and synovia (tissues around joints). Forty-seven percent of all childhood soft tissue sarcomas have a histology (how the cells look under a microscope) that is different from rhabdomyosarcoma. As a group, these soft tissue sarcomas comprise only 3 percent of all malignant tumors in children. They include the following:

- **Synovial sarcoma.** The most common non-rhabdomyosarcoma soft tissue sarcoma in childhood. Synovial sarcoma is found most often in older children and is very rarely diagnosed in those under ten years of age. The disease occurs most frequently in the lower extremities, most often in the area of the thigh or knee. The second most common sites are the upper extremities, followed by the head, neck, and trunk.

- **Fibrosarcoma.** This soft tissue sarcoma is the most frequently occurring non-rhabdomyosarcoma soft tissue sarcoma in children under one year of age. The two incidence peaks that occur with this disease are in infants and children under five years of age, and children between ages ten and fifteen. These tumors occur most often in the extremities and the majority of children diagnosed have localized disease. Infants diagnosed with this disease tend to respond to treatment better than do older children.

- **Malignant peripheral nerve sheath tumor (also known as neurofibrosarcoma or malignant Schwannoma).** An aggressive malignancy that accounts for approximately 5 to 10 percent of all non-rhabdomyosarcoma soft tissue sarcomas of childhood. The disease often occurs in association with neurofibromatosis. The most common site of origin is the extremities.

- **Malignant fibrous histiocytoma.** This form of soft tissue sarcoma most frequently occurs in the lower extremities and the trunk area. Other sites include the upper limbs, scalp, and kidney.

There are other extremely rare forms of childhood soft tissue sarcomas. Young children with these diseases are generally treated on protocols based on those used for childhood rhabdomyosarcoma. Teens are usually treated on protocols similar to those used for adults with soft issue sarcomas. These rare soft tissue sarcomas include:

- **Leiomyosarcoma.** Leiomyosarcoma, which arises from smooth muscle, most often occurs in the gastrointestinal tract, especially the stomach.

- **Liposarcoma.** Liposarcoma arises in fatty tissue and is found most frequently in early adolescents. The most common sites of origin are the legs or trunk.

- **Hemangiopericytoma.** Hemangiopericytoma is a tumor of the blood and lymph vessels that occurs most frequently in infants.

- **Alveolar soft part sarcoma.** This is a rare sarcoma found most often in older children. The tumor arises from skeletal muscle of the extremities, head, and neck, and presents as an asymtomatic, slow-growing mass.

Signs and symptoms

Typically, soft tissue sarcomas are first noticed as a painless mass, with symptoms, if present, caused by the tumor pressing on surrounding structures. For example, a soft tissue sarcoma in the head can cause paralysis of nerves. Invasion of the disease into peripheral nerves can cause pain or weakness in the pelvis and extremities. Tumors that arise on the chest wall can cause difficulty in breathing and an abdominal mass can block the gastrointestinal or genitourinary tract.

Treatment overview

Treatment for non-rhabdomyosarcoma soft tissue sarcomas is usually surgery and sometimes radiation therapy. Chemotherapy is sometimes used to shrink large tumors to make them operable.

Surgery is the cornerstone of treatment for soft tissue sarcomas (see Chapter 18). Ideally, the surgeon will attempt to completely remove the mass with wide margins (portions of the surrounding tissue) to ensure that no microscopic disease remains. This is often followed by radiation, given every day for five to six weeks. The total dose is usually 4000 to 5500 cGy.

Although medical science has made advances in treating soft tissue sarcomas while reducing the side effects and long-term impact to the child, amputation is sometimes necessary. Limb-sparing procedures have made this less common.

Since these malignancies are so rare in children, treatment for non-rhabdomyosarcoma soft tissue sarcomas are based on experience with the adult population. Generally, the size and location of the tumor, as well as tumor histology, are more significant than the actual type of sarcoma when determining prognosis. The most important prognostic factor with each is the ability to completely remove the primary tumor.

The Intergroup Rhabdomyosarcoma Study Group studies 3 and 4 demonstrated that children with non-rhabdomyosarcoma soft tissue tumors do as well on IRSG studies as do children with rhabdomyosarcoma. Since the number of children with these tumors is small, these results need to be verified with additional multi-institutional studies.

Newest treatment options

New treatments for rhabdomyosarcoma and other soft tissue sarcomas are being developed using immunotherapy and other biologic modifiers. These include antitumor immune responses and methods to interrupt specific growth factor loops. Research into the basic biology of soft tissue sarcomas has made these advances possible.

To learn of the newest treatments available, call (800) 4-CANCER and ask for the PDQ (physicians data query) for "sarcoma, rhabdomyosarcoma, childhood" or "sarcoma, soft tissue, childhood." These free statements explain the disease, state-of-the-art treatments, and ongoing clinical trials. There are two versions available: one for patients, which uses simple language and contains no statistics, and one for professionals, which is technical, thorough, and includes citations to scientific literature. The PDQ can also be read on the Internet at *http://cancernet.nci.nih.gov/*.

Kenny was the most beautiful baby. He laughed a great deal and
very rarely cried until the age of two when he was diagnosed with stage
IV, embryonal rhabdomyosarcoma. Kenny had tumors from his pelvis up

to his aorta. *Because of the extensive disease, our surgeon couldn't remove them. He began chemotherapy the day after Christmas and continued until July when he began radiation. He had 27 rounds of radiation throughout July, all under anesthesia. It was very difficult and draining, but toward the end, Kenny would set up all the equipment, hook his pulse oximeter up, turn his oxygen on, and hold his mask to be anesthetized. He was just shy of his third birthday.*

In September of 1997, we began to see the light at the end of the tunnel. Kenny's tumors seemed to disappear and a biopsy of the scar tissue found no cancer, but he continued chemotherapy until January 1998. Kenny recently celebrated his fourth birthday. He whooped with delight as he put on his new helmet, gloves, and kneepads and took off down the hill on his new bright blue skateboard.

CHAPTER 11

Bone Sarcomas

*To reach a port we must sail, sometimes with
the wind, and sometimes against it. But we
must not drift or lie at anchor.*

—Oliver Wendell Holmes

BONE SARCOMAS COMPRISE A group of several different cancerous tumors of the bone. The most common bone sarcomas diagnosed in children and teens are osteosarcoma and Ewing's sarcoma. There are more than 1000 children diagnosed each year in the United States with some form of bone cancer.

There are distinct differences in how different bone sarcomas are treated. This chapter first covers osteosarcoma. Ewing's sarcoma, extraosseous Ewing's sarcoma (EES) and peripheral primitive neuroectodermal tumor (PPNET) are then discussed. Together, these three malignancies are called the Ewing's sarcoma family of tumors (ESFT).

The chapter first looks at the structure and function of the skeletal system. Then it examines who gets bone sarcomas, what the signs and symptoms are, how they are diagnosed, and how doctors determine the prognosis. The chapter then discusses current and future treatments for osteosarcoma and ESFT.

The skeletal system

The human skeleton contains 206 bones, all held in place by connective tissues such as ligaments and tendons. There are several types of bone which make up the skeletal system, each classified according to its shape: long, short, irregular, and flat. Together, they provide several different functions. The skeleton gives structure to the body and protects the internal organs. It determines our size and shape. The skeleton also works as a factory, since various blood cells are manufactured in the marrow of the bones. Bones also act as a storage depot holding calcium and phosphorus compounds for later use by the body.

The structure of bones is continuously changing. The skeleton of the fetus in the womb is made up mostly of cartilage. As pregnancy continues, bone develops, but even when the child is born, there are still areas that are a combination of bone and cartilage. These areas are called the growth plates. In the long bones, such as the arms and legs, there are growth plates at each end. Growth plates have a high level of activity until the child stops growing. By the time a child reaches age twenty, the 270 softer bones she was born with will have fused to form the 206-bone structure of the skeleton.

Osteosarcoma

Osteosarcoma is a malignant tumor of the bone. It is the most common of the bone sarcomas. Scientific advances over the past 25 years have dramatically improved outcome. Advancements in surgery have also improved the quality of life for children and teens diagnosed with osteosarcoma.

Who gets osteosarcoma?

The peak incidence for osteosarcoma occurs between the ages of 10 and 25 years. This has led researchers to believe that there is an association between the disease and the rapid period of bone growth experienced in adolescents. In adolescents, osteosarcoma is the fourth most common cancer, following leukemias, lymphomas, and brain tumors. The disease is almost twice as common in males than in females and is slightly more common in white children than in black children.

In children and teens, 80 percent of these tumors arise in either the end of the thigh bone (femur) closest to the knee or the end of the shin bone (tibia) closest to the knee. It also sometimes appears in the end of the upper arm bone (humerus) nearest the shoulder. Other less common sites are the pelvis, jaw, and ribs. Twenty percent of children diagnosed with this bone tumor have metastases (cancer which has spread to other places in the body) at the time their cancer is found. Of this group, approximately 85 percent have tumors in the lungs.

> Our daughter was just ten years old when she was diagnosed with osteosarcoma. Unfortunately, I was sick with a fever of 103° and had to stay home when her dad took her to the appointment. My husband told me it was the worst day of his life when she looked up at him and asked

him if she was going to die. Both he and the doctor immediately responded
that we were all going to do everything to keep that from happening. She
trusted that we would take care of the cancer and she would recover.

Genetic factors

The cause of osteosarcoma is not known. However, persons with Li-Fraumeni syndrome, a rare, inherited disorder, have a higher risk of developing cancers including soft tissue and bone sarcomas.

A rare eye cancer of childhood, called retinoblastoma, is also associated with osteosarcoma. Children who have the inherited form of retinoblastoma have a substantial risk of developing osteosarcoma. The risk appears to be increased by treatment with radiation to the bones of the eye socket. But the increased frequency of osteosarcoma in non-irradiated sites, e.g., arms and legs, indicates a genetic abnormality predisposing the child to these two cancers. When scientists examine osteosarcoma cells from patients who had retinoblastoma, they find that both copies of a gene called RB1 are mutated. The RB1 gene is the same gene that is mutated in retinoblastoma. For more information on this gene, see Chapter 13, *Retinoblastoma*.

Environmental factors

Radiation is the only known environmental factor believed to lead to increased risk of osteosarcoma. About 3 percent of children diagnosed with the disease have had previous irradiation of the site. Treatment for prior malignancies with certain chemotherapy drugs, such as alkylating agents, may also contribute to the development of secondary osteosarcoma.

Osteosarcoma signs and symptoms

Osteosarcoma occurs most frequently in the long bones. Symptoms usually include pain, with or without an associated swelling. The affected area may have an increased temperature. Osteosarcoma is often noticed after the child or teen has an incidental injury. It is important to note that the injury did not cause the tumor, it only brought it to attention. Often, the child will be limping, since about 80 percent of these tumors are located near the knee. The range of motion of joints may be decreased.

Leeann was ten years old when she was diagnosed with osteosar-
coma in the left femur. I remember feeling total and utter shock. She had
been complaining of pain in her knee for a month or so, but since she was
physically active playing basketball, baseball, and gymnastics, I assumed
it was something minor like a pulled ligament. I also told her more than
once that it was just "growing pains."

Fortunately, she persisted and we took her to a local orthopedist. The
orthopedist asked us to make an appointment with a pediatric orthope-
dist two and a half hours from home. I knew at this point it was some-
thing much more serious than a pulled muscle. Once the initial diagnosis
was made, we went into a fog.

Symptoms that may indicate the presence of metastatic disease are fever and
weight loss. Metastatic disease in the lung is most often asymptomatic. Occasionally, it may cause shortness of breath, chest pain, and coughing.

Diagnosis of osteosarcoma

Before a diagnosis of osteosarcoma can be reached, specific tests and procedures are performed. This always begins with the physician obtaining the
child's medical history and performing a complete physical examination. A
complete blood count (CBC) and differential is ordered (see Appendix B,
Blood Counts and What They Mean), along with other bloodwork and a
urinalysis.

The first imaging studies done are often x-ray films of the area suspected of
having a malignancy. Because these tumors have a distinct appearance when
viewed on plain films, a radiologist may suspect that osteosarcoma is present
based on x-ray alone. In addition, an MRI of the affected bone is almost
always done prior to biopsy. MRIs provide accurate information that is used
by the surgeon to plan the appropriate surgical intervention. They are also
excellent scans for detection of "skip lesions." Skip lesions are areas of disease occurring at different sites, but within the same bone as the primary
tumor.

A definitive diagnosis of osteosarcoma can only be made based on actual
tumor tissue. An open biopsy or a needle biopsy removes samples of the
mass which are then examined by a pathologist under a microscope. The
biopsy should be performed by a physician who has experience in surgery
for osteosarcoma.

I was a sixteen-year-old cheerleader preparing for a national competition when my knee started to hurt. I thought it was just a sports injury and I put ice on it. When it didn't improve, I went to physical therapy and then to a specialist in sports medicine. He took an x-ray and then sent me for an MRI. That night he called to say, "I'm so sorry, but you have a tumor." I had a biopsy the next day. It was osteosarcoma.

Staging

Once osteosarcoma has been diagnosed, more tests are done to determine if the cancer has spread to other parts of the body. Imaging studies that may be performed to check for metastases are computed tomography (CT) of the chest and a bone scan.

> *My daughter Shoshana is now nineteen. She was diagnosed with osteosarcoma just before her sixteenth birthday in 1995. The tumor was located in her right fibula. She also had lung metastasis. Pain was her basic symptom, especially at night. We started out at the pediatrician, then an orthopedic doctor, and finally an orthopedic oncologist who did a biopsy. We were then passed on to a pediatric oncologist, who is our primary doctor. The latter two are a great team!*

A bone scan that uses a radiopharmaceutical, called technetium-99m, is frequently ordered to provide the physician with clear images of the entire skeleton. Technetium-99m is very sensitive to osteosarcoma, therefore, these bone scans are particularly helpful in detecting the presence of metastatic disease and skip lesions. It is, however, sensitive to many other normal events, for example, minor strains and injuries to the bone. So an abnormality on the bone scan does not always mean tumor spread.

There are two stages for osteosarcoma:

- **Localized.** These tumors are limited to the bone of origin, although skip lesions may exist in the same bone.
- **Metastatic.** These tumors are found in other parts of the body, including the lungs, other bones, or distant sites.

Prognosis

Since the 1970s, the treatment of osteosarcoma has dramatically improved. The majority of children and teens now survive the disease, many with limbs still intact. The prognosis and best treatment for each child with osteosarcoma is determined by analysis of several clinical and biologic features.

The most significant of all factors used to determine prognosis for the child with osteosarcoma is the extent of the disease at diagnosis and whether it has metastasized or not. For children or teens with localized disease, the following factors are considered: resectability of the tumor determined by location and tumor size, and response of the tumor to chemotherapy.

The prognoses of children or teens with metastatic disease at diagnosis depend on the site of the metastases and the resectability of the metastatic tumors (either at diagnosis or after chemotherapy). Osteosarcoma is much harder to cure if there is metastatic disease.

Treatment of osteosarcoma

The majority of children and teens with osteosarcoma who receive optimal treatment are cured of the disease. At diagnosis, many parents are confused about how to find the best doctors and treatments for their child. State-of-the-art care is available from physicians who participate in the Children's Cancer Group (CCG) and the Pediatric Oncology Group (POG). These study groups, composed of pediatric surgeons and oncologists, urologists, radiation oncologists, researchers and nurses, establish the standard of care for patients worldwide, conduct new studies to discover better therapies, and establish follow-up for survivors. They are in the process of merging into one entity called the Children's Oncology Group (COG). If the treatment center you are referred to is a member of one of these groups, you can rest assured that your child will have access to the best thinking on the treatment of pediatric cancers.

The oncologist will choose the best treatment or clinical trial (see Chapter 5, *Clinical Trials*) based on many factors. For most patients, treatment is chemotherapy, followed by surgery and then more chemotherapy. Osteosarcoma is not very responsive to radiation.

Surgery

The improvements that have been made in surgical management of osteosarcoma over the past several years have significantly improved the long-term survival rate and the quality of life for children diagnosed with this disease.

Surgery is usually undertaken after a period of pre-operative chemotherapy, although some protocols may call for initial surgical resection. Successful surgical resection of the primary tumor most often consists of either limb-salvage surgery or amputation. A surgical procedure called a thoracotomy (opening the chest cavity) is also used to treat children with metastases to the lungs.

> Eric was diagnosed in September 1996 at age fifteen with osteosar-coma in his left femur. He's had chemotherapy and successful limb salvage surgery. Before cancer he was a baseball player, aggressive in-line skater, and a real on-the-go kid. I'm proud to say, he took his new limitations very well. He was able to remain very active despite his reconstructed leg. Although high impact activities were discouraged, he continued to ride his bicycle, go canoeing, and hiking and camping in the mountains. He played softball with his friends, but preferred to let someone else do his base running.

The surgeon chooses the best surgery after considering several factors, including the size, location, and extent of the primary tumor, the presence or absence of distant metastases, the age of the child, skeletal development, and patient and family preferences. This surgery is best done by surgeons who have a great deal of experience treating osteosarcoma.

> Shoshana had limb-sparing surgery after weeks of chemotherapy (all high-dose through a Broviac line). The surgery took nine hours. She got back onto her chemotherapy protocol about four weeks later. We did the wheelchair, then crutches (for a long time) then a cane, then walking, dancing, running! She had a sternocotomy for the lung tumors later that same year.

Amputation

In recent years many advances have been made in the surgical management of osteosarcoma. However, some children still require amputation of the affected limb. Amputation involves removal of all or a portion of an arm or a leg. Children with large tumors involving the nerves and blood vessels may not be candidates for limb-salvage procedures. Very young children with lower extremity tumors, as well as those who do not respond well to chemo-therapy, may need amputation. In most instances, amputation allows removal of all gross and microscopic disease.

In the past, it was felt by many surgeons that removal of the entire affected bone was the safest approach to lasting control of the disease. This was because of a significant rate of recurrence in the remaining stump. However, improved imaging techniques using CT and MRI allow surgeons to view areas of disease with greater accuracy, permitting aggressive surgery while still preserving as much of the affected limb as possible.

Children who require amputation need a great deal of rehabilitation and psychological support. While it is traumatic to deal with at any age, osteosarcoma typically occurs during the teenage years, when appearance is especially important to the adolescent's emotional well-being. State-of-the-art prosthetic limbs allow great mobility as well as cosmetic appeal. Studies have been done which show no difference in the quality of life between patients who had amputation and those who had limb-salvage surgery.

Limb-salvage surgery

Advances made in limb-salvage procedures have enabled this technique to be used with an increasing number of children. The challenge for the surgeon is to remove all evidence of disease while maintaining surrounding nerves and blood vessels. The structural integrity of the bone is then restored through the use of bone grafts or metallic devices. With successful, complete resection, the outcome is equivalent to that of amputation.

The benefits of limb-salvage procedures are both functional and psychological. However, limb-sparing surgery is not used if there is any doubt that the surgeon will be able to completely remove the tumor. The first priority is complete surgical excision, even if that requires amputation.

Children who have a broken bone at the time of diagnosis may not be good candidates for limb-salvage surgery. Chemotherapy before surgical intervention may cause poor healing of the fracture, which creates added obstacles when attempting limb-sparing techniques. Tumor location, as well as the age of the child, can also dictate amputation as a more suitable curative approach.

> Leeann's limb salvage surgery kept her leg in an immobilizer for six
> weeks, day and night. There was a big problem getting her flexibility
> back, even with a year of painful physical therapy. The pain was manage-
> able with the help of morphine, but getting her around was very difficult.
> Even the three-hour car ride home was a trial. Once at home, we rented a

wheelchair for the first month until she felt comfortable on crutches. I
spent many hours on the floor of the bathroom, holding her leg up while
she used the toilet. She became a real pro on those crutches!

There are several different approaches to structural reconstruction in limb-salvage surgery. Autologous grafts involve removing a healthy bone from another area of the child's body to replace the diseased bone. Allografts use bone from cadaver donors. Endoprostheses employ a manufactured replacement for the diseased bone, usually made of steel or titanium.

My daughter was sixteen when she was diagnosed with osteosar-
coma. During her surgery, they wrapped a muscle from the back of her
calf around to the front to hold the bone graft in place. It left a large open
area that was covered by a skin graft from her thigh. It certainly worked
in holding her graft in place, but left her leg looking pretty awful (even
though we had a plastic surgeon assist with that part of the surgery) and I
haven't seen a scar like it on anyone else. They also put small bone sliv-
ers from her own bones around the graft sites in hopes of faster grafting
and that apparently worked as well. She walks much better than they
expected, a slight limp but no braces necessary. She never did regain feel-
ing in the bottom of her right foot. Sometimes she thinks amputation
would have been better because with a prosthesis she'd be able to run and
jump and roller blade and participate in sports, things she can't do now
with the bone graft and complete knee replacement.

Tumor removal without replacement by a graft or endoprotheses

Sometimes the surgeon will perform a procedure known as rotationoplasty when the tumor involves the knee region. This method still requires use of a prosthetic device, but the benefit is that it allows greater functional use of the limb in children requiring removal of the knee. In this procedure, the surgeon removes the affected femur and knee joint, but maintains the connection of the lower leg to the upper thigh. The lower portion of the leg is then rotated 180 degrees, and attached to the remaining thigh bone. The ankle serves as a replacement for the surgically removed knee. An artificial limb is then designed to fit over the foot and ankle.

This surgery can cause cosmetic and psychosocial difficulties because of the appearance of the reconstructed limb. However, the increased function of the limb after using this technique should be considered. In addition, rotationoplasty can allow a more aggressive surgical removal of a diseased bone, making it a possible alternative to amputation in some cases.

Chemotherapy

Chemotherapy has greatly improved the long-term survival of children with osteosarcoma. Before the use of chemotherapy, the prognosis was very poor for a child diagnosed with osteosarcoma, despite amputation. This is because many children, including those with no obvious signs of metastatic disease, had microscopic involvement to the lungs at the time of diagnosis.

> *All in all, this cycle of chemo went very well for Shoshona in terms of side-effects. The only time she threw up was when she gagged on a pill! The neutropenia and fever came on like clockwork, but the hospital stay was very short. She never actually "bottomed-out" and despite low platelets and anemia, she had no nose bleeds, bruising, or low energy. She used the treadmill on the floor and was doing two miles a day at two and a half miles per hour. Her biggest problem was gingivitis, so we brought our blender and pureed food. She is eating a very nutritious diet (fish, beans, tofu, nuts, seeds, whole grains, fresh fruits and vegetables, miso soup, etc.). She is learning yoga, relaxation, and visualization techniques.*

The list of chemotherapy drugs that are used against the disease is shorter than that of many other malignancies. Doxorubicin, high-dose methotrexate with leucovorin rescue, cisplatin, and ifosfamide were among the first combination of chemotherapeutic drugs to improve long-term survival. The use of anticancer drugs as an adjuvant, or addition, to surgery, has led to a survival rate of approximately 70 percent in children with non-metastatic disease at diagnosis.

> *Overall, Leeann survived chemotherapy without too many side effects. She gained weight and even grew a couple of inches during the year she received treatment. The usual nausea was controlled with Zofran and Benedryl. The hardest part was losing her hair. She was at such a critical time in her growing up that showing up at a new school wearing a wig caused a lot of anxiety.*

> *As for lasting physical side effects, there don't seem to have been any. They ran a battery of tests on her heart, hearing, vision, and lungs*

immediately following the completion of chemo and declared her totally
healthy. In fact, the audiologist said she had never tested someone with
hearing that perfect after completing chemotherapy.

Chemotherapy is given in most instances before and after surgery. Administration of chemotherapy before surgery has been shown to facilitate limb-salvage procedures by allowing tumor shrinkage prior to removal. It can also be used as a prognostic indicator; children who respond well to presurgical chemotherapy have a better prognosis.

Other treatments

Studies are currently underway that attempt to use the child's immune system to fight osteosarcoma. One of these includes the use of a biologic response modifier known as liposome-encapsulated muramyl tripeptide-phosphatidylethanolamine, or MTP-PE. This biologic agent is used in children with non-metastatic osteosarcoma to treat microscopic disease that may be present in the lungs. MTP-PE activates certain cells of the immune system which attack and destroy osteosarcoma cells.

Monoclonal antibodies are also being investigated as a potential therapeutic approach against the disease. It is hoped that this method will allow delivery of anti-cancer drugs directly to the tumor cells.

These treatments are still in the early stages, and it will be some time before their long-term efficacy will be shown.

Ewing's sarcoma family of tumors

Ewing's sarcoma gets its name from the physician who first described it in 1921, Dr. James Ewing. He noted that this bone cancer was different from osteosarcoma because it was particularly sensitive to radiation. For several years it was felt that Ewing's sarcoma occurred only within the bone, however, other tumors were found within soft tissues and determined to be similar under the microscope. These include extraosseous Ewing's sarcoma (EES) and peripheral primitive neuroectodermal tumor (PPNET). Together, these malignancies are called the Ewing's sarcoma family of tumors (ESFT).

Who gets ESFT tumors?

Each year, about 150 children are diagnosed in the United States with a ESFT malignancy. Ewing's sarcoma of the bone accounts for 87 percent of these diagnoses, while 8 percent are extraosseous Ewing's sarcoma, and 5 percent are peripheral primitive neuroectodermal tumors.

Most ESFT tumors occur between the ages of ten to twenty years. Only 27 percent will be diagnosed before the age of ten years. Boys tend to be diagnosed with this disease more often than girls, and there is a much higher incidence in white children compared to those of any other race. Ninety-six percent of all ESFT tumors are found in white children.

The most common areas in which these tumors occur are the pelvis, the thigh bone (femur), the upper arm bone (humerus), and the ribs.

Genetic factors

ESFT tumors usually don't occur in association with childhood congenital diseases. However, when scientists look at the genetic material (DNA in chromosomes) of an ESFT tumor, more than 90 percent have a translocation between chromosomes 11 and 22 called t(11:22). This shifts a portion of one chromosome to the other, and produces a new protein from the fusion of the two chromosomes. Scientists are studying this protein to try to learn more about ESFT tumors.

Environmental factors

No environmental factors have been associated with development of ESFT tumors.

ESFT signs and symptoms

The symptoms of ESFT tumors depend very much on the location of the disease. Almost all children diagnosed with Ewing's sarcoma of the bone will have pain, and more than half will have swelling of the affected area. Approximately 16 percent will have a fracture at the site of disease, and 21 percent will have a fever. A diagnosis is sometimes delayed because the symptoms of a ESFT tumor can be very similar to those of an infection. It is not unusual for several months to pass, once the onset of symptoms has occurred, before the disease is discovered. Children with metastatic disease may seem tired and have unexplained weight loss. If the cancer has spread to areas around the spine, symptoms may include back pain or paralysis.

In November 1997, our nine-year-old daughter was diagnosed with Ewing's sarcoma. She had been sick on and off for about a year previous to diagnosis and had constantly complained of extreme pain in her left side. The pain was always coming and going, so the pediatrician figured it might have something to do with her intestinal tract (as the pain was always in the lower left side near to this area.). He scheduled her for an ultrasound in late November, but I guess you could say the cancer beat him to it. My mother came to visit in early November and found a rather large suspicious lump in my daughter's back near the left shoulder blade. I took her in to the children's hospital that evening and we were told to see the pediatrician in the morning and be prepared for an admission to the hospital. I managed to hold myself together until I got home. No one had mentioned the "C" word, but I knew that it wasn't good.

Diagnosis of ESFT

For a diagnosis of a ESFT tumor to be reached, the physician will order several tests and procedures. This process always begins with the doctor obtaining the child's medical history and performing a complete physical examination. Several blood tests will be ordered (see Appendix B), including a complete blood count (CBC) and differential. Other laboratory studies include the measurement of lactate dehydrogenase (LDH). If there is suspicion that the disease may be neuroblastoma, a urinalysis to measure catecholamine levels may be ordered.

Imaging studies will generally begin with x-ray films of the site that is suspected of having a malignancy.

A definitive diagnosis of a ESFT tumor cannot be made unless the doctor has confirmation with actual tumor tissue. This may be accomplished with either an excisional biopsy, in which the surgeon will remove the mass completely, an incisional biopsy, in which only a small portion of the tumor is removed for evaluation, or a needle biopsy. For further reading on these tests, see Chapter 2, *Coping with Procedures*.

Staging

Once a diagnosis is made, other tests are done to determine if the disease has spread. This process is called staging. Computed tomography (CT) of the chest, abdomen, and pelvis are usually done to stage the tumor. Magnetic resonance imaging (MRI) provides detailed images which help define the extent of the disease. Radionuclide scanning, or scintigraphy, with technetium-99m methylene diphosphonate (tTc 99m MDP) is used to determine the extent of the primary tumor, and also helps to determine the presence of metastatic disease in bone. The doctor may order a gallium scan, since Ewing's sarcoma accumulates this radiopharmaceutical very well. The doctor does bilateral bone marrow biopsies and aspirates to determine if the disease has spread to the bone marrow.

There are only two stages for ESFT tumors:

- **Localized.** These tumors have not spread to distant sites.
- **Metastatic.** These tumors have spread to other parts of the body, including the lungs, bones, and bone marrow.

Prognosis

Treatment for childhood ESFT has steadily improved in the last two decades. In the 1960s, virtually all children with ESFT died, but by the 1990s, the majority of children with localized disease who receive optimal treatment are cured.

Like many cancers, the most important prognostic factor for ESFT tumors is the presence or absence of metastatic disease at diagnosis. In those children with localized tumors, the location of the primary site has also been shown to be of prognostic significance. Those with a tumor originating in the pelvic area have a less favorable prognosis than those with tumors originating in the distal bones and ribs.

> On November 5, 1997, we received a prognosis. Metastatic Ewing's sarcoma of the bone. If left untreated, Elizabeth would have two months to live. We were advised to put her on a new form of treatment designed by the Children's Cancer Group. She would then have a little bit better than 20 percent chance of survival. We gave our consent and began our journey into the world of cancer treatment.

Treatment of ESFT

At diagnosis, many parents are confused about how to find the best doctors and treatments for their child. State-of-the-art care is available from physicians who participate in the Intergroup Ewing's Sarcoma Study, Children's Cancer Group (CCG) and the Pediatric Oncology Group (POG). These study groups, composed of pediatric surgeons and oncologists, urologists, radiation oncologists, researchers, and nurses, establish the standard of care for patients worldwide, conduct new studies to discover better therapies, and establish follow-up for survivors. They are in the process of merging into one entity called the Children's Oncology Group (COG). If the treatment center you are referred to is a member of one of these groups, you can rest assured that your child will have access to the best thinking on the treatment of pediatric cancers.

The goal of treatment for ESFT is to cure the child and to maintain as much function of the affected area as possible, as well as minimize the possible long-term effects of treatment. Treatment for a ESFT tumor includes surgery and chemotherapy, and in some circumstances, radiation. When the tumor is completely resected with good margins of normal tissue, radiation is generally not given.

> Elizabeth was treated for her metastatic Ewing's with five rounds of intense chemotherapy consisting of doxorubicin, cyclophosphamide, vincristine, ifosfamide, and etoposide. She also had mesna, ondansetron, Decadron, Septra, an NG tube, TPN, numerous blood transfusions, and morphine to help with all the side effects of treatment. She then had 24 targeted radiation treatments, consisting of twelve days of treatments to the pelvic area and ribs. After that we went to total body irradiation for six treatments, given over three days. Then she had more chemotherapy, specifically, melphalan and etoposide for three days. Finally, she had an autologous peripheral stem cell reinfusion as a rescue.

Surgery

The approach to surgical management of ESFT tumors depends largely on the location of the mass and the impact that resection will have on the function of the affected part of the body (see Chapter 18, *Surgery*). If the tumor is situated in a non-essential bone or soft tissue, it can sometimes be removed without creating deformity or resulting in loss of function. However, the primary site is often found in the extremities where this approach may not be possible.

> My son Jeremy had Ewing's in his left distal femur. He was diagnosed at age eleven. He had chemo from February to April of that year ('94) and then limb-salvage surgery in May. He was on crutches for a very long time. They were able to spare his distal growth plate in the ini-

tial surgery. However, three surgeries later (problems with the "hard-ware") they finally screwed bolts into his growth plate. Since then, he has had to have surgery once to shorten his "unaffected" leg.

Before the development of limb-salvage surgery and newer radiation techniques, most children with extremity tumors had the affected limb amputated. Many children now have limb-salvage procedures using autologous grafts, allografts, an endoprosthesis, or state-of-the-art radiation therapy to treat their tumor.

> *When we decided that amputation was the best treatment, we spent the next few weeks talking about it. It was almost as if we were mourning the loss of his leg and foot—saying goodbye to his toes. The surgery to remove his leg just below the hip took fourteen hours. Troy's femur was removed, and the tibia was moved up and flipped to act as the upper leg bone. The foot was amputated. His prosthesis was attached at the knee.*

> *I have never regarded my son as handicapped. Troy is able to do almost all things other kids his age enjoy doing. He climbs, rides a bike, skateboards, and even spends time on his boogie board. Today he is a healthy, happy thirteen year old. I have no anger about what has happened. In fact, I feel very fortunate. Troy's amputation took place at a time when he was not being treated for cancer, and when his body was disease-free. The worries of chemotherapy and its side-effects were not an issue, and we were able to deal exclusively with the amputation. My son has adjusted very well, physically and emotionally, to losing his leg. He doesn't let it slow him down.*

Tumors located in the lungs can often be removed by a procedure called thoracotomy (surgery in which an incision is made to open the chest cavity). Disease located within the ribs sometimes requires the removal of affected bones and replacement with a synthetic material to reconstruct the chest wall.

Radiation

Radiation is often needed to treat children diagnosed with ESFT tumors. Radiation is used for tumors that cannot be completely resected. Some chest wall tumors are treated with whole-lung irradiation. ESFT tumors are generally treated with doses ranging from 4000 to 5600 cGy, fractioned over a period of four to six weeks. For more information, see Chapter 17, *Radiation.*

Chemotherapy

Before chemotherapy became a standard weapon against ESFT tumors in the 1960s, very few children survived. Chemotherapy improved the long-term survival rate and also facilitated surgical management of the disease by reducing the tumor size before resection. Treatment of Ewing's now includes systemic chemotherapy for all children. This is necessary even for those children with localized disease.

The most commonly used combination of chemotherapy drugs includes vincristine, doxorubicin, cyclophosphamide, ifosfamide, etoposide, and dactinomycin. For more information, see Chapter 15, *Chemotherapy*.

> *Troy (age five) was diagnosed in October 1990 with Ewing's sarcoma. The disease was completely capsulated in his right femur. He had a total of eighteen courses of chemotherapy consisting of ifosfamide, vp-16, vincristine, and adriamycin. Less than halfway through the protocol, the doctors decided that it was time to operate to remove the tumor. He had surgery to remove the femur and the knee. He then continued on with several more months of chemotherapy. Treatment was hard on Troy, and he struggled with nausea and vomiting, along with loss of appetite.*

Newest treatment options

Much research is being conducted into new treatments for ESFT tumors. Peripheral blood stem cell transplants (see Chapter 19, *Bone Marrow and Stem Cell Transplantation*) are being performed at various centers across North America. Gene therapy is being researched as a potential therapy against ESFT tumors. Monoclonal antibodies may soon allow delivery of anti-cancer drugs directly to the tumor cells.

To learn about the standard treatment for your child's illness, call (800) 4-CANCER and ask for the PDQ (physician's data query) for osteosarcoma or Ewing's sarcoma/primitive neuroectodermal tumor. These free statements explain the disease, state-of-the-art treatments, and ongoing clinical trials. Two versions are available: one for patients, which uses simple language and contains no statistics, and one for professionals, which is technical, thorough, and includes citations to scientific literature. The PDQ can also be read on the Internet at *http://cancernet.nci.nih.gov/*.

My daughter Casey was treated for osteosarcoma by an orthopedic oncologist. As soon as she stopped vomiting from chemotherapy, she returned to her beloved cheerleading, took up jazz dancing (she claims it was the best physical therapy), and is now on the varsity springboard diving team at her high school. She sends her orthopedic oncologist photos and videotapes of her doing these things that he claims give him heart pains. But, one day, when he observed her sitting cross-legged in his examining room, he finally admitted that she has had the best physical response of any of his patients and he took a picture of her sitting that way for a brochure. I can't explain to you how wonderful it makes me feel to see this doctor actually glow when he sees Casey (now only once a year)—he calls the whole office together to behold her!

CHAPTER 12

Liver Cancers

*There are only two ways to live your life. One
is as though nothing is a miracle. The other is
as though everything is a miracle.*

—Albert Einstein

LIVER TUMORS COMPRISE LESS than 5 percent of all childhood cancers. The most
common forms of liver cancers in children are hepatoblastoma and hepatocellular carcinoma.

This chapter first looks at the structure and function of the liver. Then it
examines who gets liver cancers, what the signs and symptoms are, how
they are diagnosed, and how doctors determine the prognosis. The chapter
then discusses current and future treatments for childhood liver cancers.

The liver

The liver is the body's largest internal organ and one of the most complex.
Located beneath the rib cage in the upper right quadrant of the abdomen,
this wedge-shaped organ is divided into two main lobes—right and left—
and two smaller lobes (see Figure 12-1).

The liver is like a chemical refinery that operates 24 hours a day. It receives
blood from both the hepatic artery and the portal vein and modifies substances contained in the blood that passes through it. This includes everything that is swallowed and absorbed into the bloodstream. For example,
after food is digested by the stomach and small intestine, the liver metabo-
lizes, or chemically changes, it into forms that are easier for the rest of the
body to use.

Another major function of the liver is to filter blood. Harmful material from
food, drugs, or bacteria are removed by this unique filtration system. The
liver changes these toxic substances into forms which can be easily eliminated from the body.

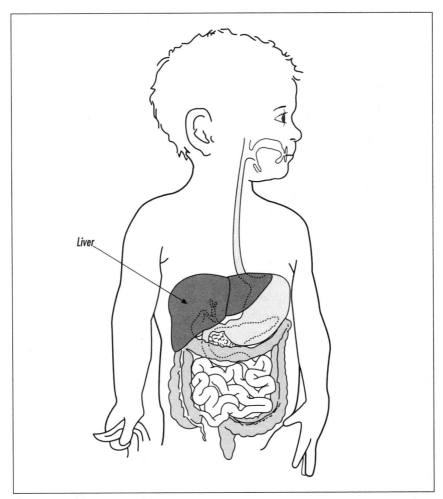

Figure 12-1. The liver

The liver produces bile, a greenish-brown fluid essential for proper digestion. Bile is stored in the gallbladder. When food is ingested, the gallbladder
contracts and releases bile into the intestine. Bile is also used to rid the body
of unwanted compounds, such as bilirubin, which is a by-product of red
blood cell turnover.

The liver produces, stores, and provides glucose to keep the body active. It
also produces, stores, and exports fat to help regulate the supply of body
fuel. The liver regulates the balance of many important hormones including
adrenal, thyroid, and sex hormones. It regulates the supply of essential minerals and vitamins, such as copper and iron. The liver produces, excretes,
and converts cholesterol into other important substances. It manufactures

key proteins, such as those used to transport other substances in the blood, and those providing resistance to infection. Other proteins made by the liver aid in the clotting of blood. These are but a few examples of the hundreds of complex functions of the liver.

Who gets liver cancer?

Approximately one child in every million will be diagnosed with a liver tumor each year in North America. Boys are affected by these malignancies more frequently than girls. Since there are different risk factors for hepatoblastoma and hepatocellular carcinoma, they are discussed separately.

Hepatoblastoma

Hepatoblastoma is a rare form of liver cancer most often diagnosed in children under the age of three. Premature infants have a higher risk of developing hepatoblastoma than children who were not born prematurely. Children with Beckwith-Wiedemann syndrome, familial adenomatous polyposis, and Aicardi syndrome also have a higher risk of developing hepatoblastoma than the general population. However, most children with these syndromes do not develop hepatoblastoma, and most children with hepatoblastoma do not have one of these syndromes.

Hepatocellular carcinoma

Hepatocellular carcinoma is seen most often in children under the age of four and those between twelve and fifteen years of age. This form of liver cancer has been associated with several other conditions, including some rare metabolic diseases. The strongest association has been with hepatitis B and C, and other conditions that lead to cirrhosis of the liver.

Hepatitis B is an infectious disease of the liver caused by the hepatitis B virus (HBV) that results in acute or chronic hepatitis. Hepatitis C is an infectious disease of the liver caused by the hepatitis C virus (HCV) that results in chronic hepatitis. Many children who develop hepatocellular carcinoma have been previously infected with hepatitis B or sometimes hepatitis C.

Biliary atresia is a disease diagnosed in infants in which there is inflammation and obstruction of the ducts carrying bile from the liver. The disease causes cirrhosis, which places the child at an increased risk of hepatocellular carcinoma.

Other causes of cirrhosis that may in time lead to hepatocellular carcinoma include alpha-1-antitrypsin deficiency, von Gierke disease, and ataxia telangiectasia.

Signs and symptoms

Hepatoblastomas are usually found when a parent notices a painless, upper right quadrant or midline abdominal mass. The abdomen may appear distended and 15 to 20 percent of children have abdominal pain. A small number of children have jaundice, a yellowing of the skin and the whites of the eyes. The child may have a poor appetite (anorexia) and recent weight loss. Nausea and vomiting, in addition to weakness, may also be present.

> In December 1994, I noticed something unusual when changing her diaper before bedtime. It looked as if someone had taken an orange crayon and colored the inside of her diaper. I called her pediatrician who suggested we bring her in the next day, along with the diaper, just to check her over before the holidays. I wasn't too worried, because I thought that maybe it was just food coloring from something that she ate coming out in her urine. When we saw the doctor the next day, he immediately found a lump, and asked if she had received any blows or falls injuring the stomach area recently. We were sent to the hospital and she was given some blood tests and a CT scan, which showed the tumor.

The signs and symptoms of hepatocellular carcinoma are very similar to those of hepatoblastoma. A parent may find a lump or mass in the upper right or middle of the abdomen, with or without distension of the abdomen. The child may complain of abdominal pain and general weakness. Fifteen to twenty percent of children have jaundice or fever. Poor appetite and weight loss are frequently present. Bleeding into the abdominal cavity (hemoperitoneum) may occur because of tumor rupture.

Diagnosis

Several tests and procedures are necessary to diagnose liver cancer. Most of these procedures are the same for both hepatoblastoma and hepatocellular carcinoma. In addition to completing a history and physical examination of the child, the doctor will order a complete blood count (CBC). The doctor also orders bloodwork to evaluate liver enzymes, alfa fetoprotein (AFP), and bilirubin levels. AFP is elevated in 90 to 95 percent of all children with hepatoblastoma. Though not to the same degree, it may also be elevated in children with hepatocellular carcinoma. AFP provides a convenient way of monitoring tumor response to treatment and is regularly checked. Liver function tests, such as AST, ALT, LDH, and alkaline phosphatase, are also usually ordered. For more information, see Appendix B, *Blood Counts and What They Mean*.

Ultrasonography (US) and computed tomography (CT) of the liver and abdomen are performed. The doctor may also order a magnetic resonance imaging (MRI) of the liver.

> Logan had been sick for three months prior to the diagnosis with severe vomiting, weight loss, a hard abdomen, and irritability. He cried day and night and was very clingy. He had a lot of trouble sleeping. Four different doctors saw Logan and said it was just a stomach bug. When his testicle became enlarged and purple, he was diagnosed as having hydrocele (accumulation of fluid in the testicle). He was taken to surgery and the hydrocele was repaired.
>
> He continued to have all the same symptoms after that, but only worse. I took Logan to the emergency room three weeks later because I had enough. Scans were performed and we were told that Logan had a mass in his liver and they were 99.9 percent sure it was cancer.

The definitive test is a liver biopsy, which is a diagnostic procedure used to obtain a small amount of cancerous liver tissue. This may be done during an open surgical biopsy or by a fine needle biopsy guided by CT or US. For more information about these tests, see Chapter 2, *Coping with Procedures*.

Staging

Once liver cancer has been diagnosed, the oncologist will order more tests and scans to determine the extent (stage) of the disease. An imaging study, such as a CT, MRI, or bone scan, may be performed to check for metastases.

Staging is very important because it has a direct impact on prognosis and choosing the most appropriate therapy. The following staging system is based on the extent of tumor involvement and its ability to be removed surgically:

- Stage I. The tumor is able to be completely removed.
- Stage II. The tumor is removed surgically, but there are microscopic traces of disease still present.

- Stage III. The tumor is not able to be removed surgically at diagnosis or is partially removed. Lymph nodes are positive for disease or there is tumor spill during surgery.
- Stage IV. The disease has spread to distant areas in the body, regardless of the extent of liver involvement.

Ten percent of patients with hepatoblastoma have metastatic disease in the lungs at diagnosis. Rare areas of spread can include the central nervous system and the abdomen. Common areas of metastases in children with hepatocellular carcinoma include the lungs, bone marrow, and lymph nodes.

Logan was nineteen months old when he was diagnosed with hepatoblastoma. At diagnosis, the tumor was the size of a grapefruit and had spread to his lymph nodes and also the right atrium of his heart.

Prognostic indicators

Treatments for childhood liver cancers have improved in the last two decades. The appropriate treatment for liver cancer is determined by analysis of many clinical and biologic features.

To choose the best treatment for children with hepatoblastoma, doctors consider the child's age, health, stage of disease, type of cancer cells, and the level of alpha fetoprotein in the blood. Long-term survival for hepatoblastoma is approximately 60 to 70 percent with a survival rate of 90 percent in early stage disease.

The prognosis for children with hepatocellular carcinoma is much worse than for those with hepatoblastoma because hepatocellular carcinoma cancer cells are very aggressive. These tumors often involve all lobes of the liver, making surgery difficult. Doctors, therefore, carefully consider the child's age, stage of disease, and the cellular characteristics of the tumor to choose the treatment that provides the best chance for cure.

Treatment

At diagnosis, many parents are confused about how to find the best doctors and treatments for their child. State-of-the-art care is available from physicians who participate in the Children's Cancer Group (CCG) and/or the Pediatric Oncology Group (POG). These study groups, composed of pediatric surgeons and oncologists, urologists, radiation oncologists, researchers and nurses, establish the standard of care for patients worldwide, conduct new studies to discover better therapies, and establish follow-up for survivors. They are in the process of merging into one entity called the Children's Oncology Group (COG). If the treatment center you are referred to is a member of one of these groups, you can rest assured that your child will have access to the best thinking on the treatment of pediatric cancers.

All children with liver tumors have all or part of their tumor removed surgically, and many children require chemotherapy. Liver transplantation is also necessary in some cases. The aggressiveness of treatment is based on the type of liver cancer and its histology (how it looks under a microscope), the extent of tumor involvement and stage of disease, as well as the child's age and overall health. The AFP levels of children with liver cancer are followed throughout treatment to evaluate the effectiveness of therapy and later to screen for recurrence.

Surgery

Surgery is the cornerstone therapy for both hepatoblastoma and hepatocellular carcinoma. Complete removal of the tumor provides the best chance for a cure. Large portions of liver can be removed, because the liver regenerates itself rapidly. Generally, surgery occurs very soon after diagnosis. However, some oncologists feel that preoperative chemotherapy is the best approach because it can minimize the amount of healthy liver that will need to be removed along with the tumor.

Sometimes it isn't possible to completely remove the tumor at diagnosis due to extensive tumor involvement of the liver or because the disease has spread to other organs. In some cases, the CT or MRI suggests that more than one lobe of the liver is involved, making surgery not possible. In these instances, preoperative chemotherapy can shrink the tumor to a size that will allow resection. Surgery is also used to remove tumors that have metastasized to the lungs.

The types of surgery for childhood liver tumors are:

- **Wedge resection.** Removal of part of one lobe of the liver.
- **Lobectomy.** Removal of a whole lobe of the liver.
- **Trisegmentectomy.** Removal of an entire lobe and part of the other.
- **Thoracotomy.** Removal of tumors from the lungs.

Coley's surgery was very scary, I think more for us than for her. She has been my role model for bravery throughout the entire process. The surgery took a few hours and has left her with a large scar that goes from one side of her stomach to the other in an upside down U. I was very scared to see her in intensive care, because I was afraid that I would break down when I saw her with all those tubes. But after waiting all those hours, when we were finally able to see her, she looked so beautiful. She had made it!

The doctors told us she would be out for a day or so, but while they were telling us this, she was trying to say "waffle" with the tube still down her throat. The doctors were shocked, and they took the tube out a day earlier than they expected.

• • • • •

Just ten days after his second birthday, Logan had a five-hour operation to remove the entire right lobe of his liver and his gallbladder. During surgery he lost quite a lot of blood and was given five units while in the operating room. He was transferred to ICU and was given another unit of blood and platelets. He remained there for only 36 hours and was transferred to the oncology floor.

By the third day, he was walking around. He had very little pain and he never complained. By the fourth day, he was running up and down the hall feeling wonderful. You would never guess that he had just had a major operation. On the fifth day, we were able to take him home. Two weeks after the operation, he went back to have one more round of chemotherapy and then we were done.

A child with a previously damaged liver who is diagnosed with hepatocellular carcinoma may not be eligible for surgery. For example, a child with liver damage from hepatitis B or C could not survive if large portions of his liver were surgically removed. Consequently, only small tumors are removed under these circumstances.

Chemotherapy

Chemotherapy is almost always used to treat both forms of liver cancer. It is considered systemic therapy because the anticancer drugs are injected into the bloodstream to reach all areas of the body. This method of treatment not only attacks the disease located in the liver, but it also destroys cancerous cells that may have spread to other areas.

Hepatoblastoma is very sensitive to chemotherapy. Effective chemotherapy agents include cisplatin, vincristine, fluorouracil, and doxorubicin. Other drugs, such as ifosfamide, dactinomycin, and etoposide may be used for more advanced stages of disease. For more information on these drugs, see Chapter 15, *Chemotherapy*.

> *The doctor went over the protocol and told us that Logan's chance of survival was 70 percent. The chemotherapy was hung and dripping within two hours of the pathology report. Logan received cisplatin, vincristine, and 5-FU. He had chemotherapy every three weeks that usually took an average of two days. Logan had many reactions to chemotherapy—vomiting, diarrhea, nickel-sized blisters on his bottom, thrush, rashes, hair loss, loss of appetite, blotchy skin color, severe high frequency hearing loss, seizures (he was put on phenobarbitol), leg and hand/arm pain. After Logan received the first round, there was a small decrease in the tumor. After the second, there was a little more. Since his tumor was responding, we decided to stay on the protocol. After the fifth course, Logan was admitted for surgery to have the tumor removed.*

Hepatocellular carcinoma is not as sensitive to chemotherapy as hepatoblastoma. Initial treatment for hepatocellular carcinoma usually includes the drugs cisplatin and doxorubicin. For more advanced disease, vincristine and fluorouracil may be used.

Radiation

Radiation therapy is not commonly used to treat tumors of the liver because normal, healthy liver tissue is extremely sensitive to the damaging effects of radiation. However, radiation may be used to treat tumors that have spread to other areas in the body.

Liver transplantation

Liver transplantation is used to treat children with hepatoblastoma and hepatocellular carcinoma whose tumors are unresectable because of involvement in both lobes of the liver or who have relapsed. Advances made in transplantation include transferring portions of a liver from a child's parent to the child, where it regenerates and becomes fully functional.

Removing the entire liver, called hepatectomy, and then transplanting a new, healthy organ from a donor is considered by some to be experimental. However, long-term survival rates following this procedure are improving.

Other treatments

Researchers are constantly working to find new methods for treating liver cancer to increase survival rates. Currently, there are some phase I and phase II clinical trials taking place across North America which try to improve the quality of life for children with liver cancer, as well as strive for the ultimate goal of a cure (see Chapter 5, *Clinical Trials*).

Some of these experimental treatments follow:

- Cryosurgery is a technique that involves freezing cancerous cells to kill tumors.

- Ethanol ablation involves injecting concentrated alcohol directly into the tumor via the hepatic artery.

- High-dose chemotherapy followed by stem cell transplantation (see Chapter 19, *Bone Marrow and Stem Cell Transplantation*) is being used by some institutions in an attempt to improve long-term survival in children with a poor prognosis.

- Hepatic arterial chemoembolization is being researched, using new drugs such as floxuridine.

- Chemotherapy drugs, such as tamoxifen, are being used in phase II studies along with a combination of other anticancer agents.

- A new form of therapy, called antiangiogenesis, which attempts to destroy tumors by starving them of their blood supply, is also being tested in phase I studies.

Newest treatment options

To learn of the newest treatments available, call (800) 4-CANCER and ask for the PDQ (physicians data query) for hepatoblastoma or hepatocellular carcinoma. You can also access the PDQ on the Internet at *http:// cancernet.nci.nih.gov/*. These free statements explain the disease, state-of-the-art treatments, and ongoing clinical trials. There are two versions available: one for patients, which uses simple language and contains no statistics, and one for professionals, which is technical, thorough, and includes citations to scientific literature.

Matthew was diagnosed with hepatoblastoma in June of 1993. His only symptom was an enlarged belly. He seemed to be a normal, active eighteen-month-old. His medical team estimated that his tumor was initially the size of a grapefruit. Four months of chemotherapy shrank the tumor to about the size of an egg, making surgery safer and more likely to be successful. Two additional months of chemotherapy were used as follow-up after his surgery. His alfa feta protein level returned to normal following the surgery in September of 1993 and remained normal until spring of 1996, when it started to slowly climb. After ruling out all other possible causes, we knew it would only be a matter of time before our fears were confirmed. A CT scan found the liver mass.

Surgery was scheduled right away to attempt to resect the tumor. We tried several different chemotherapy protocols in the next five months, but Matthew was not improving. We met with the liver transplant team and Matthew was placed on the list. As the clock continued to tick and his AFP continued to climb, he continued on chemotherapy.

In April of 1997, Matthew had his liver transplant. It was thrilling for us to see him recover from major surgery so quickly! Matthew has only had two episodes of rejection, and both responded well to treatment with high doses of steroids.

At almost two years following his transplant, his AFP has remained normal and our hospital visits are not so frequent. Matthew played ball this past summer, completed his kindergarten year with very few absences and is now a first grader learning to read!

CHAPTER 13

Retinoblastoma

The potential possibilities of any child are the
most intriguing and stimulating
in all creation.

—Ray L. Wilbur

RETINOBLASTOMA IS A CANCEROUS tumor of the eye. It is the most common eye cancer of childhood and occurs in both hereditary and non-hereditary forms. The disease primarily affects very young children, and may be present in one or both eyes. There may be one or more than one tumor in either eye.

This chapter first looks at the structure and function of the eye. Then it examines who gets retinoblastoma, what the signs and symptoms are, how it is diagnosed, and how doctors determine the prognosis. The chapter ends with a discussion of the current treatments and looks ahead to new treatment options.

The eye

The eyes have often been called the windows to the world. Each structure within the eye has a specific task to help transmit information from the outside world through the optic nerve to the brain (see Figure 13-1).

The cornea is the convex outer portion of the eyeball that transmits light to the retina. Behind the cornea is the iris, which is the colored portion of the organ. The iris controls the amount of light entering into the eye by making the opening at the center, called the pupil, either larger or smaller.

As light rays pass through the curved surface of the cornea, they are bent and then passed through the pupil. Inside the eye, sitting behind the pupil, is a disc-shaped structure called the lens. The lens is clear in the healthy eye, and has two curved surfaces which refract the light two more times on its journey to the back of the eye. As light rays are passed from the front to the

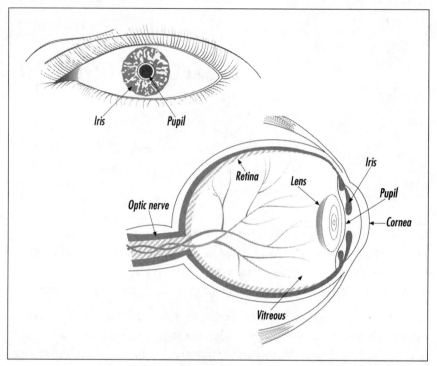

Figure 13-1. The anatomy of the eye

back of the organ, they pass through a colorless, jelly-like material, called the vitreous, that fills the eyeball behind the lens.

The inside lining of the eyeball consists of a structure called the retina. It is the retina that converts light energy into electrical impulses that are transmitted to the brain through the use of its sensory receptors, the rods and cones. The retina is a collection of nerve tissue in the eye and its job is to form the images that we see. The retina cells in babies and very young children are called retinoblasts.

Retinoblastoma originates in the retina of the eye.

Who gets retinoblastoma?

Each year approximately 200 children in the United States and 20 children in Canada are diagnosed with retinoblastoma. This relatively uncommon childhood cancer accounts for about 2 percent of all childhood malignancies. There is no higher incidence in any particular race, and boys are affected as often as girls. There is a hereditary and non-hereditary form of this disease (see "Genetic factors").

> *John Allen was fifteen months old when he was diagnosed with unilateral retinoblastoma. The doctor didn't give us any information other than it was a fast growing cancer and that it needed to be taken care of right away. We couldn't see the specialist for another five days, so we cried and prayed. We didn't know whether we were going to lose our baby or not. When we saw the specialist, she answered all of our questions in detail. We were then referred to a pediatric oncologist and pediatric ophthalmologist surgeon. They, too, were fantastic. We were relieved when they explained the enucleation to us. What mattered most was that our little boy had an excellent chance of beating his disease.*

Retinoblastoma is usually diagnosed in very young children, and may be present at birth. Although it may occur at any age, 90 percent of cases are diagnosed before the age of five. Those with more than one tumor or a tumor in both eyes (usually the hereditary form) are diagnosed at a younger age than those with only one tumor and one eye involved (usually the non-hereditary form).

Genetic factors

As with most types of childhood cancer, the exact cause of retinoblastoma is not known. However, more is known about the genetics and inheritance of this tumor than any other kind of childhood cancer. Because the tumor occurs at a very young age and within paired organs (eyes) and the gene involved is known, retinoblastoma is considered the model for genetic studies into childhood cancer. Scientists hope to use this model to learn more about other forms of childhood cancer.

A change in a gene called RB1 is involved in the development of retinoblastoma. This change is called a mutation. Genes are located inside the body's cells. They are passed from parent to child through the egg and the sperm. Children get one copy of each gene from their mother and the other copy from their father. The genes contain material called DNA. The DNA tells the cells what proteins to make. These proteins determine such things as eye color, skin color, and blood type. These proteins plus other factors such as diet and lifestyle can affect such things as body weight and the risk of certain diseases such as diabetes or heart disease.

The RBI gene is located on chromosome 13. In about 60 percent of cases, there is a change in both copies of the RB1 gene but only in the retinoblast cells that make up the retinoblastoma tumor in the eye. If you look at cells from any other area in the body, chromosome 13 is completely unchanged with no mutation in the RB1 gene. It is not known what causes the mutation in this gene. Most of the time, these children develop one tumor only in one eye. This is called the non-hereditary form of the disease.

> *Thirty years ago I was diagnosed with retinoblastoma when I was eighteen months old. I had one tumor in just one eye. The eye was surgically removed and I had no chemotherapy or radiation. I have no late effects other than wearing a prosthesis and having vision in only one eye.*

In the other 40 percent of cases, the children are born with one variant RB1 gene that has a mutation. This mutated copy of the RB1 gene is found in all the cells of the body. In 85 percent of these cases, there is no one else in the family with retinoblastoma; the mutation happened in the egg or the sperm. This new or spontaneous mutation is passed on to the child.

The remaining 15 percent of the children have a family member with the disease (usually a parent). In these instances, the parent had an abnormal copy of the RB1 gene in every cell in the body and passed it on to the child through the egg or sperm. This time it was not a new (or spontaneous) mutation. All of these children start their life with one variant copy of the RB1 gene in every cell, including all the retinoblasts in the eye. After conception, something happens to the copy of the RB1 gene in one or more than one retinoblast in one or both eyes. Now, in these eyes, both copies of the gene are mutated and retinoblastoma occurs. In these children, the disease can occur in one or both eyes. There may be one or more than one tumor. New tumors may form in the first five years of life. This is called the hereditary form of retinoblastoma even if there is no one else in the family with the disease.

It is not known what causes the changes in the RB1 gene in either of these forms of retinoblastoma. It is known that there is nothing parents can do to change these risks.

No simple blood test is available to tell whether your child has the hereditary form or the non-hereditary form of retinoblastoma. The genetics are very complicated. Currently, oncologists decide on whether the disease is hereditary or non-hereditary based on a number of factors, including family history, age at diagnosis, number of tumors, and whether one or both eyes are involved. If your oncologist has not told you which type of retinoblastoma your child has, ask. Your oncologist can then explain how your child and other family members need to be followed. This affects treatment decisions, risk for having another child with retinoblastoma, risk of your child having a child with retinoblastoma, and the risk of your child getting other cancers later in life.

> *Because I had bilateral retinoblastoma, the doctors told my mother long ago that I had a high chance of passing it on to any offspring. When I got married, my wife and I chose not to have any kids.*

Environmental factors

No clear environmental factors have been linked to increased risk of retinoblastoma.

Signs and symptoms

In North America, most cases of retinoblastoma are diagnosed while the tumor remains within the eye. The most frequently observed sign of this malignancy is a white appearance of the pupil when exposed to light—called leukokoria. This is often referred to as "the cat's eye reflex." It is usually noticed when a flash picture is taken and is especially noticeable when only one eye is affected.

Another frequently seen symptom of retinoblastoma is strabismus—when the affected eye drifts inward (esotropia), or outward (exotropia). However, most children who have strabismus do not have retinoblastoma. Since young children generally do not complain of vision problems, vision loss is rarely noted by the parents. Pain is not common, and apart from the above noted symptoms, the child appears otherwise healthy.

> *It took a few days to get a diagnosis. On a Friday morning, at Noah's two-month checkup, the pediatrician noticed a white reflex in one of his pupils and showed me the difference between the eyes. When I asked what would cause it he was vague and said he would call an ophthalmologist for an appointment for us. When the ophthalmologist's office called asking us to come in that same day we began to realize that something quite serious must be going on.*

The ophthalmologist said Noah either had cancer or another pro-
gressive condition and he would need to be seen by a retina specialist in
Seattle (a 1 hour and 45 minute drive away). When we asked if he would
be able to see out of the eye, he very matter-of-factly informed us that
there was no question that he could not see and would not again from that
eye.

On Monday morning we were told that Noah had retinoblastoma,
that the tumor was very large, and the eye would need to be removed. We
were in shock and scared of the tests and surgery he would need. It was
hard to imagine what it would be like for him to lose his eye, and we were
worried about the possibility of metastases. Everything seemed very
unreal, but we just did what had to be done.

Diagnosis and staging

After a parent or doctor notices the abnormality in a child's eye(s), the child is examined by an ophthalmologist. After an examination is done in the office, the child is then examined under anesthesia (EUA). An ultrasound is usually also done at this time. After a diagnosis of retinoblastoma is made, the child should be referred to a pediatric oncologist. The oncologist takes a full history, does a thorough examination, and together with the ophthalmologist decides on the best treatment plan.

Staging the tumor is done to find out the extent of the disease. It is usually done by the oncologist, but part may also be done by the ophthalmologist. Computerized tomography (CT) or magnetic resonance imaging (MRI) is used to examine for disease in both eyes, orbits, optic nerves, and the brain. Rarely, retinoblastoma can go to the pineal gland in the brain. Even more rarely, it can spread to other places in the brain or the bone marrow. For this reason, a complete blood count (CBC) is done. If the CT, MRI, or CBC suggests that the disease has spread outside the eye, a lumbar puncture (spinal tap) and a bone marrow test will be done. These tests are rare, however.

From the beginning, we always talked to our son about what was
happening, about what he might be feeling, about how sorry we were that
we couldn't avoid having him go through a specific procedure. He under-
stood our love and concern. We always felt it was important to be honest
with him about what was happening because he had a right to know. We
bought him a doctor kit, a Playmobile operating room, and kept one of his

anesthesia masks for him to play with. We gave him empty dilating drop
bottles so he could be the one to put the eye drops in a willing patient
(stuffed animal).

Successful treatment of retinoblastoma depends largely on the size of the tumor and the extent of the disease. The staging system most widely used is the Reese-Ellsworth staging classification of retinoblastoma. This system allows the ophthalmologist and oncologist to better plan therapy. Children are grouped into very favorable, favorable, doubtful, unfavorable, or very unfavorable categories regarding the preservation of their vision based on several factors, such as tumor size, the location and number of lesions, and the presence of disease within the layers of the retina (seeding).

Children with retinoblastoma should be followed closely for recurrence or spread outside the eye from diagnosis through age five. The intervals at which exams are done depends on many factors including whether the disease is in one or both eyes, the number, size, and location of tumors, family history, and the type of treatment. After age five, the chance of recurrence or spread is very low, but children should still be seen at least once a year by an ophthalmologist and an oncologist to monitor for late effects.

Prognosis

The prognosis for cure from retinoblastoma is excellent (close to 95 percent). In most cases, the child will be able to lead a very good life despite visual impairment or blindness in one or both eyes. Vision may be spared if the disease is diagnosed early and newer treatments are used.

Treatment

At diagnosis, many parents are confused about how to find the best doctors and treatments for their child. State-of-the-art care is available from physicians who participate in the Children's Cancer Group (CCG) and/or the Pediatric Oncology Group (POG). These study groups, composed of pediatric surgeons and oncologists, urologists, radiation oncologists, researchers and nurses, establish the standard of care for patients worldwide, conduct new studies to discover better therapies, and establish follow-up for survivors. They are in the process of merging into one entity called the Children's Oncology Group (COG). If the treatment center you are referred to is a member of one of these groups, you can rest assured that your child will have access to the best thinking on the treatment of pediatric cancers.

It is also important that your child be followed by a pediatric ophthalmologist who has experience treating retinoblastoma. He needs to work closely with the child's oncologist throughout treatment. The ophthalmologist and oncologist together choose the best treatment or clinical trial (see Chapter 5, *Clinical Trials*) based on the extent of the tumor within and outside the eye. Treatment goals are both cure and preservation of sight.

Depending on the situation, treatment may include surgery, radiation, chemotherapy, and local eye treatments.

> We relied on the opinions of the surgeon, retina specialist, two pathologists, a retinoblastoma specialist from Canada, parents of children with retinoblastoma, and material from the medical journals when deciding on treatment for Hailee (fourteen months old). They all offered pieces of the puzzle, which allowed us to make an informed decision. Hailee had her eye enucleated, and since all the cancer was removed, further treatment wasn't necessary. She is followed every six months with EUA (exam under anesthesia) and MRI, and has done very well. She has coped well with the enucleation, and she looks beautiful.

Surgery and local eye treatments

There are several types of procedures used to treat retinoblastoma: enucleation, cryotherapy, photocoagulation, and thermotherapy. The most appropriate treatment is chosen on an individual basis.

Enucleation

Enucleation is the surgical removal of an eye. The procedure may be used for the following situations:

- If the tumor is very large and there is no hope that the eye will have useful vision.
- If the tumor has spread to the optic nerve, choroid, or orbit.
- If other treatment methods have failed to eradicate the disease.
- If the retina is not able to be examined because of vitreous hemorrhage or cataract.

The enucleation procedure is a relatively simple operation that is done under general anesthesia. In addition to removing the eye, the surgeon will also remove a section of the optic nerve. An orbital implant is placed into the socket immediately after the eyeball is removed. The child will be fitted for an artificial eye four to six weeks after the procedure.

We were very worried about how we would react to seeing John Allen without an eye, but the doctors prepared us, and when the time came, we were okay. It has been an interesting process dealing with his prosthesis. When the ocularist was making his artificial eye, my wife and I both almost began to cry, because it looked so real. It was almost as if nothing had happened. But, deep inside, we knew that this was only the beginning of a long journey for us and our son. We have had a difficult time learning how to take his eye out and put it back in. He cries, because he doesn't like anyone to mess with it. At first, it was heartbreaking, because he would take the eye from us, and try to put it back in himself. Of course, he couldn't do it, and we would have to continue to hold him and try to put it in.

· · · · ·

Hailee (fourteen months) never experienced any difficulties with her prosthetic eye. We spent a great deal of time preparing Hailee when the eye was about to be enucleated. We read her My Fake Eye [see Appendix D, Books and Online Sites], which helped a great deal with the prosthesis. She took the book to daycare and the caregiver read it to the other children. It has never been a big deal for her. She is now four years old and continues to do well.

After the enucleation, a pressure patch is placed over the eyelid. When the patch is removed, the child is started on antibiotic drops which are put into the socket. The eyelid is usually swollen and bruised for the next few days.

Noah had his left eye enucleated at age two months. We were able to take him home a couple of hours later. The most difficult part for me was handing him over to the nurse who took him into the operating room, and not getting to see him until he had awakened. We were impressed that he recovered quickly from anesthesia, and, when the bandages were removed three days later, that there was virtually no bruising.

Children who have one or both eyes removed before the age of three may have an altered facial appearance when they mature due to the slowing of the growth of the orbit. After enucleation, a prosthesis needs to be placed and replaced periodically to foster orbital growth.

> *I am a long-term survivor of bilateral retinoblastoma, diagnosed when I was ten months old. My first enucleation (surgical removal of the eye) was the left eye in May 1971, with radiation to the right eye. The enucleation of the right eye was in March 1972. I have had no subsequent treatment since then. Due to my loss of sight at such an early age, I had no traumatic adjustment period that losing sight later in life might have caused. I really can think of no significant effects that my retinoblastoma has had on my adult life other than the usual adaptations required for dealing with blindness.*

Cryotherapy

Cryotherapy, also sometimes called cryosurgery, is used to treat small primary tumors or new tumors that develop. It is now often used in combination with chemotherapy. It can also be used after radiation therapy.

Cryotherapy uses extreme cold applied by a small probe placed directly on the tumor. The surgeon uses ultrasound to guide the probe to ensure that healthy tissue around the tumor remains unharmed. The procedure is conducted under general anesthesia and may be repeated on several occasions if necessary.

One advantage of this procedure is that it may help prevent the need for enucleation or radiation therapy. The major disadvantages are that larger tumors cannot be treated sufficiently, and the procedure may leave a retinal scar which damages vision.

> *Zachary was ten months old when he was diagnosed with unilateral retinoblastoma in the left eye. He had several eye exams since birth because I had retinoblastoma when I was a child. He was treated with cryotherapy and radioactive plaques. Zachary did well, so our experience with cryotherapy was pretty positive. Of course, being so young, he didn't really know what was going on.*

Thermotherapy

Thermotherapy is a method of delivering heat to the eye using ultrasound, microwaves, or infrared radiation. Like cryotherapy, it is only useful for very small tumors and can be combined with chemotherapy or radiation therapy. It leaves a relatively small scar, preserving more vision.

Photocoagulation

Photocoagulation, also called light coagulation, is another method for treating small tumors. This technique cauterizes tissues with focused light from an argon laser while the child is anesthetized. The light is delivered through an ophthalmoscope and is used to kill the tumor by destroying its blood supply. Photocoagulation is sometimes used in combination with chemotherapy.

Radiation

Retinoblastoma is a radiosensitive tumor. Radiation is used to destroy local disease while attempting to maintain vision. The two methods of radiotherapy that are used to treat retinoblastoma are external-beam radiation and radioactive plaques.

External beam radiation

External beam radiation is used most frequently with large tumors, multiple tumors, tumors that are very close to the optic nerve or fovea (a tiny area on the retina), or those with extensive seeding into the vitreous. Because of the need to sedate young children and the importance of precise delivery, the child should be treated only by professionals who specialize in pediatric radiation therapy.

Radiation is produced by a linear accelerator and targeted at the tumor. While doses may vary, use of 180 to 200 cGy fractions given over four and a half to six weeks to a total dose of 3500 to 4600 cGy is common. Investigators are looking into the possibility of using lower doses in combination with other treatments. Since precise delivery is vital, most children are anesthetized. The actual treatment takes approximately two or three minutes; the preparation, however, takes significantly longer. For more information, see Chapter 17, *Radiation*.

> The doctor had been optimistic that he would be a unilateral case, so
> we were all quite devastated to learn five months later that Noah had
> new tumors in his remaining eye. Both were small enough to treat with
> laser, but unfortunately one was adjacent to the optic nerve so Noah had
> to have radiotherapy. The treatment was very localized. His white count

dropped some, but not seriously. He experienced a mild radiation burn on the opposite side of the eye being treated and some eyebrow hair loss.

Late effects that may develop after external beam radiation are cataracts, slowed growth of the bones in the orbit, vision loss, abnormal tear production, chronic conjunctivas, damage to retina and optic nerve, and second cancers in the radiation field. Children who have had radiation to the eye need expert follow-up evaluations on a routine basis.

Radioactive plaque therapy

Radioactive plaque therapy, also called brachytherapy, is used primarily to treat small, single tumors in children with unilateral, early-stage disease or if the disease returns after external beam radiation. It is also used in combination with chemotherapy if local eye treatments don't work. This technique, which uses radioactive iodine, cobalt, or ruthenium, can only be used on tumors that are of a certain size and distance from the area of central vision. Children who get radioactive plaque therapy are isolated for one to three days, depending on the actual dose of radiation that is administered. Parents and hospital staff can spend only short periods of time in the child's room. Pregnant women and children are not permitted to visit the child in isolation.

Chemotherapy

Chemotherapy is being used with increased frequency to treat some children with retinoblastoma. Until recently, chemotherapy was used only to treat retinoblastoma that had spread outside the eye. Now, in order to prevent the long-term problems that can occur after enucleation or radiation, more doctors are using chemotherapy to treat retinoblastoma in the eye. The decision to use chemotherapy is complex and depends on a number of factors, including your child's age, the number, size and location of tumors, ability of the ophthalmologist to use local treatments, family history, and other medical problems. It is almost always given together with local eye treatments, so it may require visits as often as every three weeks. Chemotherapy works better for lower stage tumors and for tumors without seeding.

Usually chemotherapy is used to destroy the tumor. In retinoblastoma, it is used to shrink the tumor and help prevent new ones from growing. This is called chemoreduction therapy.

The chemotherapy drugs that are most commonly used in retinoblastoma are vincristine, carboplatin, and etoposide. Cyclosporine A is also used in some centers. For more information on these drugs, see Chapter 15, *Chemotherapy*. All of these chemotherapy protocols are being done in clinical trials to evaluate their effectiveness in treating retinoblastoma (see Chapter 5).

Newest treatment options

To learn about the standard treatment for your child's illness, call (800) 4-CANCER and ask for the PDQ (physician's data query) for retinoblastoma. This free statement explains the disease, state-of-the-art treatments, and ongoing clinical trials. Two versions are available: one for patients, which uses simple language and contains no statistics, and one for health professionals, which is technical, thorough, and includes citations to scientific literature. The PDQ can also be read on the Internet at *http://cancernet.nci.nih.gov/*.

I am a long-term survivor of bilateral retinoblastoma. I think that parents can be very instrumental in their child's recovery. Even though it may not be easy, I feel that it is important to be strong and positive. Seek all of the information possible, and don't hesitate to ask questions. Times will be tough, so please find support, whether it be family counseling focusing on cancer or corresponding with other parents who have had similar experiences. Don't hold all of your feelings in. Have the same expectations for your child with retinoblastoma as you would for any other. Don't set limitations for your child, there are already plenty of those out there.

Although I am blind, when I was a child I tap danced, rode horses, and I was a competitive roller skater. Now I ride in mountain bike competitions. I attend college full-time and have many good friends. I have matured into a woman with strong character, spirit, and motivation, and this has helped me overcome many challenges.

CHAPTER 14

Sources of Support

The effort to "put up a front" is draining,
isolating, and counterproductive.

—David Spiegel, MD
Living Beyond Limits

THE DIAGNOSIS OF CANCER can be a frightening and isolating experience. Every parent of a child with cancer has a story to tell of lost or strained friendships. Yet we are social creatures, reliant on a web of support from family, friends, neighbors, and church. We need the presence of people who not only care for us, but try hard to understand what we are feeling. Many parents experience deep loneliness after the first rush of visits, cards, and phone calls end, when the rest of the world goes back to normal life.

Members of families struck by childhood cancer—parents, the child with cancer, and siblings—are turning increasingly to support groups and various other methods of psychological help. Families join support groups to dispel isolation, share suggestions for dealing with the illness and its side effects, and talk to others who are living through the same crisis. Individual and family counseling can help address shifting responsibilities within the family, explore methods to improve communication, and help find ways to channel strong feelings constructively.

The various methods of support described in this chapter can help return to families a sense of control over their lives as well as provide a setting for making wonderful new friends.

Hospital social workers

While the need for skilled pediatric social workers is widely recognized, shrinking hospital budgets often prevent adequate staffing. If you bring your child to a children's hospital well-staffed with social workers, child life specialists, and psychologists, consider yourself lucky. Sadly, millions of dollars are spent on technology, while programs which help people cope emotionally are often the first to be discarded. If your pediatric center offers no support, explore the other methods described later in the chapter to get help in dealing with the pain of childhood cancer.

Pediatric social workers usually have a master's degree in social work, with additional training in oncology and pediatrics. They serve as guides through unfamiliar territory by mediating between doctors and families, helping with emotional or financial problems, locating resources, and easing the young patient back into school. Many social workers form close, long-lasting bonds with families, and continue to answer questions and provide support long after treatment ends.

> Over the course of my son's treatment, I became very close to the hospital's social worker. I came to see her as not only a person who was very good at her job and providing me with wonderful support, but also as a friend. She was very much "in tune" with my personality, and seemed to sense when I was having a rough day, even if I had been doing my best to hide it. So many times she would stop by my son's room and invite me to join her for coffee in the cafeteria, her treat. And we would sit and talk about anything and everything. She seemed to have a natural talent for making me laugh when I really needed to most. And she never expressed discomfort when I needed to cry or curse the unfairness of the situation we were in. She was a very good listener.

· · · · ·

> We went to a children's hospital which was renowned in the pediatric cancer field. The medical treatment was excellent, but psychosocial support was nonexistent. The day after diagnosis, we were interviewed for twenty minutes by a psychiatric resident, and that was it. I never met a social worker, and the physicians were so busy, they never asked anything other than medical questions. If I started crying, they usually left the room. I didn't know Candlelighters existed; I didn't know that there was a local support group; I didn't know that there was a summer camp for the kids. I felt totally isolated.

In addition to social workers, some hospitals have on-staff child life specialists, psychiatric nurses, psychiatrists, psychiatric residents, and psychologists who can help deal with problems while your child is an inpatient.

After I relapsed, I had a hard time with nausea, so I went to learn
self-hypnosis. The doctor who taught the hypnosis also counseled me, and
that was very helpful. He was somebody that I could relate to and talk to
about what was going on. Talking about how I felt about having cancer,
and how that affected my life, was very helpful to me.

Support groups for parents

Support groups offer a special perspective for all parents of children with
cancer, as well as fill the void left by the withdrawal or misunderstanding of
family and friends. Parents in similar circumstances can share practical information learned through personal experience, provide emotional support,
give hope for the future, and truly listen. The Seattle Candlelighters sum up
their beliefs in the following statement:

> *We believe children with cancer are normal children with special*
> *needs. We believe a unique bond exists among families who are experi-*
> *encing childhood cancer that allows for friendship and support through*
> *treatment, the uncertainties of daily life, the grief, and the triumphs. We*
> *believe in enjoying every day to its fullest and in providing a loving envi-*
> *ronment to all families facing childhood cancer.*

Coping with life-threatening illness requires perspective—the ability to
accept the gravity of the situation while not blowing it out of proportion.
Many families find this frame of reference in support groups, where there are
always those with more severe problems than theirs, as well as families
whose children have completed treatment and are thriving. Just meeting
people who have lived through the same situation is profoundly reassuring.

> *The group was a real lifeline for us, especially when Justin was so*
> *sick. We looked forward to the meetings and were there for every one. It*
> *was a real escape; it was a place to go where people were rooting for us.*
> *People from the group would always swing by to see us whenever they*
> *were bringing their own kids in for treatment. They always stopped by to*
> *visit and chat. We amassed a tremendous library of children's books that*
> *the group members would drop off. The support was wonderful. But it*
> *came from the people more than it came from the group experience itself.*

· · · · ·

> *I felt like I was always putting up a front for my family and friends. I*
> *acted like I was strong and in control. This act was draining and counter-*

productive. With the other parents, though, I really felt free to laugh as well as cry. I felt like I could tell them how bad things were without causing them any pain. I just couldn't do that with my family. If I told them what was really going on, they just looked stricken, because they didn't know what to do. But the other parents did.

Many people find comfort in formal support groups, while others get support from informal groups, such as those in Ronald McDonald Houses. Cancer can be a very isolating experience. The issues of all the other moms on the street are light years away from the mother of a kid with cancer. But the moms in the kitchen at Ronald McDonald can just look at a child on prednisone wolfing down a complete second dinner, and tell the new mom how fast the appetite goes when the prednisone is tapered. They understand each other's feelings and emotions because they are sharing the same experience. The understanding of a mother or father of a child with cancer cuts across all social, economic, and racial barriers.

My two-year-old daughter was diagnosed one week after I gave birth to a new baby girl. I remember early in her treatment, I was sitting with Gina on my lap, and my husband sat next to me, holding the new baby. The doctor breezed in and said in a cheerful voice, "How are you feeling?" I burst into sobs and could not stop. He said just a minute and dashed out. A few minutes later a woman came in with her eight-year-old daughter who had finished treatment and looked great. She put her arms around me and talked to me. She told me that everyone feels horrible in the beginning, and it might be hard to believe, but treatment would soon become a way of life for us. She was a great comfort, and of course, she was right.

In addition to Candlelighters—the international support organization—there are dozens of different types of support groups ranging from those with hundreds of members and formal bylaws to three moms who meet for coffee once a week. Some groups deal with only the emotional aspects of the disease while others may focus on education, advocacy, social opportunities, or crisis intervention. Some groups are facilitated by trained mental health practitioners while others are self-help groups of parents only. And, naturally, as older members drop out and new families join, the needs and interests of the group may shift. Several of these groups are listed in Appendix C, *Resource Organizations*.

Our group is very informal. We do have two social workers who are considered the facilitators, and are there as resource persons. We just talk about whatever anyone wants to discuss. Occasionally we have invited speakers in. I remember having a psychiatrist discuss stress management, and we also had a talk on therapeutic massage. We have formed close friendships from the group, and we still go twice a month even though our daughter is a year off treatment and doing great. I think our presence comforts the new families.

Parents from small, isolated communities may have a difficult time finding a support group in their area that fits their needs. For those families, finding emotional support is possible via their computer. Several online discussion groups exist for families dealing with childhood cancer. These groups provide parents with the understanding that only another parent of a child with cancer can give. Topics might include various coping skills that have been effective for families, or other helpful medical information that you can use in your fight against childhood cancer. Participants in on-line discussion groups, just like those in face-to-face groups, may provide incorrect or upsetting information. Take any concerns or questions you have to your physician or nurse practitioner.

The support that I have gained through online discussion groups is priceless. I have received a great deal of comfort from my participation in these groups. They have enabled me to connect with families from all over the world, many of which are fighting the exact same disease. I have often come to my computer in the middle of the night, when everyone else in the house is asleep. I can express my fears at 3 a.m., and know that someone will always be there to hold my hand and reassure me with the knowledge that they have felt these things, too. That's one of the most beautiful things about these groups. Someone is always there, even in the middle of the night.

• • • • •

Going online enabled me to find answers to many questions. I spent countless hours searching out hopeful stories about other kids who had been through what Leeann was dealing with, and walked away with more optimism. It didn't take me long to realize that I had to be choosy about what information I took to heart and what I should disregard. I found another mother who had posted to one of the groups with a daughter in the same circumstances as Leeann, and we began to write each other about their treatments, day to day lives, etc. We became very good friends and still write on a daily basis four years later. She's always picked me up when I've gone into a panic and her sense of humor and experience grounds me. We've never met in person even though we only live two states apart, but getting input from her means the world to me.

These groups are not intended to replace the support system you may have available in your area, but they may be beneficial to you. Use Appendix D, *Books and Online Sites*, and look under "Emotional support" for further information on Internet support groups.

In person-to-person support groups, or those online, you need to exercise caution. If the information given sounds different from what you have been told or if it is distressing to you, you should discuss these issues with your child's doctor and/or social worker for clarification.

Support groups for children with cancer

Many pediatric hospitals also have ongoing support groups for children with cancer. Often these are run by experienced pediatric social workers, who know how to balance fun with sharing feelings. For many children, these groups are the only place where they feel completely accepted, where most of the other kids are bald and have to take lots of medicine. The group is a place where children or adolescents can say how they really feel, without worrying that they are causing their parents more pain. Many children form wonderful and lasting friendships in peer groups.

> *All four of my kids have been going to the support groups for over seven years now. We have one group for the kids with cancer which is run by a social worker. The sibs group is run by a woman who specializes in early childhood development. Both groups do a lot of art therapy, relaxation therapy, playing, and talking. They meet twice a month, and I will continue to take them until they ask to stop. I think it has really helped all of them. We also have two teen nights out a year. All of the teenagers with cancer get together for an activity such as watching a hockey game or basketball game, or going bowling, to the movies, or out for pizza. They also see each other at our local camp for children surviving cancer (Camp Watcha-Wanna-Do) each year.*

For children who are too ill or shy to join a group, there are alternatives. There are hundreds of kids who use computers to contact and chat with other kids in similar situations. Use Appendix D to access some of the available computer groups.

Support groups for siblings

Many hospitals have responded to the growing awareness of siblings' natural concerns and worries by creating hospital visiting days for them. This allows not only one-on-one parent time for the siblings, but gives them the opportunity to explore and become familiar with the hospital environment. Sibling days allow interaction with staff, a time to have questions answered and concerns addressed. Some hospital staffs have expanded these one-day programs into ongoing support groups aimed not just at siblings who are having problems, but also at improving communication, education, and support for all siblings.

> *Annie went to Club Goodtimes long after her brother stopped going and attended camp as many years as they would allow. She intends to be on the staff at camp next summer.*

Parent-to-parent programs

Some pediatric hospitals, in conjunction with parent support groups such as Candlelighters, have developed parent-to-parent visitation programs. The purpose of these visits is for veteran parents to provide one-on-one support for newly diagnosed families. The services provided by the veteran parent can be informational, emotional, or logistical. The visiting parent can also:

- Empathize with the newly diagnosed parents.
- Help notify family and friends.
- Help overcome loneliness.
- Ease feelings of isolation.
- Provide hospital tours.
- Write down parents' questions for the medical team.
- Advise on sources of financial aid.
- Explain unfamiliar medical terms.

- Be available by phone for any problems that arise.

- Supply lots of smiles and hugs, but most of all, hope.

Newly diagnosed families can ask if the hospital has a parent-to-parent program. If not, ask to speak to the parent leader of the local support group. Often, this person will ask a veteran parent to visit you at the hospital. Many, many veteran parents are more than willing to visit, as they know only too well what those first weeks in the hospital are like. They are often accompanied by their child who has completed therapy, rosy-cheeked and full of energy—a living beacon of hope.

> *I am the parent consultant for our region. Among the services I provide are: meet with all newly diagnosed families; give a packet of info to each child or teen with cancer; continue to visit the families whenever they return to the hospital; educate families about the various local resources; provide moral support; stay with children during painful procedures if the parents can't; organize and present all the school programs; liaise with schools for school re-entry; organize and send out monthly reminders for meetings; send out birthday cards to kids on treatment; serve as activities director at the summer camp; and generally try to help out each new family in any way possible.*

For step-by-step suggestions on how to create, organize, recruit volunteers, and work with the hospital to create a parent-to-parent visitation program, obtain the booklet *Making Contact* from Candlelighters (see Appendix C).

Clergy

Religion is a source of strength for many people. Many parents and children find that their faith is strengthened by the cancer ordeal, while some begin to question their beliefs. Others, who have not relied on religion in the past, turn to it now.

Most hospitals have staff chaplains who are available for counseling, religious services, prayer, and other types of spiritual guidance. Often, the chaplain visits families soon after diagnosis and is available on an on-call basis. As with any mental health encounter, approaches that work well for one family may not be helpful to others.

> *When Shawn was first diagnosed, Father Ron came in, and we all just really bonded with him. Shawn was in the hospital most of the first year, so we had a chance to become very close. Often Shawn would ask*

for Father Ron before he had to have a painful procedure. Father Ron would talk to him, give him a little stuffed animal and a big hug, and then Shawn would feel fine.

When Shawn was very ill, I began to worry about the fact that he had never been baptized, and I asked Father Ron to baptize him in the chapel. We ended up going to his own little church nearby, and we had a private service with just godparents and family because Shawn's counts were so low. It was a wonderful, special service; I'll never forget it.

· · · · ·

When our son was first diagnosed, we didn't feel as if we could discuss any of our fears with the hospital chaplain. I believe it was simply because our personalities didn't "click" well together, and we would feel more uncomfortable than anything else whenever he would visit. Several months into treatment, the hospital had a new chaplain, and we hit it off immediately. It was a joy to see him walking down the hall toward my son's room. He seemed to have a natural gift for making me feel better, even when things seemed to be crumbling around me.

Parents who were members of a church, synagogue, or mosque prior to the diagnosis of their child's cancer often derive great comfort from the clergy and members of their home church. Members of the congregation may rally around the family, providing meals, babysitting, prayers, and support. Regular visits from the priest, minister, or rabbi provide spiritual sustenance throughout the initial crisis and subsequent months of treatment.

We belong to a Bible study group that has met weekly for eight years. In our group during that time there have been three cancer diagnoses and one of multiple sclerosis. We have all become an incredibly supportive family, and we share the burdens. I cannot begin to list the many wonderful things these people have done for us. They consistently put their lives on hold to help. They fill the freezer, clean the house, support us financially, parent our children. They do the laundry covered with vomit. They quietly appear, help, then disappear. I can call any one of them at 3 a.m. in the depths of despair and find comfort.

Individual and family counseling

Cancer is a crisis of major proportions for even the strongest of families. Parents do not need to face this crisis alone and unassisted. Many find it helpful to seek out sensitive, objective mental health care professionals to explore the difficult feelings—fear, anger, depression, anxiety, resentment, and guilt—that cancer arouses. Family responsibilities and authority undergo profound changes when a child is diagnosed with cancer. Sometimes members of the family have difficulty adjusting to the changes. While some families discuss the uncomfortable changes and feelings openly and agree on how to proceed, many need help.

Seeking professional counseling is a sign of strength, not failure. In dealing with children with cancer, problems often become too complex for families to deal with on their own. Seeking advice sends children a message that the parents care about what is happening to them and want to face it together.

One of the first questions that arises is, "Who should we talk to?" There are a number of resource people in the community who can make referrals and valuable recommendations, including:

- Pediatrician
- Oncologist
- Nurse practitioner
- Clinic social worker
- School psychologist or counselor
- Health department social worker
- Other parents who have sought counseling

Ask each of the above for a short list of highly regarded mental health care professionals who have experience working with your issues (for example, traumatized children, marital problems, stress reduction, or family therapy). Generally, the names of the most well-respected clinicians in the community will appear on several of the lists.

> *The cancer experience put an enormous strain on our marriage. My wife has always been easy to excite, whereas I've always been very "laid back." There were moments when I was afraid that it would completely fall apart. We managed to survive, and I think in many ways, it has even brought us closer together.*

In making your decision, it helps to understand the different levels of training and education of the various types of mental health care professionals. You will be able to choose from individuals trained in one of these fields:

- Psychology (EdD, MA, PhD, PsyD). Marriage and family psychotherapists have a master's degree, clinical and research psychologists have a doctorate (in some states, the use of the title "psychologist" may also be allowed for those with only a master's degree.)

- Social work (MSW, DSW, PhD). Clinical social workers have either a master's degree or a doctorate in a clinically emphasized program.

- Pastoral Care (MA, MDiv, DMin, PhD, DDiv). Some laymen and members of the clergy have received specialized training in counseling.

- Medicine (MD, RN). Psychiatrists are medical doctors (and only they are able to prescribe medications). In addition, some nurses obtain postgraduate training in psychotherapy.

The designations LCSW (Licensed Clinical Social Worker), LSW (Licensed Social Worker), LMFCC (Licensed Marriage and Family Child Counselor), LPC (Licensed Professional Counselor), LMFT (Licensed Marriage and Family Therapist) refer to licensure by state professional boards, not academic degrees. These initials usually follow others that indicate an academic degree. If they don't, inquire about the therapist's academic training.

You may hear all of the above professionals referred to as counselors or therapists. Many jurisdictions require licensure or certification in order for professionals to practice independently; unlicensed professionals are allowed to practice only under the supervision of a licensed professional (typically as an intern or assistant in a clinic or licensed professional's private practice).

When seeking a good counselor, ask the professional how long she has been in practice. A licensed marriage and family therapist who has been seeing patients for ten years may be a much finer clinician for your needs than a licensed psychologist or psychiatrist in their first year of practice.

Another way to find a suitable counselor is to call The American Association for Marriage and Family Therapy, in Washington, DC, (202) 452-0109. This is a national professional organization of licensed/certified marriage and family therapists. It has more than 20,000 members in the U.S. and Canada, and its membership also includes licensed clinical social workers, pastoral counselors (who are MFCC/LMFTs), psychologists, and psychiatrists.

To find a therapist, a good first step is to call two or three therapists who appear on several of your lists of recommendations. During your telephone interview, the following are some suggested questions to ask:

- Are you accepting new clients?

- Do you charge for an initial consultation?

- What training and experience do you have working with ill or traumatized children?

- How many years have you been working with families?

- What is your approach to resolving the problems children develop from trauma? Do you use a brief or long-term approach?

- What evaluation and assessment procedures will be used to define the problem?

- How and when will treatment goals be set?

- How will both parents be involved in treatment?

- What are your fees? Will the insurance company be billed directly?

The next step should be to make an appointment with one or two of the therapists who you think might be able to best address your needs. Be honest about the fact that you are interviewing several therapists prior to making a decision. The purpose of the introductory meeting is to see if you feel comfortable with the therapist. After all, credentials do not guarantee that a given therapist will work for you. Compatibility, trust, and a feeling of genuine caring are essential. It is worth the effort to continue your search until you find a good match.

> I called several therapists out of desperation about my daughter's withdrawal and violent tantrums. I made appointments with two. The first I just didn't feel comfortable with at all, but the second felt like an old friend after one hour. I have been to see her dozens of times over the years, and she has always helped me. I wasn't interested in theory; I wanted practical suggestions of how to deal with the behavior problems. My four-year-old daughter asked why I was going to see the therapist, and I said that Hilda was a doctor, but instead of taking care of my body, she helped care for my feelings. She asked to go to the "feelings" doctor, but was concerned about whether her conversations would be private. I asked the counselor to explain about the limits of confidentiality. So that began a very helpful course of therapy for my very traumatized daughter. To this day I don't know what was said, nor would I ever ask my daughter or Hilda. I do know that they did a lot of art therapy, and I know that it helped immensely.

· · · · ·

We went into family therapy because every member of my family experienced misdirected anger. When they were angry they aimed it at me—the nice person who took care of them and loved them no matter what. But I was dissolving. I needed to learn to say "ouch," and they needed to learn other ways to handle their angry feelings.

Children need to be prepared for psychological intervention as for any unknown procedure. The following are several parents' suggestions on how to prepare your child:

- Explain who the therapist is, and what you hope to accomplish. For instance, you might be taking the whole family to improve communication or resolve conflicts. If you are bringing your child in for therapy, explain why you think talking to an objective person might benefit him.

- Older children should be involved in the process of choosing a counselor. Younger children's likes and dislikes should be respected. If your young child does not get along well with one counselor, change.

- Make the experience positive rather than threatening.

- Reassure young children that the visit is for talking, drawing, or playing games, not for anything that is physically painful.

- Ask the therapist to explain the rules of confidentiality to both you and your child. Do not quiz your child after a visit to the therapist.

David had a very difficult time dealing with his brother's cancer. Realizing that we were unable to provide him with the help that he needed, we sought professional help for him. I think the reason that he feels so comfortable with his therapist is that he is aware of the rules of confidentiality. After his sessions, I'll always ask him how it went. Sometimes he'll just grin and say that it was fine, and other times he might share a little of his conversation with me. I never push or question him about it. If it is something he needs to discuss, I wait until he decides to broach the subject.

- Make sure that your child does not think that she is being punished; instead assure her that therapists help both adults and children understand and deal with feelings.

- Go yourself for counseling or to support group meetings to model the fact that all ages and types of people need help from time to time.

In the beginning of treatment, my son had terrible problems with going to sleep and then having nightmares, primarily about snakes. We took him to a counselor, who worked with him for several weeks and completely resolved the problem. The counselor had him befriend the snake, talk to it, and explain that it was keeping him awake. He would tell the snake, "I want you to stop bothering me because I need to go to sleep." The snake never returned.

In *Armfuls of Time*, Barbara Sourkes quotes Jonathan, a boy with cancer, who told her, "Thank you for giving me aliveness." She discusses the importance of psychotherapy for the child with a life-threatening illness:

Even when life itself cannot be guaranteed, psychotherapy can at least "give aliveness" to the child for however long that life may last. Through the extraordinary challenges posed by life-threatening illness, a precocious inner wisdom of life and its fragility emerges. Yet even in the struggle for survival, the spirit of childhood shines through.

Camps

Summer camps for children with cancer, and often their siblings as well, are becoming increasingly popular. These camps provide an opportunity for children with cancer and their siblings to have fun, meet friends, and talk with others in the same situation. Counselors are typically volunteers, many of whom are cancer survivors or their siblings. Sometimes oncology nurses, residents, social workers, and child life specialists are camp counselors. Supervised by experts, children can have their concerns addressed without involving their parents. These camps provide a carefree time away from the sadness of the family or the all too frequent hospital visits.

Of all the ways to get support, I think the camp really helps the most. You are all there together for enough time to break down the barriers. Although camp does not focus on cancer, many times we really got down to talking about how we really felt. I have been a counselor at the camp for eight summers now. Most of the campers know that I relapsed three times and I'm doing great many years later. They see the many other long-term survivors who are counselors, and it gives them what they need the most—hope. The best support is meeting survivors, because nobody else truly understands.

We are one family
  you and I—
Not by birth or legal joining
Not by choice, and definitely not by desire
    But by a commonality given to us by the unseen
        Seeking peace with uncertainty
            Needing the support of another
                who has known.

We are one family
  you and I—
We fight the beast hungry for our child
    and battle for their lives
Striving to plan for tomorrow
    explaining, educating, researching
Assertiveness and occasional aggression
To fight with
    and for
        Our child.

We are one family
  you and I—
With the same questions and fears
    Why my child? Did I do something to cause this horror?
    Am I weak because I still cry?
Will the beast return? When?
    Am I missing an early sign?
What late effects of this battle will we see?
    How do we deal with them? Where do we get help?
What about my other children?
    Will the beast find them too?

We are one family
  you and I—
We share a bond that we wish did not exist
    and yet since it does exist
        we are glad it is there
We gather strength
    and rejoice in today
We accept the tears, acknowledge the fears

love and are loved
We walk the road together
 not knowing where it leads
  on our common journey we are not alone,
   Thus we are blessed.

We are one family
 you and I—
Not by birth or legal joining
Not by choice, and definitely not by desire
 But by a commonality given to us by the unseen
  Seeking peace with uncertainty
   Needing the support of another
    who has known.

—Mary Riecke

CHAPTER 15

Chemotherapy

In the depths of winter I finally learned there
was in me an invincible summer.

—Albert Camus

THE WORD CHEMOTHERAPY is derived from a combination of "chemical" and "treatment." It means using drugs, singly or in combination, to destroy or disrupt the growth of cancer cells without permanently damaging normal cells.

This chapter describes the most common drugs that are used to kill cancer cells as well as drugs that prevent nausea and pain. Numerous stories are included that show the range of responses to different chemotherapy drugs.

Reading about potential side effects of chemotherapy can be disturbing. However, it is important to be aware of the possibilities in order to recognize symptoms early and report them to the doctor so that swift action can be taken to make your child more comfortable. On rare occasions, side effects may be life-threatening and some can persist throughout life. However, most are merely unpleasant and subside soon after treatment ends. Remember that your child or teen may experience several, a few, or none of the side effects discussed here.

How chemotherapy drugs kill cancer cells

Normal, healthy cells divide and grow in a well-established pattern. When normal cells divide, an identical copy is produced. The body makes only the number of normal cells that it needs at any given time.

Cancer cells, on the other hand, reproduce uncontrollably and grow in an unpredictable way. They invade surrounding tissue and can travel in the blood or lymphatic system to lodge in other parts of the body.

There are several groups of chemotherapy drugs that act on cancer cells in very different ways:

- **Alkylating agents.** All cells use building blocks (DNA and RNA) to make exact copies of themselves. Alkylating agents poison cancer cells by interacting with DNA to prevent cell reproduction.

- **Antimetabolites.** These drugs starve cancer cells by replacing essential cell nutrients.

- **Antibiotics.** This type of drug prevents cell growth by blocking reproduction.

- **Alkaloids.** These drugs, derived from plants, interrupt cell division.

- **Hormones.** These drugs create a hostile environment that slows cell growth.

- **Enzymes.** These interfere with cancer cells' ability to reproduce.

How chemotherapy drugs are given

The most common ways drugs are given during treatment for cancer are:

- **Intravenous (IV).** Medicine is delivered directly into the bloodstream via a right atrial catheter or IV needle in the arm or hand.

- **Oral (PO).** Drugs taken by mouth in liquid, capsule, or tablet form, are absorbed into the blood through the lining of the stomach and intestines.

- **Intramuscular (IM).** Drugs that need to seep slowly into the bloodstream are injected into a large muscle such as the thigh or buttocks.

- **Intrathecal (IT).** Doctors perform a spinal tap and inject the drug directly into the cerebrospinal fluid (the fluid surrounding the brain and spinal cord), circumventing the barrier between the blood and brain.

- **Intraperitoneal (IP).** Drugs are delivered directly into the abdominal cavity.

- **Intracavitary.** Drugs are delivered directly into a body cavity through a catheter.

- **Arterial perfusion.** Blood is removed from the child and chemotherapy drugs are added. The blood is then returned through a major artery in the area that is being treated. Sometimes chemotherapy is delivered via an arterial catheter.

Dosages

Dosages vary among protocols; however, most are based on your child's weight or body surface area (BSA). BSA is calculated from your child's weight and height and is measured in meters squared (m²).

> My son's protocol required that his height and weight be measured each time chemotherapy was to start. When we would arrive in clinic, the nurses would take his measurements, then calculate his body surface area using those figures. His weight fluctuated considerably over the course of his treatment, so the actual dosage of the drugs that he received was never quite the same.

Chemotherapy drugs and their possible side effects

The following drug information contains not only common and infrequent side effects, but also parent and survivor experiences and suggestions. You may be overwhelmed by reading the potential side effects of each drug. Please remember, each child is unique and will handle most drugs without any problems. Most side effects are unpleasant, not serious, and subside when the medication stops. Parent experiences are included to alert new parents to possibilities and provide comfort and suggestions should their child have an unusual side effect. Consult your child's pediatrician or oncologist should any concerns arise from the following information. Remember to keep all chemotherapy drugs in a locked cabinet away from children and pets.

> The chemotherapy made Rachel's tastes change, so we adapted to what she liked or would eat. She lived on bland or very salty foods, like pickles and bacon. Basically, we gave her whatever she wanted, whenever she wanted.

Questions to ask the doctor

Prior to giving your child any drug, you should be given basic information including answers to the following:

- What is the dosage? How many times a day should it be given?
- What are the common, and the rare but serious, side effects?

- What should I do if my child experiences any of the side effects?
- Will the drug interact with any over-the-counter drugs (e.g., Tylenol) or vitamins?
- Will my teen be given detailed counseling on avoiding risks such as drinking alcohol, smoking cigarettes or marijuana, and pregnancy?
- What should I do if I forget to give my child a dose?
- What are both the trade and generic names of the drug?
- Should I buy the generic version?

Guidelines for calling the doctor

Sometimes parents are reluctant to call their child's physician with questions or concerns. Here are general guidelines for when calling is necessary:

- Temperature above 101°F (38.5°C)
- Shaking or chills
- Shortness of breath
- Severe nausea or vomiting
- Unusual bleeding, bruising, or cuts that won't heal
- Pain or swelling at chemotherapy injection site
- Exposure to chicken pox or measles
- Severe headache or blurred vision
- Constipation lasting more than two days
- Severe diarrhea
- Painful urination or bowel movements
- Blood in urine
- Whenever child appears sick and parent is concerned

Chemotherapy drug list

Drugs used for chemotherapy are known by a variety of names. You may hear the same drug referred to by its generic name, abbreviation, or one of several brand names, depending on which doctor, nurse, or pharmacist you are talking to. The list below gives various names of chemotherapy drugs, and what name to look under in this chapter:

Name	Look Under
Adriamycin	Doxorubicin
Alkeran	Melphalan
ARA-C	Cytarabine
Blenoxane	Bleomycin
Camptosar	Irinotecan
Carboplatin	Carboplatin
Cerubidine	Daunorubicin
Cosmegen	Dactinomycin
Cyclophosphamide	Cyclophosphamide
Cytarabine	Cytarabine
Cytoxan	Cyclophosphamide
Cytosar	Cytarabine
Cytosine arabinoside	Cytarabine
Daunomycin	Daunorubicin
Daunorubicin	Daunorubicin
DTIC-Dome	Dacarbazine
Doxorubicin	Doxorubicin
Droxia	Hydroxyurea
Etoposide	Etoposide
Hycamtin	Topotecan
Hydroxyurea	Hydroxyurea
Idamycin	Idarubicin
Ifex	Ifosfamide
Ifosfamide	Ifosfamide
Methotrex	Methotrexate
Methotrexate	Methotrexate
MTX	Methotrexate
Myleran	Busulfan
Oncovin	Vincristine
Paraplatin	Carboplatin
Platinol	Cisplatin
Thiotepa	Thiotepa
Velban	Vinblastine

Name	Look Under
VePesid	Etoposide
VCR	Vincristine
Vinblastine	Vinblastine
Vincristine	Vincristine
VP-16	Etoposide
5-FU	5-Fluorouracil

Bleomycin (Blee-oh-MY-sin)

Also called: Blenoxane, BLM

How given: Intramuscular (IM), subcutaneous (SQ), intravenous (IV), intracavitary

How it works: Bleomycin binds with DNA in order to stop cell growth.

Precaution: A small percentage of children may be allergic to this drug. Lung function tests are used to detect possible lung toxicity.

Common side effects:

Hair loss (alopecia)
Mouth sores (stomatitis)
Nausea and vomiting
Weight loss
Darkening of skin
Rash
Thickening of skin of palms and fingers
Fever (after first dose)
Loss of appetite (anorexia)

Infrequent side effects:

Lung toxicity (potentially permanent)
Allergic reactions
Joint swelling

Busulfan (Byoo-SUL-fan)

Also called: Myleran, busulphan

How given: Pills by mouth (PO)

How it works: Busulfan is an alkylating agent that interferes with DNA to prevent cell division.

Precaution: The child should have lung function tests for early detection of possible toxicities.

Common side effects:

    Low blood counts (myelosuppression)
    Darkening of the skin
    Diarrhea
    Abdominal pain
    Fever
    Weakness
    Loss of appetite (anorexia)
    Dry mouth
    Mouth sores (stomatitis)
    Gout

Infrequent side effects:

    Lung toxicity
    Cataracts (when used over long periods of time)
    Seizures
    Nausea and vomiting

Carboplatin (CAR-bo-plat-un)

Also called: Paraplatin

How given: Intravenous (IV)

How it works: Carboplatin is a platinating agent that inhibits DNA replication, RNA transcription, and protein synthesis.

Precaution: The child should be given extra fluids to prevent possible kidney toxicity.

Common side effects:

    Low blood counts (myelosuppression)
    Nausea and vomiting
    Loss of appetite (anorexia)

Altered taste

Infrequent side effects:

Tinnitus (ringing in the ears)
Hearing loss
Diarrhea
Constipation
Mouth sores (stomatitis)
Hair loss (alopecia)
Peripheral neuropathy (numbing or tingling in fingers or toes)
Kidney toxicity

Cisplatin (sis-PLAT-un)

Also called: CDDP, cisplatinum, Platinol

How given: Intravenous (IV), intra-arterial

How it works: Cisplatin is a platinating agent that inhibits DNA replication, RNA transcription, and protein synthesis.

Precaution: The child should drink lots of water or be given large amounts of IV fluids while receiving cisplatin to prevent damage to the kidneys. A diuretic drug, called Mannitol, may also given to decrease the risk of kidney damage. The child should be monitored for possible hearing loss.

Common side effects:

Nausea and vomiting
Low blood counts (myelosuppression)
Loss of appetite (anorexia)
Loss of taste
Hearing loss
Tinnitus (ringing in the ears)
Mineral imbalance
Gout
Kidney toxicity

Infrequent side effects:

Central nervous system toxicity
Hypotension (low blood pressure)

Tachycardia (fast heart rate)

Color blindness

Muscle weakness

Poor coordination

Liver toxicity

Missy's protocol for neuroblastoma required her to have both cisplatin as well as carboplatin (for her stem cell transplant). Both of these drugs, over the course of her treatment, damaged her high-pitch frequency hearing so much that her speech development took a turn for the worse. She needed hearing aids to help correct the problem.

Cyclophosphamide (Sye-kloe-FOSS-fa-mide)

Also called: Cytoxan

How given: Pills by mouth (PO), intravenous (IV)

How it works: Cyclophosphamide is an alkylating agent that disrupts DNA in cancer cells, preventing reproduction.

Precaution: The child should drink lots of water or be given large amounts of IV fluids while taking cyclophosphamide to prevent damage to the bladder. Mesna is given as a precaution to prevent bladder irritation. Antinausea drugs should be given before and for several hours after this drug is administered.

Common side effects:

Low blood cell counts (myelosuppression)

Nausea and vomiting

Loss of appetite (anorexia)

Mouth sores (stomatitis)

Diarrhea

Hair loss (alopecia)

Infrequent side effects:

Hemorrhagic cystitis causing blood in the urine

Abdominal pain and diarrhea

Cough or dyspnea (shortness of breath)

Dizziness and difficulty walking

Skin rash and itching

Menstrual periods in teenage girls may temporarily stop

Sterility (rare even for children who receive high doses)

Secondary leukemia

Christine breezed through the Cytoxan infusions. She would go to Children's in the afternoon, they would give her lots of IV fluids, and then ondansetron a half hour before the Cytoxan. She would sleep through the night with absolutely no nausea because they were so good about giving her the ondansetron all night and the next morning. It was harder on me because I had to wake up every two hours to change her diaper so that the nurse could weigh it to make sure she was passing enough urine.

• • • • •

Preston took cyclophosphamide in pill form, and it made him very ill. He even started to try to hide the pills. I tried to make him drink lots of water. He knew it was important, but it was very difficult.

Cytarabine (Sye-TARE-a-been)

Also called: ARA-C, Cytosar, cytosine arabinoside

How given: Intravenous (IV), intrathecal (IT), subcutaneous (SQ)

How it works: Cytarabine kills cancer cells by disrupting DNA.

Common side effects:

Low blood counts (myelosuppression)

Nausea and vomiting

Diarrhea

Loss of appetite (anorexia)

Hair loss (alopecia)

Mouth sores (stomatitis)

Rash

Infrequent side effects:

Jaundice (yellow skin or eyes)

Joint and bone pain

Fever or chills

Pneumonia

Peripheral neuropathy (numbing or tingling in fingers, toes, or face)
Headache
Seizures
Temporary loss of balance

> *I told my daughter's oncologist how happy I was that she had not had any severe nausea after her first few doses of ARA-C. His only reply was, "It's cumulative." Within an hour, on the long drive home, she was vomiting constantly. We became ensnared in a two-hour traffic jam. She ran out of clean clothes, so for two hours, I repeatedly carried her to the side of the road, a naked, bald, 25-lb. four-year-old with tubing hanging from her chest, and supported her as she dry-heaved. The people in the cars around us were in tears, and kept asking if there was anything they could do to help. I just focused on comforting her, and getting her home to that vial of ondansetron in our fridge.*

Dacarbazine (Da-KAR-ba-zeen)

Also called: DTIC-Dome

How given: Intravenous (IV)

How it works: Dacarbazine is an alkylating agent that prevents cancer cell reproduction.

Precaution: The child should be given an antinausea drug prior to infusion. Dacarbazine causes severe skin reactions if it leaks outside the IV.

Common side effects:

Low blood counts (myelosuppression)
Nausea and vomiting
Hair loss (alopecia)
Photosensitivity (extreme sensitivity to the sun)
Loss of appetite (anorexia)
Mouth sores (stomatitis)
Diarrhea
Lightheadedness
Itching
Fatigue, aching, and low-grade fever

Liver dysfunction

Peripheral neuropathy (numbing or tingling in fingers or toes)

Dactinomycin (dack-tin-o-MY-sin)

Also called: Actinomycin D, Act D, Cosmegen

How given: Intravenous (IV)

How it works: Dactinomycin interferes with DNA and RNA.

Precaution: Severe skin reaction occurs with IV leakage.

Common side effects:

Nausea and vomiting

Hair loss (alopecia)

Low blood cell counts (myelosuppression)

Loss of appetite (anorexia)

Infrequent side effects:

mouth sores (stomatitis)

Diarrhea

Fever and chills

Rash

Difficulty in swallowing (dysphagia)

Temporary impairment of liver function (may be severe)

Daunorubicin (Daw-no-ROO-bi-sin)

Also called: Daunomycin, Cerubidine

How given: Intravenous (IV) or infusion over several days

How it works: Daunorubicin is an antibiotic which prevents DNA from forming, thus preventing cancer cells from multiplying.

Precaution: Daunorubicin is a red color, and may turn urine red for a day or two after each dose. This is normal.

Common side effects:

　　Low blood counts (myelosuppression)
　　Nausea and vomiting
　　Hair loss (alopecia)
　　Mouth sores (stomatitis)
　　Diarrhea

Infrequent side effects:

　　Burning pain and swelling if any drug leaks into skin
　　Heart damage
　　Shortness of breath (dyspnea)
　　Skin rash

> *My son didn't have any problems, but I sure worried about heart damage. I went to a conference and learned that the cut-off dose was below what he had on the protocol. I requested an echocardiogram, and his heart function was normal.*

Doxorubicin (Dox-o-ROO-bi-sin)

Also called: Adriamycin, Doxil, Rubex

How given: Intravenous (IV) or infusion

How it works: Doxorubicin is an antibiotic that prevents DNA from forming, thus preventing cancer cells from multiplying.

Precaution: Doxorubicin is a red color, and may turn urine red for a day or two after each dose. This is normal.

Common side effects:

　　Low blood cell counts (myelosuppression)
　　Nausea and vomiting
　　Hair loss (alopecia)
　　Mouth sores (stomatitis)

Infrequent side effects:

　　Loss of appetite (anorexia)
　　Diarrhea
　　Burning pain and swelling if any drug leaks into skin

Heart damage (at high doses)
Shortness of breath (dyspnea)
Fever and chills
Abdominal pains
Dark or bloody stools
Darkening or ridging of nails

The Adriamycin just burned right through my son. He never got mouth sores, but he sure had problems at the other end. They had him lie on his stomach with the heat lamp on his bare bottom. His whole bottom was blistered so badly that it looked like he'd been in a fire. They used to mix up what they called "Magic Butt Paste," and I'll never forget the recipe: one tube Nystatin cream, one tube Desitin, and Nystatin powder. It was like spackle that they would just slather on. He had a lot of gastrointestinal bleeding, too, so he was continuously getting platelets.

• • • • •

Other than red urine and the expected low counts, hair loss, and nausea, Christine had no problems from her many doses of Adriamycin.

Etoposide (E-TOE-poe-side)

Also called: VP-16, VePesid, Etopophos, Toposar

How given: Intravenous (IV), pills by mouth (PO)

How it works: Etoposide prevents DNA from reproducing, and also causes death of dividing cells.

Common side effects:

Low blood cell counts (myelosuppression)
Loss of appetite (anorexia)
Nausea and vomiting
Hair loss (alopecia)
Fatigue

Infrequent side effects:

Hypotension (low blood pressure)
Shortness of breath (dyspnea)
Difficulty in walking

Peripheral neuropathy (numbing or tingling in fingers or toes)

Fever or chills

Rash

Secondary cancers (new cancers that occur later in life)

5-Fluorouracil (5-Floor-ROAR-ah-sill)

Also called: 5-FU, Adrucil

How given: Intravenous (IV) and intracavitary

How it works: 5-Fluorouracil is an antimetabolite that prevents DNA synthesis and blocks RNA translation.

Precaution: The child should be monitored for possible liver toxicity.

Common side effects:

Nausea and vomiting

Mouth sores (stomatitis)

Diarrhea

Blurred vision

Darkening of the skin

Low blood cell counts (myelosuppression)

Infrequent side effects:

Hair loss (alopecia)

Brittle nails

Photosensitivity (extreme sensitivity to the sun)

Rash

Itching

Watery eyes

Soreness and redness of the soles of the feet and palms of the hands

Coley received several different chemotherapy drugs to treat her hepatoblastoma, including 5-FU. She lost a lot of weight and her hair fell out. She also had a lot of vomiting, but the antinausea drugs helped a great deal.

Hydroxyurea (Hi-DROX-ee-yoo-REE-ah)

Also called: Droxia

How given: Pills by mouth (PO)

How it works: Hydroxyurea has an action that is not well understood, but it is thought to work by stopping DNA production.

Common side effects:

> Low blood cell counts (myelosuppression)

Infrequent side effects:

> Nausea and vomiting
> Loss of appetite (anorexia)
> Fever and chills
> Rashes
> Drowsiness
> Diarrhea
> Convulsions
> Headache or dizziness
> Stomach pain
> Confusion or hallucinations

Idarubicin (Eye-dah-ROO-bah-sin)

Also called: Idamycin

How given: Intravenous (IV)

How it works: Idarubicin is an anthracycline that works to destroy cancer cells by changing the shape of their DNA.

Precaution: The child should have his heart tested prior to starting this drug, and after each course.

Common side effects:

> Low blood cell counts (myelosuppression)
> Nausea and vomiting
> Abdominal pain
> Diarrhea

Hair loss (alopecia)

Mouth sores (stomatitis)

Infrequent side effects:

Heart damage

Ifosfamide (Eye-FOSS-fah-mide)

Also called: Ifex, IFF

How given: Intravenous (IV)

How it works: Ifosfamide is an alkylating agent that disrupts DNA in cancer cells, preventing reproduction.

Precaution: The child should be given extra fluids by mouth or intravenously during infusion. Mesna, a drug that protects the bladder, should also be given.

Common side effects:

Hair loss (alopecia)

Low blood cell counts (myelosuppression)

Nausea and vomiting

Sleepiness or disorientation

Dizziness

Infrequent side effects:

Kidney toxicity

Lung scarring

Bladder irritation (hemorrhagic cystitis)

Liver toxicity

Swelling of feet or lower legs

Irinotecan (Eye-rin-oh-TEE-can)

Also called: Camptosar, CPT-11

How given: Intravenous (IV)

How it works: Irinotecan is a plant alkaloid that disrupts the structure of DNA, preventing cell reproduction.

Common side effects:

Loss of appetite (anorexia)
Low blood cell counts (myelosuppression)
Nausea and vomiting
Diarrhea
Abdominal cramping
Excessive sweating
Excessive salivation
Watery eyes
Hair loss (alopecia)
Tiredness and weakness

Infrequent side effects:

Mouth sores (stomatitis)
Muscle cramps
Temporarily impaired liver function
Rash
Itching

Melphalan (MEL-fa-lan)

Also called: Alkeran

How given: Pills by mouth (PO)

How it works: Melphalan is an alkylating agent that interferes with DNA, RNA, and nucleic acid function.

Precaution: The child should drink lots of water or be given large amounts of IV fluids while receiving Melphalan to prevent damage to the kidneys and the bladder.

Common side effects:

Low blood cell counts (myelosuppression)
Menstrual irregularities

Infrequent side effects:

Nausea and vomiting
Skin rashes

Shortness of breath (dyspnea)

Mouth sores (stomatitis)

Gout

Lung scarring

Methotrexate (Meth-o-TREX-ate)

Also called: Methotrex, MTX

How given: Pills by mouth (PO), intravenous (IV), intrathecal (IT)

How it works: Methotrexate is an antimetabolite which replaces nutrients in the cancer cell, causing cell death.

Precautions: Children should not be given extra folic acid in vitamins or the methotrexate will not be effective.

Common side effects:

Low blood cell counts (myelosuppression)

Photosensitivity (extreme sensitivity to the sun)

Diarrhea

Fatigue

Skin rashes

Headache, backache, spinal cord irritation (when given intrathecally)

Infrequent side effects:

Mouth sores (stomatitis)

Alopecia (hair loss)

Nausea and vomiting

Loss of appetite (anorexia)

Dry cough caused by lung damage

Chills and fever

Dizziness

Jaundice (yellow skin and eyes)

Shortness of breath (dyspnea)

Neurotoxicity (which can cause learning disabilities)

> *My son developed learning disabilities from his high-dose methotrexate protocol. He received tutoring through high school and is doing extremely well in college.*

My daughter had serious problems with rashes during treatment with methotrexate. The doctors thought that she had developed an allergy. She often would be covered with rashes which looked like small, red circles with tan, flaky skin inside. They were extremely itchy.

Thiotepa (Thigh-oh-TEE-pah)

Also called: Thioplex

How given: Intramuscular (IM), intrathecal (IT), intravenous (IV)

How it works: Thiotepa is an alkylating agent that disrupts DNA, inhibiting protein synthesis, causing cell death.

Precaution: The child should be encouraged to drink extra fluids to flush the bladder since thiotepa can irritate its lining. A small percentage of children have an allergic reaction to this drug.

Common side effects:

Low blood cell counts (myelosuppression)
Nausea and vomiting
Loss of appetite (anorexia)
Headache
Dizziness

Infrequent side effects:

Hair loss (alopecia)
Darkening of the skin
Allergic reaction
Bone marrow changes (after long-term use)
Soreness and redness of the soles of the feet and palms of the hands
Kidney toxicity

Topotecan (Toe-poe-TEE-can)

Also called: Hycamtin

How given: Intravenous (IV)

How it works: Topotecan is a derivative of a plant alkaloid and interferes with a cellular enzyme involved in maintaining the structure of DNA.

Precaution: Dose may need to be adjusted for those children with kidney damage.

Common side effects:

Low blood cell counts (myelosuppression)
Nausea and vomiting
Loss of appetite (anorexia)
Hair loss (alopecia)

Infrequent side effects:

Mouth sores (stomatitis)
Diarrhea

> Matthew tolerated the topotecan very well. He had the usual nausea and vomiting that he experienced with other chemotherapy drugs, though. He wouldn't eat much during the treatments, but within a day or two he was usually back to his old self again.

Vinblastine (vin-BLAS-teen)

Also called: VLB, Velban

How given: Intravenous (IV)

How it works: Vinblastine is an alkaloid derived from the periwinkle plant that causes cells to stop dividing.

Precaution: Care should be taken to prevent leakage of vinblastine from the IV site. The child may need to start on a program to prevent constipation.

Common side effects:

Low blood cell counts (myelosuppression))
Nausea and vomiting
Loss of appetite (anorexia)
Abdominal discomfort
Constipation
Pain and blisters if drug leaks into tissues

Infrequent side effects:

Hair loss (alopecia)
Mouth sores (stomatitis)

Diarrhea

Headaches

Pain at the tumor site

Peripheral neuropathy (numbing or tingling in fingers or toes)

Rash

Vincristine (Vin-CRIS-teen)

Also called: Oncovin, VCR

How given: Intravenous (IV)

How it works: Vincristine is an alkaloid derived from the periwinkle plant that causes cells to stop dividing.

Precaution: Care should be taken to prevent leakage of vincristine from IV site. The child may need to be started on a program to prevent constipation.

Common side effects:

Constipation

Pain in jaw, face, back, joints, bones (may be severe)

Foot drop (child has trouble lifting front part of foot)

Peripheral neuropathy (numbing or tingling in fingers or toes)

Extreme weakness and loss of muscle mass

Blurred or double vision, drooping eyelids

Hair loss (alopecia)

Pain and blisters if drug leaks into tissues

Infrequent side effects:

Loss of appetite (anorexia)

Nausea and vomiting

Weight loss

Headaches, dizziness, lightheadedness

Convulsions

Difficulty urinating (dysuria)

Rash

Difficulty sleeping

Itchiness

Erica (diagnosed at one year old) once had a vincristine burn on her arm at the IV site. It was red when we went home from the clinic, but by the second day it was badly burned. She developed a blister as big as a half dollar, which left a bad scar. It hurt and was sensitive for a long time. She also developed severe foot drop (she could not lift up the front part of her foot) and fell a lot. This went away when treatment ended.

· · · · ·

Stephan is a very tough boy who rarely complains, but he cries when he gets the vincristine because it gives him severe bone pain. I insisted that he get a strong pain killer, and we give him Tylenol with codeine when the pain starts. It usually only lasts a few days.

Colony-stimulating factors

Colony-stimulating factors play an important role in cancer therapy. High-dose chemotherapy reduces the number of white blood cells used by the body to fight infections. The administration of colony-stimulating factors, such as granulocyte colony-stimulating factor (G-CSF) and granulocyte-macrophage colony-stimulating factor (GM-CSF), can reduce the severity and duration of low white blood counts, reducing the chance of infection.

Kenny was only two years old when he was receiving G-CSF, so he was too young to understand why he needed the shots. He would cry and beg us not to hurt him, that he was sorry. My heart would break, but I would have to stick him. We finally developed a really good system. Right before being discharged after a round of chemo, we would put EMLA on Kenny's arm and then have the nurse place an insulflon. It was a small catheter that Kenny didn't even notice was in his arm. It was good for seven to ten days, which was the duration of his G-CSF for the entire month. We would draw up the amount needed for injection, then place it in the insulflon and inject very slowly. Kenny never felt it and no longer begged us not to do the G-CSF. Oh, how I wished we had done this from the beginning! Kenny's counts would usually start to decline about four days after his chemo. At about day ten the G-CSF would kick in and his counts would skyrocket.

Erythropoietin (Epogen and Procrit are the brand names) is a protein normally produced by the kidneys that stimulates red blood cell production. It is manufactured using recombinant DNA technology and is sometimes used in chemotherapy patients to reduce anemia and, hence, the need for blood transfusions. It is given as an injection, usually three times a week.

Oprelvekin (Neumega is the brand name) is a copy of a protein called IL-11, that stimulates the formation of platelets. It is manufactured using recombinant DNA technology. It is used to lessen the degree of thrombocytopenia (low platelets) associated with chemotherapy. It is given as a daily subcutaneous injection, usually starting after chemotherapy is complete and continuing until the platelet count recovers.

Antinausea drugs used during chemotherapy

Antinausea drugs, also referred to as antiemetics, make chemotherapy treatments more bearable, but can potentially cause side effects. The following section lists some commonly used antinausea drugs.

Antinausea drug list

As with chemotherapy drugs, several different names can be used to refer to each of the antinausea medications. You may hear the same drug referred to by its generic name, abbreviation, or one of several brand names, depending on which doctor, nurse, or pharmacist you are talking to. The list below gives various names of antinausea drugs, and what name to look under in this chapter:

Name	Look Under
Ativan	Lorazepam
Benadryl	Diphenhydramine
Compazine	Prochlorperazine
Decadron	Dexamethasone
Dexamethasone	Dexamethasone
Hexadrol	Dexamethasone
Kytril	Granisetron
Lorazepam	Lorazepam
Ondansetron	Ondansetron
Phenergan	Promethazine
Prochlorperazine	Prochlorperazine
Zofran	Ondansetron

Dexamethasone (dex-a-METH-a-sown)

Also called: Decadron, Hexadrol

How given: Intravenous (IV), usually given in combination with other antinausea drugs

Common side effects:

Euphoria
Restlessness
Confusion

Side effects are different than those experienced when it is given in high doses for long periods of time.

Diphenhydramine (Die-fen-HIGH-dra-meen)

Also called: Benadryl

How given: Liquid by mouth (PO), intravenous (IV)

When given: Diphenhydramine is usually given every six to eight hours.

Common side effects:

Drowsiness
Dizziness
Impaired coordination

Granisetron

Also called: Kytril

How given: Intravenous (IV), pills by mouth (PO)

When given: Kytril is usually given one half hour prior to the start of chemotherapy infusion.

Common side effects:

Headache

Infrequent side effects:

Diarrhea
Constipation

Sarah got Zofran at first, then the clinic switched to liquid Kytril.
Sarah usually hates liquid meds (she much prefers pills) but she loves
Kytril. She thinks it's really yummy. And it works, too!

Lorazepam (lor-AZ-a-pam)

Also called: Ativan

How given: Pills by mouth (PO), intravenous (IV), or intramuscular (IM)

When given: This is a tranquilizer and is generally given in combination with other antinausea drugs.

Common side effects:

  Drowsiness or sleepiness
  Forgetfulness
  Impaired coordination
  Low blood pressure (hypotension)

Ondansetron (on-DAN-se-tron)

Also called: Zofran

How given: Intravenous (IV), liquid or pills by mouth (PO)

When given: Ondansetron is usually given 30 minutes prior to chemotherapy drugs, and every four to eight hours until nausea ends, or in a higher dose once a day.

Infrequent side effects:

  Mild headache
  Constipation

After Jeremy had his first inpatient treatment, he was allowed to go
on an outpatient basis, wearing a cad pump at home. He felt fine, but
every couple hours he would vomit for no reason. The next morning,
when his oncologist asked him how it had gone, Jeremy was hesitant to tell
him about the vomiting. When he did, the doctor asked us if the Zofran
hadn't helped. I gave him a confused look and asked him what a Zofran

was. I can laugh about it now, but it was an oversight. Everyone thought someone else had taken care of it! We rarely had any problems with nausea after that.

Prochlorperazine (pro-chlor-PAIR-a-zeen)

Also called: Compazine

How given: Pills or long-acting capsule by mouth (PO), rectal suppository, intramuscular (IM), or intravenous (IV)

When given: Prochlorperazine is used alone if only mild nausea is expected.

Common side effects:

Drowsiness
Low blood pressure (hypotension)
Nervousness and restlessness
Tightness in the muscles of the jaw and face

Promethazine (Pro-METH-ah-zeen)

Also called: Phenergan

How given: Pills by mouth (PO), rectal suppository, intramuscular (IM), or intravenous (IV)

When given: Promethazine is usually given every four to six hours.

Common side effects:

Drowsiness
Dizziness and incoordination
Fatigue
Blurred vision
Euphoria
Insomnia

Drugs used to relieve pain

As with other drugs, medications used for pain relief can be given by various methods and can cause side effects. The following section lists some of the commonly used drugs to relieve pain.

Pain medication list

Several different names can be used to refer to each of the pain medications. You may hear the same drug referred to by its generic name or one of several brand names, depending on which doctor, nurse, or pharmacist you are talking to. The list below gives various names of pain medications, and what name to look under in this chapter:

Name	Look Under
Codeine	Codeine
Demerol	Meperidine
Dilaudid	Hydromorphone
EMLA cream	EMLA cream
Methadone	Methadone
Morphine	Morphine
Numby Stuff	Numby Stuff
Percocet	Oxycodone

Codeine

How given: Intramuscular (IM), pills or liquid by mouth (PO)

How it works: Codeine is an alkaloid obtained from opium.

Common side effects:

> Lightheadedness
>
> Dizziness
>
> Sedation
>
> Euphoria
>
> Constipation

Infrequent side effects:

> Nausea
>
> Vomiting

Meperidine

Also called: Demerol

How given: Intravenous (IV), liquid or pill by mouth (PO)

How it works: Meperidine is a narcotic similar to morphine.

Common side effects:

Sedation

Constipation

Infrequent side effects:

Dizziness

Nausea and vomiting

Sweating

Rashes

Respiratory depression

Decreased blood pressure

Seizures

Headaches

Visual disturbances

EMLA Cream

How given: Applied to the skin and covered with an airtight dressing one to two hours before procedures such as spinal taps, bone marrow aspirations, or injections

How it works: EMLA cream is an emulsion that contains two anesthetics, lidocaine and prilocaine.

Note: It may take longer than an hour to achieve effective anesthesia in dark-skinned individuals.

> We use EMLA for everything: finger pokes, accessing port, shots, spinal taps, and bone marrows. I even let her sister use it for shots because it lets her get a bit of attention, too. Both of my children have sensitive skin which turns red when they pull off tape, so I cover the EMLA with saran wrap held in place with paper tape. I also fold back the edge of each piece of tape to make a pull tab so the kids don't have to peel each edge back from their skin.

Hydromorphone

Also called: Dilaudid

How given: Intravenous (IV), pill by mouth (PO), rectal suppository

How it works: Hydromorphone is a narcotic pain reliever.

Precautions: Hydromorphone can cause respiratory depression.

Common side effects:

Lightheadedness and dizziness
Sedation
Nausea
Vomiting
Sweating
Euphoria
Alterations of mood
Headache
Respiratory depression

Infrequent side effects:

Circulatory depression
Hallucinations and disorientation
Respiratory arrest
Shock
Cardiac arrest

Methadone

Also called: Dolophine

How given: Intravenous (IV), pill or liquid by mouth (PO)

How it works: Methadone is a narcotic pain reliever.

Common side effects:

Lightheadedness and dizziness
Sedation
Nausea and vomiting
Sweating
Euphoria
Loss of appetite (anorexia)

Infrequent side effects:

Respiratory depression
Circulatory depression
Shock

Morphine

How given: Intravenous (IV), pill or liquid by mouth (PO)

How it works: Morphine is a narcotic derived from the opium plant.

Common side effects:

> Euphoria
> Nausea and vomiting
> Drowsiness
> Constipation

Infrequent side effects:

> Reduction in body temperature
> Respiratory depression
> Allergic reactions (including hives)
> Seizures

> *Zachary's first surgery was fairly easy to recover from. His second,
> however, had a horrible three-week recovery period, involving painful
> bladder spasms, extreme diarrhea, an infection in his Hickman line, and
> massive weight loss. It took a lot of morphine to help him feel comfortable.*

Numby Stuff

How given: Numby Stuff provides a needle-free method of delivering pain
medication through the use of low level electric currents applied to the skin.

How it works: Numby Stuff is an emulsion that contains two anesthetics,
lidocaine and prilocaine.

Note: It anesthetizes skin and tissue in ten to fifteen minutes. Some children
and teens do not like the electrical sensation that goes from the site to the
battery pack.

Oxycodone

Also called: Percocet, oxycotin

How it works: Oxycodone is a narcotic derived from opium.

Common side effects:

Lightheadedness

Dizziness

Sedation

Nausea and vomiting

Infrequent side effects:

Respiratory depression

Skin rash

Adjunctive treatments

In recent years there has been increasing research on mind-body medicine and its effect on coping with the side effects of illness. Adjunctive therapies are those that can be expected to add something beneficial to the ongoing treatment program. For example, the use of imagery and hypnosis are widely used in established treatment programs to help children and teens prepare for or cope with medical procedures. Other helpful adjunctive therapies are relaxation, biofeedback, massage, visualization, acupuncture, meditation, aromatherapy, and prayer. Chapter 2, *Coping with Procedures*, discusses adjunctive therapies and how to obtain information about them.

Alternative treatments

Alternative treatments can be defined as those that are used in place of conventional medical treatment or, if used in addition to treatment, may have unknown or adverse effects. Sometimes these therapies are illegal or unavailable in the United States or Canada, and patients travel to other countries to obtain them.

Alternative treatments are usually based on word-of-mouth endorsements called anecdotal evidence. Medical therapy is based on scientific studies using large groups of patients. In treating cancer, these large clinical trials have resulted in increases in survival rates in the past three decades.

Many alternative treatments can help parents and children feel that they are aiding the healing process. Even with a good prognosis for your child, it is difficult to ignore the advice of friends and relatives extolling the virtues of various alternative treatments. Parents just want to help their children in every way possible; they often feel helpless, and they agonize over the pain and misery that their child endures for many months while on conventional therapy. Conventional treatment can be brutal, but it is effective in many cases.

It is extremely important that any therapy that involves ingestion or injection into the body (herbs, vitamins, special diets, enemas) only be given with the oncologist's knowledge. The involvement of the physician is necessary to prevent giving something to your child that could lessen the effectiveness of the conventional chemotherapy. For instance, folic acid (a B vitamin) replaces methotrexate in cells and reduces or eliminates its effectiveness, allowing cancer cells to flourish. The oncologist will be much more knowledgeable about these potential conflicts than a parent, herbalist, or health food store salesperson.

Despite the effectiveness of childhood cancer treatment, you may wish to research one or more alternatives. Parents of children who have relapsed one or more times often are drawn to exploring alternative treatments. To help you evaluate claims made about alternative treatments, here are several ways to collect enough information to make an educated judgment:

- Go to or call your local American Cancer Society or Canadian Cancer Society's division office and ask for their information on the therapy you are considering. They have compiled information on many therapies describing the treatment, its known risks, side effects, opinion of the medical establishment, and any lawsuits that have been filed. The American Cancer Society has an online database at *http://www.cancer.org/* with information about many alternative treatments.

- Check the National Institutes of Health's Office of Alternative Medicine to see if any scientific evidence exists on the treatment that interests you. The office can be reached at (301) 443-3170, or online at *http://altmed.od.nih.gov/*.

- Ask specifically what this treatment is expected to do for your child; ask what is in it; ask what tests will be done to ascertain whether your child needs it and whether your child is benefiting from it.

- Collect and study all available objective literature on the treatment. Ask the alternative treatment providers if they have treated other children with cancer, what results have been achieved, how these results have been documented, and where they have reported their results. Ask for the reports so that your doctor can review them.

- Talk with other people who have gone through the treatment. Inquire about the training and experience of the person administering the treatment. Be sure to find out how much the therapy costs, as your insurance company may not pay for alternative treatments.

- Beware of any practitioner who will give your child the alternative therapy only if you stop taking the child in for conventional treatments.

Take all the information you have gathered to your child's oncologist to discuss any positive or negative impact that it may have on your child's current medical treatment. Do not give any alternative treatment or over-the-counter drugs to your child in secret. Some treatments negate the effectiveness of chemotherapy while other substances, such as those containing aspirin or related compounds, can cause uncontrollable bleeding in children with low platelet counts.

> At one point, we decided to try some alternative therapies with our son. Our plan was to use it in conjunction with his conventional treatment. I scheduled a meeting with his oncologist and discussed the alternatives with him. I wouldn't dare attempt to start anything, not even vitamin supplements, without first talking it over with the doctor, because I was scared that I would cause him more harm than good. I was grateful that he was willing to listen to what I had to say and offer his opinion.

> We both agreed that the alternative therapy we had in mind wouldn't do any damage or interfere with the chemotherapy he was receiving. Two months later, we decided that it was doing absolutely nothing for him, so we stopped. I figured the money would be better spent at the toy store than on a useless alternative therapy. I learned a valuable lesson from that experience. I'm much more skeptical now than I used to be. My new motto is "show me the proof."

· · · · ·

> I gave my son echinacea when he received chemotherapy. I checked with his doctor first. He didn't think it would hurt, but didn't think it would help, either. Still, all the nurses in emergency swore by the stuff. We got good results, too. We started the echinacea after lots of treatment, and it was the first time that he didn't have to be readmitted three days after

chemo for febrile neutropenia. I'm convinced that it helped him during the recovery period when his counts would bottom out.

If, after thorough investigation, you feel strongly in favor of using an alternative treatment in addition to conventional treatment and your child's oncologist adamantly opposes it, listen to his reasoning. If you disagree, go get a second opinion. Remember, the child is the most important person here. Don't give the treatment in secret or your child may be the loser.

When Zack (age six) was treated for neuroblastoma, he always developed a fever after chemotherapy. I could tell when his counts were dropping because the fever would start off low and go up to around 102°. When his fever went over 101°, the doctor would put him on IV antibiotics and draw blood cultures every day. His fevers usually started about seven days after the first day of chemo. His counts would drop real fast. For us, it became normal. He'd always need platelet and red blood cell transfusions after chemotherapy, also. It was a scary time but we became used to it.

I thank God daily for sustaining Zack this long. Yesterday was just a horrible day. But today I arose with positive thoughts. I will take care of my son and live life for we have been blessed to be his parents.

CHAPTER 16

Common Side Effects of Chemotherapy

*Take the first step in faith. You don't have to
see the whole staircase, just take the first step.*

—Martin Luther King, Jr.

CHEMOTHERAPY DRUGS interfere with cancer cells' ability to grow or reproduce. Because rapidly dividing cells are more susceptible to chemotherapy
drugs, cancer cells are severely affected. Unfortunately, healthy cells that
multiply rapidly can be damaged as well. These normal cells include those of
the bone marrow, mouth, stomach, intestines, hair follicles, and skin.

This chapter explains the most common side effects of chemotherapy drugs,
and explores ways to effectively deal with them. Chemotherapy side effects
that prevent good nutrition are discussed in Chapter 21, *Nutrition.*

Hair loss

Chemotherapy drugs destroy not only cancer cells, but also normal cells that
are produced at a rapid rate. Because hair follicle cells reproduce quickly,
chemotherapy causes some or all body hair to fall out. The hair on the scalp,
eyebrows, eyelashes, underarms, and pubic area may slowly thin out or may
fall out in big clumps.

Hair regrowth usually starts one to three months after intensive chemotherapy ends. The color and texture may be different from the original hair.
Straight hair may regrow curly; blond hair may be brown.

Parents suggest the following ways to deal with hair loss:

- When hair is thin or breaking, use a brush with very soft bristles.

- Avoid bleaches, permanents, curlers, blow dryers, or hair spray, as these
  may cause additional damage.

- If hair is thin, use a mild shampoo specifically designed for overtreated or damaged hair.

- A flannel receiving blanket placed on the pillow at night will help collect hair that is falling out.

- Recognize that hair loss is traumatic for all but the youngest children. It is especially hard on teenagers.

- Emphasize to your child that the hair loss is temporary and that it will grow back.

- Try to have your child meet children who have completed therapy so that they can see for themselves that hair will regrow soon.

- Allow your child or teen to choose a collection of hats, scarves, or cotton turbans to wear. These are tax-deductible medical expenses, and may be covered by insurance.

- To order several styles of reversible all-cotton headwear for girls seven to twelve and women, contact Just In Time in Philadelphia, (215) 247-8777.

- If your child expresses an interest in wearing a wig, take pictures of her hairstyle prior to hair loss. Also cut snippets of hair to take in to allow a good match of original color and texture. The cost of the wig may be covered by insurance if the doctor writes a prescription for a "wig prosthesis." This should include the medical reason for the wig such as "Alopecia due to cancer chemotherapy." To find a wig retailer, look in the yellow pages of your phone book under "Hair Replacements, Goods, and Supplies." The American Cancer Society (800) ACS-2345, the Canadian Cancer Society (888) 939-3333, and some local cancer service organizations offer free wigs in some areas. Another source for a free wig is Hair Club for Kids, sponsored by Hair Club for Men in New York, (212) 462-1400 ext. 3085.

- Advocate that school-age children be permitted to wear hats or other head coverings to school.

- Separate your feelings about baldness from your child's feelings. Many parents rush out to buy wigs and hats without discussing with their child how he wants to deal with his baldness.

- Allow your child to choose whether to wear head coverings or not. Let it be okay to be bald.

Hair loss is quite variable for children being treated for cancer. Some only lose part of their hair, some have hair that thins out, and some quickly lose every hair on their body.

> *Preston never completely lost his hair, but it became extremely thin and wispy. When he was first diagnosed, a friend bought him a fly-fishing tying kit, and he became very good at tying flies. He even began selling them at a local fishing shop. When his hair began to fall out, we would gather it up and put it in a plastic bag. He started tying flies out of his hair, and they were displayed in the shop window as "Preston's Human Hair Flies." He was only eleven, but the shop owner hired him to help around the shop. He became very popular with the clientele, because everyone wanted to meet the boy who tied flies from his own hair. He really turned losing his hair into something positive.*

Nausea and vomiting

The effects of anticancer drugs vary from person to person and dose to dose. A drug that makes one child violently ill often has no effect on other children. Some drugs produce no nausea until several doses have been given, while others cause nausea after a single dose. Because the effects of chemotherapy are so wildly variable, each child's treatment must be tailored to her individual needs. There is no relationship between the amount of nausea and the effectiveness of the medicine.

The following is a list of suggestions for helping children and teenagers cope with nausea and vomiting:

- Give your child antiemetic (antinausea) medications as prescribed. Do not skip any doses.

- Your child should wear loose clothing because it is both more comfortable and easier to remove if soiled.

- Parents should always have at least one change of clothes for their child in the car.

- Carry a bucket, towels, and baby wipes in the car in case of vomiting.

- Keep your child in a quiet, well-ventilated room after chemotherapy.

- Smells can trigger nausea. Try not to cook in the house when your child feels ill. If possible, open windows to provide plenty of fresh air.

- If your child is nauseated by smells, use a covered cup with a straw for liquids.

- Do not serve hot foods, as the odor can aggravate nausea.

- Serve dry foods such as toast, pretzels, or crackers in the morning or whenever the child is feeling nauseated.

- Serve several small meals rather than three large ones.

- Have the child keep his head elevated after eating. Lying flat can induce nausea.

- Serve plenty of clear liquids such as water, juice, Gatorade, or ginger ale.

- Avoid serving sweet, fried, or very spicy food. Instead, serve bland foods such as potatoes, cottage cheese, soup, or toast.

- Watch for any signs of dehydration. These include dry skin and mouth, sunken eyes, dizziness, and decreased urination. Call the physician if your child appears dehydrated.

- Use distractions such as TV, videos, music, games, or reading aloud to divert attention from nausea.

- After the child vomits, rinse his mouth with water or a mixture of water and lemon juice to remove the taste.

- If your child develops a metallic taste in her mouth, chewing gum or sucking on popsicles may help.

> Mikey went through chemotherapy with minimal side effects. In the beginning, his dad would stay with him during his infusions and I would leave. I couldn't bring myself to watch what the doctors said "might" happen (nausea, vomiting, etc). I thought it would happen immediately after chemotherapy entered his body.

If the various antinausea medications do not work well for your child, investigate the Relief Band. This wrist band gives an electrical stimulation (too faint to feel) to an acupuncture point in the wrist that affects the portion of the brain which controls nausea. After ten years of study, the band has been approved by the FDA.

Low blood counts

Bone marrow, the spongy material that fills the inside of the bones, produces red cells, white cells, and platelets. Chemotherapy drugs destroy the cells inside the bone marrow and dramatically lower the number of cells circulating in the blood. Frequent blood tests are crucial in determining whether the child needs transfusions. Many children treated for cancer require transfusions of red cells and platelets. Consequently, when the number of infection-fighting white cells is low, the child is in danger of developing serious infections.

What is an ANC? (also called AGC)

The activities of families of children with cancer revolve around the sick child's white count, specifically the absolute neutrophil count (ANC). This is sometimes called an absolute granulocyte count (AGC). The ANC (or AGC) provides an indication of the child's ability to fight infection.

When a child has blood drawn for a complete blood count (CBC), one section of the lab report will state the total white blood cell (WBC) count and a "differential," in which each type of white blood cell is listed as a percentage of the total. For example, if the total WBC count is 1500 mm^3, the differential might appear as in the following table:

White blood cell type	Percentage of total WBCs
Segmented neutrophils (also called polys or segs)	49%
Band neutrophils (also called bands)	1%
Basophils (also called basos)	1%
Eosinophils (also called eos)	1%
Lymphocytes (also called lymphs)	38%
Monocytes (also called monos)	10%

To calculate the ANC, add the percentages of neutrophils and bands, and multiply by the total WBC. Using the example above, the ANC is 49% + 1% = 50%. 50% of 1500 (.50×1500) = 750. The ANC is 750.

> Erica ran a fever whenever her counts were low, but nothing ever grew in her cultures. They would hospitalize her for 48 hours as a precaution. She was never on a full dose of medicine because of her chronically low counts. She's five years off treatment now and doing great.

How to protect the child with a low ANC

Generally, an ANC over 1000 provides the child enough protective neutrophils to fight off exposure to infection due to bacteria and fungi. With an

ANC this high, you can allow your child to attend all normal functions such as school, athletics, and parties. However, it is wise to keep close track of the pattern of the rise and fall of your child's ANC. If you know that the ANC is 1000, but is on the way down, it should affect your decision on what activities are appropriate. Each hospital has different guidelines concerning appropriate activities for children with low ANCs.

The following are parents' suggestions for detecting and preventing infections:

- Insist on frequent, thorough hand washing for every member of the family. Use soap and warm water, lather well, and rub all portions of the hands. Children and parents need to wash before preparing meals, before eating, after playing outdoors, and after using the bathroom.

    We always had antibacterial baby wipes in our car. We washed Justin's hands, and our own, after going to any public places such as parks, museums, or restaurants. They can also be used to wipe off tables or high chairs at restaurants.

- Make sure that all medical personnel at the hospital or doctor's office wash their hands before touching your child.

- Keep your child's diaper area and skin creases clean and dry.

- When your child's ANC is low, make arrangements with your pediatrician to use a back entrance to the office to avoid exposure to sick kids in the waiting room. It sometimes helps to make all appointments for early morning so that your child can be seen in a room that hasn't had several sick children in it.

- Whenever your child needs a needle stick, make sure that the technician cleans your child's skin thoroughly with both betadine and alcohol.

- Protect your child if she has a low ANC.

    When my son's ANC was low, we took extra care to avoid situations that increased his risk of infection. We kept him home from school and restricted the number of visitors to our home. Little things that many people take for granted were dependent upon whether his ANC was high enough. For example, we wouldn't take him to see a movie if his ANC was low. Sitting in an enclosed theater with so many people would have definitely been a bad idea without enough neutrophils.

- If your child gets a small cut, wash it with soap and water, rinse with hydrogen peroxide, and cover with a clean Band-Aid.

- Take your child's temperature every day at the same time. When your child is ill, take his temperature every two to three hours.

- Do not take the temperature rectally (in the anus) or use rectal suppositories, as this may cause anal tears and increase the risk of infection and bleeding.

- Do not use a humidifier as the stagnant water can become a reservoir for contamination.

- Apply sunscreen whenever your child plays outdoors. Children taking certain chemotherapy drugs, such as methotrexate, are sun sensitive, and a bad sunburn can easily become a site for infection.

- Your child should not be vaccinated while on chemotherapy.

- Siblings should not be vaccinated with live polio virus (OPV). They should get the killed polio virus (IPV). Verify that your pediatrician is using the appropriate vaccine for the siblings.

> Katy was diagnosed just a week after her younger sister Alison had been given the live polio vaccine. Because there was a small risk that Alison could infect any immunosuppressed child with polio, we were not allowed to stay on the cancer floor of the hospital.

- If your child's ANC is low, an infected site may not become red or painful.

> My daughter kept getting ear infections while on chemo. They would find them during routine exams. I felt guilty because she never told me her ears were hurting. I told her doctor that I was worried because she didn't complain of pain, and he reassured me by telling me that she probably felt no pain because she didn't have enough white cells to cause swelling inside her ear.

- Never give aspirin, Motrin, or ibuprofen for fever. They may interfere with blood clotting. If your child has a fever, call the doctor before giving any medication.

- Ask your child's oncologist about using a stool softener if she has problems with constipation. Stool softeners can help prevent anal tears.

- Call the doctor if any of the following symptoms appear: fever above 101°F (38.5°C), chills, cough, shortness of breath, sore throat, severe diarrhea, bloody urine or stool, or pain or burning while urinating.

Whenever my daughter (diagnosed when one year old) was on anti-biotics (frequently), she developed a vaginal yeast infection. It was very painful for her and a nightmare for me.

· · · · ·

My son's big toes became large and red from ingrown toenails while on treatment. He had several surgeries to remove the corners of each nail to prevent infection. That was several years ago, and his toes look bad but are not painful.

Two serious infections that plague children during treatment for cancer are pneumonia and chicken pox.

Pneumonia

Pneumonia is inflammation of the lungs caused primarily by bacteria or viruses. The symptoms of pneumonia are rapid breathing, chills, fever, chest pain, cough, and bloody sputum. Children with low blood counts can rapidly develop a fatal infection, and must be treated quickly and aggressively.

My son received chemotherapy just days before he was scheduled to go to the American Cancer Society's camp. His ANC was 1200 and he looked so sick, but he begged to go and I let him. It was early in his treatment and I didn't realize the pattern of his blood counts. They called me from camp on Friday to say he had a temperature of 103°F (39.5°C) and needed to go to the hospital. He was very weak and feverish; his WBC was 140, and his ANC was 0. Both lungs were full of pneumonia. I was furious at the doctor for giving him permission to go to camp and at myself for not paying closer attention to how quickly his counts dropped. I'm sure he had the pneumonia before he even went to camp. They started him on five different antibiotics, and his fever went up to 106°F (41.1°C) that night. We didn't know if he would live or die. He started to gradually improve the next morning and was completely recovered in a week.

Chicken pox

Chicken pox is a common childhood disease caused by a virus called varicella zoster. Its symptoms are headache, fever, and malaise, rapidly followed by eruptions of pimple-like red bumps. The bumps typically start on the stomach, chest, or back. They rapidly develop into blister-like sores which break open, then scab over in three to five days. Any contact with the sores can spread the disease, and children are contagious up to 48 hours prior to breaking out.

Chicken pox can be a fatal disease for immunosuppressed children, so extreme care must be taken to prevent exposure. It will be necessary to educate all teachers and friends to be vigilant in reporting any outbreaks. The child can be kept home from school or preschool until the outbreak is over.

Chicken pox can be transmitted through the air or by touch. Exposure is considered to have occurred if a child is in direct contact or in a room for as little as ten minutes with an infected person. If your child has never had chicken pox, it is better to take him to beaches or parks rather than indoor play areas.

Untreated chicken pox or shingles can result in life-threatening complications including pneumonia, hepatitis, and encephalitis. Parents must make every effort to prevent exposure and be vigilant in watching for signs of the diseases while their child is on treatment.

If an immunosuppressed child is exposed to chicken pox, call the doctor immediately. If the doctor is able to administer a shot called VZIG (Varicella Zoster Immune Globin) within 72 hours of exposure, it may prevent the disease from occurring or minimize its effects.

> We knew when Jeremy was exposed, so he was able to get VZIG. He did get chicken pox, but only developed a few spots. He didn't get sick; he got bored. He spent two weeks in the hospital in isolation. We asked for a pass, and we were able to go outside for some fresh air each day.

If a child develops chicken pox while on chemotherapy, the current treatment is hospitalization or, if possible, home therapy for IV administration of acyclovir, a potent antiviral medication. This drug has dramatically lowered the complication rate of chicken pox.

> Kristin broke out with chicken pox on the Fourth of July weekend. Our hospital room was the best seat in the house for watching the city fireworks. She did get covered with pox, though, from the soles of her feet to the very top of her scalp. We'd just give her gauze pads soaked in calamine lotion and let her hermetically seal herself. They kept her in the hospital for six days of IV acyclovir, then she was at home on the pump (a small computerized machine that administers the drug in small amounts for several hours) for four more days of acyclovir. She had no complications.

A child who has already had chicken pox may develop herpes zoster (shingles). If your child develops eruptions of vesicles similar to chicken pox which are in lines (along nerves), call the doctor. The treatment for shingles is identical to that of chicken pox.

> Kristin also got a herpes zoster infection, this time on Thanksgiving. It looked like a mild case of chicken pox, limited to her upper right arm, her upper right chest, and her right leg. They kept her overnight on IV acyclovir and then let her go home for nine more days on the pump.

An immunization for chicken pox has been developed and is likely to be given to children with cancer in the future. Currently, there is insufficient data to indicate its usefulness or safety in these children.

Can pets transmit diseases?

It is very unlikely that your child will be harmed from living with a household pet, but several common sense precautions are needed to protect a child with a low ANC from disease, worms, or infection:

- Make sure that the animal is vaccinated against all possible diseases.
- Have pets checked for worms as soon as possible after your child is diagnosed, and then every year thereafter (more often for puppies).
- Do not let pets eat off plates, or lick your child's face.
- Keep children away from the cat litter box and any animal feces outdoors.
- Have children wash hands after playing with the pet.
- Make sure that your pet has no ticks or fleas.
- If you have a pet that bites or scratches, consider finding another home for it. On the other hand, if you have a gentle, well-loved pet, do not give it up.

> I think parents should know that you should not automatically get rid of your dog because your child has a low ANC. We went through a small crisis trying to decide whether to give away our large but beloved mongrel. The doctors wouldn't really give us a straight answer, but a parent in the support group said, "DO NOT get rid of your dog. Your son will need that dog's love and company in the years ahead." She was right. The dog was a tremendous comfort to our son.

If your child wants to buy a pet while undergoing treatment for cancer, here are some suggestions:

- Do not get a puppy. All puppies bite while teething, increasing the chance that your child may contract an infection.

- Do not get a parrot or parakeet as these species can transmit psittacosis.

- Do not get a turtle or other reptile (snake, iguana) as they sometimes carry salmonella.

- Avoid buying any animal that is likely to bite or scratch.

If you have any concerns or questions about pets you already own or are thinking of purchasing, ask your oncologist for advice.

> We had an odd situation when Christopher (age three) was diagnosed with neuroblastoma. Our oncologist told us about not letting Christopher around any birds or animals with a lot of fur. The problem was I am a farmer. Not just cattle, but I also raise turkeys. When the houses are full, we hold about 60,000 at a time.
>
> Even before Christopher could walk he would go to work with me. He especially enjoyed helping me feed baby birds. Christopher had a huge plastic dump truck he would put feed in and push around while I fed with a wheelbarrow. We would take our shirts off and be silly together—a very special time. When Christopher was diagnosed, I told the doctors I had no problem selling or shutting the farm down if it gave Christopher a better chance of surviving or would reduce the chance of infection. They told us to keep Christopher away from the animals and especially the turkeys and to keep him inside when his ANC was low, which we did. Every time I got baby turkeys in, I would move his truck to that house. Sometimes I would cry, sometimes I wouldn't. But I absolutely hated taking care of the little birds.
>
> In late June when Christopher was declared in remission, again we happened to get a house full of baby turkeys in. This time, Christopher didn't want his truck, but he pushed my wheelbarrow and we got silly again. I really missed that.

Diarrhea

Chemotherapy destroys cancer cells, as well as any cells that are produced at a rapid rate such as those that line the mouth, stomach, and intestines. This damage can cause diarrhea, ranging from mild (frequent, soft stools) to severe (copious quantities of liquid stool). Diarrhea during chemotherapy can also be caused by some antinausea drugs, antibiotics, or intestinal infections. After chemotherapy ends and immune function returns to normal, the lining of the digestive tract heals and the diarrhea ends.

The following suggestions for coping with diarrhea come from parents:

- Do not give any over-the-counter drug to your child without approval from the doctor. He may want to test your child's stool for infection prior to treating the diarrhea. Frequently recommended drugs for diarrhea are Kaopectate, Lomotil, or Immodium.

- It is very important that your child drink plenty of liquids. This will not increase the diarrhea, but will replace the fluids lost.

> *My three-year-old had stopped drinking from bottles months before her diagnosis. When she first began her intensive chemotherapy, she had uncontrollable, frequent diarrhea. Liquid would just gush out without warning. It was hard for her to drink from a cup, so one night she said in a small voice, "Mommy, would it be okay if I drank from a bottle again?" I said, "Of course, honey." It was a great comfort to her, and she took in a lot more fluids that way.*

- Hot or cold liquids can increase intestinal contractions, so serve plenty of room-temperature clear liquids or mild juices such as water, Gatorade, ginger ale, peach juice, or apricot juice.

- Diarrhea depletes the body's supply of potassium. Provide foods high in potassium such as bananas, oranges, baked or mashed potatoes without the skin, broccoli, halibut, mushrooms, asparagus, tomato juice, and milk (if tolerated).

- Low potassium can cause irregular heartbeats and leg cramps. If these occur, call the doctor.

- Do not serve greasy, fatty, spicy, or sweet foods.

- Do not serve roughage such as bran, fruits (dried or fresh), nuts, beans, or raw vegetables.

- Do serve bland, low-fiber foods such as bananas, white rice, noodles, applesauce, unbuttered white toast, creamed cereals, cottage cheese, fish, and chicken or turkey without the skin.

In the middle of treatment, my son had severe diarrhea for a week. He had large amounts of liquid stools twenty times a day. I felt so sorry for him. The doctor cultured a stool specimen, but they never identified a cause. It cleared up after a week of the BRAT diet (bananas, rice, applesauce, toast). He had a problem with diarrhea almost weekly throughout his treatment.

- Keep a record of the number of bowel movements and their volume to keep the doctor informed. Call the doctor if you notice any blood in the stool, or if your child has any signs of dehydration such as dry skin, dry mouth, sunken eyes, decreased urination, or dizziness.

- Keep the area around the anus clean and dry. Wash with warm water and mild soap after every bowel movement. Pat dry gently.

- If the anus is sore, check with the doctor before using any nonprescription medicine. She may recommend using Desitin or A&D ointment after each bowel movement.

While taking ARA-C my daughter had a terribly sore rectum, which was a big problem. It hurt to have bowel movements—she'd cry and have to squeeze our hands to go, then the urine would run back and burn. She was very itchy. We carried around bags with Q-tips and every known brand of rectal ointment—A&D, Preparation H, Desitin, Benadryl.

- Call the doctor if your child has significant pain with bowel movements, especially if your child has low blood counts.

Constipation

Constipation means a decrease in the normal number of bowel movements. There are many reasons that constipation occurs on chemotherapy. Some drugs, such as vincristine, slow the movement of the stool through the intestines resulting in constipation. Pain medication, decreased activity, decreased eating and drinking, and vomiting can all affect the normal rhythm of the intestine. When movement through the intestine slows, stools become hard and dry.

The following are parents' suggestions for preventing and helping constipation:

- Encourage your child to be as physically active as possible.

- Encourage your child to drink lots of liquids every day. Prune juice is especially helpful.

- Serve high-fiber foods such as raw vegetables, beans, bran, whole wheat breads, whole grain cereals, dried fruits (especially prunes, dates, and raisins), graham crackers, and nuts.

- Check with the doctor prior to using any medications for constipation. He may recommend a stool softener like colace. If the doctor suggests liquid ducosate, be aware that many kids don't like the taste. Metamucil or Citrucel increase the volume of the stool which stimulates the intestine. Milk of magnesia or magnesium citrate help the stool to retain fluid and remain soft.

- Do not give enemas or rectal suppositories. These can cause anal tears which can be dangerous for a child with a weakened immune system.

- When your child feels the need to have a bowel movement, sipping a warm drink can help.

Fatigue and weakness

Fatigue—a feeling of weariness—is an almost universal side effect of treatment for cancer. General weakness, while different from fatigue, is caused by many of the same things, and is treated the same way. Fatigue and weakness may be constant throughout therapy or intermittent. They can be minor annoyances or totally debilitating. Many parents worry that if fatigue is present, so is the cancer, but this is not the case. Fatigue and weakness can be caused by one, or a combination, of the following things:

- Your child's body working overtime to heal tissues damaged by treatment and rid itself of dead and dying cancer cells

- Medications to treat nausea or pain

- Mineral imbalances caused by chemotherapy, diarrhea, or vomiting

- Infection

- Emotional factors such as anxiety, fear, sadness, depression, or frustration

- Malnutrition caused by vomiting, loss of appetite, or taste aversions

- Anemia (low red cell count)

- Disruption of normal sleep patterns (common when hospitalized or when taking certain drugs, such as prednisone)

The following suggestions come from parents:

- Make sure that your child gets plenty of rest. Naps or quiet times spaced throughout the day help.

   Erica took a two-and-a-half hour nap every afternoon throughout therapy. She's four now and off treatment, but her endurance is low and she still tires easily.

- Limit visitors if your child is weak or fatigued.

   While in the hospital, my daughter was very weak. She had too many visitors, yet didn't want to hurt anyone's feelings. We worked out a signal that solved the problem. When she was too tired to continue a visit, she would place a damp washcloth on her forehead. I would then politely end the visit.

- Serve your child well-balanced meals and snacks, but don't get upset if he doesn't eat them (see the next point).

- Parents and children should try to avoid physical or emotional stress.

- Encourage your child to pursue hobbies or interests if he is able. For example, if your child is too weak to play on his athletic team, let him go to cheer the team or help keep score.

   My eighth-grade daughter was a fabulous athlete prior to her cancer diagnose. When she went back to school after missing a year, she wasn't very competitive, but she managed the softball team and dressed for basketball. So she was still part of the social scene and was able to do things with the teams.

- Help your child make a prioritized list of what he wants to accomplish. If he feels strongly that he wants to attend a certain activity, and you think he may run out of energy, throw a wheelchair or stroller into the car and go.

- Encourage your child to attend a kid's support group, and go to the parent group yourself. Seeing that others have the same problems and talking about how you are feeling can lighten the load.

Many children complete their chemotherapy protocols without fatigue or weakness, while other children are not so lucky.

Before Brent was diagnosed at age six, he was exceptionally well coordinated and a very fast runner. During treatment, he slowed down to about average. He played soccer and T-ball throughout, and was very competitive.

· · · · ·

Jeremy has had some major, persistent problems with weakness and loss of coordination. When he was a year off therapy (nine years old), he still could not catch a ball. When he ran, he was like a robot, and the trunk of his body stayed straight. Some kids made fun of him, and he got very frustrated with himself. He had five years of physical therapy, and now, three years off chemo, his skills have improved, but he still has to work harder than the other kids. We put him into martial arts in hopes of further increasing his motor skills and his confidence.

Bed wetting

Bed wetting, although infrequent, can be a very upsetting side effect of chemotherapy. Some drugs increase thirst, while others disrupt normal sleep patterns, both of which can make bed wetting more likely. When bed wetting is caused by a specific drug or lots of IV fluids at night, time will cure the problem. Once the drug or fluids are no longer necessary, bed wetting will stop.

There are also psychological reasons for bed wetting during chemotherapy. The trauma of the treatment for cancer causes many children to regress to earlier behaviors such as thumb sucking, baby talk, temper tantrums, and bed wetting. Punishment for this type of bed wetting only adds to the child's trauma and rarely solves the problem. The following are veteran parents' suggestions:

- Double-sheet the bed. Put down one plastic liner with fitted and flat sheets, then put on top another plastic liner with fitted and flat sheets. During the night, simply pull off the top sheets and plastic, and there are fresh sheets below.

- Keep a pile of extra-large or beach towels next to the bed. Cover the wet spot with towels, and save the bed change for the morning.

- Give the last drink two hours before bedtime, to allow your child's bladder to totally empty right before bed.

- Change sleeping arrangements.

Prednisone caused my daughter to have nightmares and frequent bed wetting. I felt if she could sleep through the night the bed wetting might stop. I told her she could sleep with me for the month that she was on prednisone, but that after that she would move back into her own bed. It calmed her to sleep with me. The nightmares and bed wetting decreased, and she moved back into her own bed without complaint when the time came.

- Adopt an attitude that lets your child know that bed wetting is "no big deal." There should be no shaming or punishment.

- If your child or teen is extremely distressed by his bed wetting, ask him if he wants you to set the alarm for the middle of the night in order to help him get up to go the bathroom.

- Give extra love and reassurance.

When my daughter started bed wetting, I didn't think it was the drugs. I thought long and hard about any additional worries that she might have, and I realized that because her dad had emotionally withdrawn from her during her illness, she might be worried that I would do the same. So I told her one night, "You know, I just realized that every day I tell you how much I love you. But I've never told you that no matter how hard life gets and no matter how mad we get at each other I will always love you. I love you now as a child, I will love you as a teenager, and I will love you when you are all grown up." She started to sob and hugged and hugged me. She has never wet the bed again.

Dental problems

Both radiation and chemotherapy can cause changes in the mouth and teeth. Awareness of the potential problems coupled with good preventive care can help your child be more comfortable during treatment.

Some anticancer drugs and radiation can cause changes in children's ability to salivate. Plaque may build up rapidly on your child's teeth, increasing the chance of both cavities and gum infections. Take your child for a cleaning and checkup every three to four months, as long as his counts are good (ANC above 1000 and platelets above 100,000/mm^3). If your child has a central venous catheter (Hickman or port), he should be given antibiotics before and after each visit to the dentist. Ask your dentist to refer to the current issue of the *Pediatric Dentistry Reference Manual* to formulate a dental plan.

Get recommendations from your child's oncologist and dentist for advice on teeth care when counts are very low. Often parents are advised to use a sponge or damp gauze to gently wipe off their child's teeth after meals instead of brushing.

> My daughter had problems with thick yellow saliva during the entire time she was treated. It coated her teeth and formed a lot of plaque. I brought her to an excellent pediatric dentist every three months to have the plaque removed. She took antibiotics half an hour before treatment and then again six hours afterward. He also put sealants on all of her molars and, even though there were many weeks when her teeth could not be brushed, she never got a cavity.

Some parents report delays in the arrival of their child's permanent teeth.

> We delayed getting my son's braces until after he completed his treatment. His orthodontist pointed out that two of his upper teeth never descended and would have to be surgically uncovered. I would not let him take any x-rays, so he sent me to an oral surgeon. I asked the surgeon if he could locate the teeth without x-rays, and he said yes. The oral surgeon removed the skin covering the two teeth, and the orthodontist banded them and attached a wire. He was able to gradually pull the teeth back into their proper position.

Mouth and throat sores

The mouth and throat are lined with cells that divide rapidly and can be severely damaged by chemotherapy drugs. This is more common for children on very intensive protocols and those having bone marrow transplants. The sores that develop are very painful and can prevent eating and drinking. Check your child's mouth periodically for sores, and if any are present, ask advice from the oncologist. Some parent suggestions are:

- To prevent infection, the mouth needs to be kept as clean and free of bacteria as possible. After eating, have your child gently brush teeth, gums, and tongue with a soft, clean toothbrush.
- Serve bland food, baby food, or meals put through the blender.
- Use a straw with drinks or blender-processed food.
- If your child is old enough, the doctor may recommend a rinse to prevent mouth sores.

When David was told to use Peridex, I asked the doctor if we could substitute 0.63% stannous flouride rinse. He said yes. As a dentist I knew Peridex killed bacteria and lasts up to eight hours, but it tastes terrible and stains teeth. Patients did not like using it. The 0.63% stannous flouride had the same bacterial killing properties and also lasts up to eight hours, but has a better taste and does not stain as badly. The flouride also helps prevent cavities and makes the teeth less sensitive. It comes in a variety of flavors like mint, tropical, or cinnamon. It is a prescription drug that a lot of dentists dispense.

One mixes 1/8 oz. of concentrate with warm water, making 1 oz. A measuring cup comes with the bottle. I have David swish with half the mixture for one minute (time it because it's longer than you think!). This can only be used by kids who are old enough to not accidentally swallow it. Six-year-old David has no problem taking this once a day before he goes to bed. If and when he starts developing mouth sores, he will take it a.m. and p.m. It's important not to eat or drink for 30 minutes after rinsing. That is why David rinses before bedtime, after he has taken his meds and brushed his teeth.

Changes in taste and smell

Chemotherapy can cause changes in the tastebuds, altering the brain's perception of how food tastes. Meats often taste bitter, and sweets can taste unpleasant. Even foods that children crave taste badly. Coupled with altered taste, the sense of smell is also impacted by chemotherapy. The sense of smell can be heightened so that smells which other family members are unaware of can cause nausea in a child on chemotherapy.

A child's ability to smell and taste can take months to return to normal after chemotherapy ends.

Once Katy begged me to make her my special double chocolate sour cream cake. Surprisingly, it smelled really good to her as it baked. She took a big bite, spit it out all over the table, and ran back to her room sobbing. She cried for a long time. She told me later that it had tasted "bitter and horrible."

Skin and nail problems

Minor skin problems are frequent while on chemotherapy. The most common problems are rashes, redness, itching, peeling, dry skin, and acne. The following are suggestions for preventing and treating skin problems:

- Avoid hot showers or baths as these can dry the skin.

- Use moisturizing soap such as Basic or Avena.

- Apply a water-based moisturizer after bathing.

- Avoid scratchy materials such as wool. Your child will feel more comfortable in loose, cotton clothing.

- Have your child use sunscreen with a sun protection factor (SPF) of at least 30. This is especially important for areas that have been irradiated.

- If your child is bald, and especially if she has had cranial radiation, insist on head coverings or sunscreen every time she goes outdoors.

- Buy your child lip gloss with sunscreen.

    .Matthew's lips would get very dry and eventually start to peel. It irritated him and he developed a habit of biting on his lips. To minimize the problem I learned that wiping a cool, wet cloth over his mouth many times a day worked well. I would then apply a light coating of Vaseline to his lips to keep them moist.

- Rub cornstarch on itchy skin. This is often soothing.

If your child has chemotherapy drugs injected into the veins (rather than a central catheter), you may notice a darkening along the vein. This will fade after chemotherapy ends. However, skin and underlying tissues can be damaged or destroyed by drugs which leak out of a vein. If your child feels a stinging or burning sensation, or you notice swelling at the IV site, call a nurse immediately.

Call the doctor anytime your child gets a severe rash or is very itchy. Scratching rashes can cause infections, so you need to get medications to control the itching.

Chemotherapy affects the growing portion of nails located under the cuticle. After chemotherapy, you may notice a white band or ridge across the nail as it grows out. These brittle bands are sometimes elevated and feel bumpy. As the white ridge grows out toward the end of the finger, the nail may break. Keeping your child's fingernails trimmed can help prevent breakage.

Learning disabilities

Some children who have been treated for cancer are at risk of developing learning disabilities as a consequence of their treatment. Those at highest risk include children under five years of age who receive cranial radiation and certain anticancer drugs, especially high-dose methotrexate. There is considerable research on the types of learning difficulties exhibited by these children. This subject is covered fully in Chapter 22, *School*.

Eating problems

Most children have major nutritional problems while on chemotherapy. Chapter 21 is devoted to explaining eating problems such as anorexia (lack of appetite), food aversions, overeating, and the myriad other problems induced by chemotherapy and radiation.

There were times during my son's protocol that I felt he suffered more from the side effects of treatment than from the disease. It was emotionally painful for me to watch him go through so much. I think one of the hardest moments for me was the day he lost all his hair. Up until that point I had been living in a semi-state of denial. His bald head was more proof of our reality—he really did have cancer.

I had to learn how to accept our situation, because I needed to be strong for my child. To get through, I reminded myself every day that the treatments were necessary and that without them he would die. It was a struggle, but the unpleasant side effects soon passed and he was able to resume his normal activities. I was constantly amazed at his resilience.

CHAPTER 17

Radiation

Nothing is so strong as gentleness, and
nothing is so gentle as true strength.

—St. Francis De Sales

RADIATION IS A LIFE-SAVING THERAPY that has dramatically improved survival rates for some types of childhood cancers. Radiation shrinks small tumors and helps decrease pain. However, radiation therapy can cause mild, short-term side effects, and sometimes permanent damage that may not be evident until months or years after treatment. The benefits and risks of treatment with radiation must be carefully weighed by both doctors and parents.

This chapter explains what radiation is, when and how it is used, and its potential side effects. It will dispel myths and alleviate concerns by clearly explaining what the parent and child can expect from radiation treatment.

What is radiation?

Radiation treatment, also called radiotherapy, directs high-energy x-rays at targeted areas of the body to destroy cancer cells. Radiation can be given internally or externally. Several different types of radiation are used to treat children with solid tumors.

External radiation

External radiation uses high-energy x-rays to kill cancer cells. A large machine called a linear accelerator directs x-rays to the precise portion of the body needing treatment. The treatment is usually given in small doses measured in units called centigrays or rads (short for radiation absorbed dose).

Radiation is usually given every day for a specific number of days, excluding weekends. This is called standard or conventional fractionation. Radiation given more than once a day is called accelerated fractionation, or hyperfractionation. Accelerated fractionation uses smaller amounts of radiation for each treatment. It reduces long-term side effects, but short-term side effects may be more pronounced.

Children do not become radioactive from these treatments.

> *I was very proud of my six-year-old son for handling his radiation treatments so well. In total, he had ten days of external radiation to destroy cancerous lesions in his skull. He never required sedation and was always cooperative. I'm convinced that it was partly because of his personality, and partly because of how the staff treated him. Every day that he received radiation, his favorite stuffed toy, Mr. Bear, was radiated, too.*

Internal radiation

Internal radiation—also called brachytherapy—is less commonly used than external radiation to treat childhood tumors. Brachytherapy involves the use of radioactive materials (called seeds) placed directly at the tumor site. Radioactive material can be placed within a body cavity (intracavitary), directly into tissue (interstitial implants), or applied to the surface of tumor sites (plaques). Brachytherapy is useful in treating solid tumors because it allows high-dose radiation to be delivered directly to the tumor site while sparing surrounding, healthy tissue. It differs from external radiation because it provides a continuous low dose of radiation to the tumor.

Internal radiation to body cavities or tissues is delivered through a catheter. The catheter remains in place for a specific number of days (usually two to five days) until the required amount of radiation has been given.

Radioactive plaques are custom-made disks that are positioned directly in a tumor. They are often used to treat retinoblastoma. Plaques are surgically inserted and removed, and remain in place for a specified number of days (usually three to seven days) until radiation therapy is complete.

Your child will become radioactive from each of these forms of internal radiation. She will need to be admitted to a special isolation room during treatment. Parents are allowed only a limited amount of time with their child. Children and pregnant women cannot visit as long as the child remains radioactive.

Other forms of radiation

There are other ways to use radiation to treat children with solid tumors:

- Intraoperative radiation uses external radiation applied directly to a tumor site during a surgical procedure. The major advantage to intraoperative radiation is that it allows the doctor to give a very high dose of radiation to a single area without damaging normal surrounding tissue.

- Radioimmunotherapy uses radiolabeled antibodies to act as radiation carriers. The antibodies are attached (labeled) to a radioactive material and then injected into the body. Once injected, the antibodies begin a "seek and destroy" mission, searching for specific tumor cells. Radiolabeled antibodies lessen the chance of radiation damage to normal cells.

- Radioactive iodine meta-iodobenzylguanidine (I-131 MIBG) is administered intravenously to some children with neuroblastoma. Cells absorb the radioactive material after it is injected into the body.

Who needs radiation treatment?

Your child's oncologist will recommend radiation treatment based on your child's type and stage of cancer. Some solid tumors do not respond to radiation, while others are especially radiosensitive. Childhood solid tumors that usually respond to radiation include neuroblastoma, Wilms tumor, rhabdomyosarcoma and other soft tissue sarcomas, retinoblastoma, and Ewing's sarcoma. Radiation is not used to treat osteosarcoma. It is not commonly used to treat liver tumors, except to treat disease that has spread to other sites. Children or teens with tumors in weight-bearing bones are sometimes treated with radiation to prevent fractures. Total body irradiation (TBI) is sometimes used to prepare a child for bone marrow transplant.

> Brock (age nine) had no radiation during his initial therapy. He had low dose total lung radiation during his first relapse, which was in the lower lobe of his left lung. The radiation came in the middle of the protocol and lasted for two weeks. Each radiation treatment lasted about five minutes, and both whole lungs were radiated, front and back. He tolerated the radiation, with no nausea at all until the last couple of days. Since he was almost ten years old, he didn't require any sedation for the treatments.

Brock relapsed a second time in December 1998 after being off treatment for about six months. The tumors were the exact same type and in the exact same place. This time his radiation will be high-dose, conformed field radiation to the tumor site in his lung only.

When is radiation treatment given?

Radiotherapy is given according to the schedule outlined in your child's treatment protocol. Radiation lasts for days or weeks depending on your child's situation. It may be the only treatment needed. It may be used to shrink the tumor prior to surgery or to prevent the spread of disease after surgery.

In rare situations, radiation is given to children during life-threatening emergencies. If disease or pressure from a tumor causes spinal cord compression, radiation may be used. Superior vena cava syndrome—an obstruction or narrowing of the body's major artery in the chest—may be treated with emergency radiation.

Questions to ask about radiation treatment

If radiation has been recommended as a treatment for your child, you should ask the oncologist the following questions:

- Why does my child need radiation?
- What type of radiation does she need?
- What part of her body will be treated with radiation?
- What is the total dose of radiation that she will receive?
- How many treatments of radiation will be necessary?
- How much experience does this institution have in administering this type of radiation to children?
- How will she be positioned on the table?
- Will any restraints be used?
- Will anesthesia or sedation be used?
- How long will each treatment take?

- What are the possible short-term and long-term side effects?
- Could this type and dosage of radiation cause cancer later?
- What are the alternatives to radiation?

Where should your child go for radiation treatment?

To have optimal treatment, children should receive radiation therapy only at major medical centers with experience in treating children with cancer. All treatments should be supervised by physicians who are experienced in pediatric radiation oncology. State-of-the-art equipment, expert personnel, and vast experience with pediatric cancers are what you should look for when choosing a center.

Radiation oncologist

A radiation oncologist is a medical doctor with years of specialized training in using radiation to treat disease. In partnership with the pediatric oncologist, the radiation oncologist develops a treatment plan tailored specifically for each individual child.

The radiation oncologist will explain to both child and parents what radiation is, how it will be administered, and any possible side effects. She will answer all questions regarding the proposed treatment. Parents will be given a consent form to review prior to signing (ask to take it home if you need more time to read it over). Parents should not sign the consent form until they thoroughly understand all benefits, risks, and possible side effects of the radiation. The radiation oncologist will meet at least weekly with child and parents to discuss how the treatment is going and to address concerns or answer questions.

Radiation therapist

The radiation therapist is a specially trained technologist who operates the machine that delivers the dose of radiation prescribed by the radiation oncologist. This member of the medical team will give the child a tour of the radiation room, explain about the equipment, and position the child for treatment. The technologist will operate the x-ray machine, and will monitor the child via closed-circuit TV and a two-way intercom.

> When three-year-old Katy was being given the tour of the radiation room by her technologist, Brian, he was just wonderful with her. He gave her a white, stuffed bear which he used to demonstrate the machine. He immobilized the bear on the table using Katy's mask (device to hold the head still during treatment), then moved the machine all around it so that she could hear the sounds made by the equipment. He then took a Polaroid picture of the bear on the table, in the mask, for Katy to take home with her.

Immobilization devices

Different institutions use a variety of devices to immobilize children (and adults) to ensure that the radiation beam is directed with precision. Some of the products used are custom-made plaster of paris casts, thermal plastic devices, vacuum-molded thermoplastics, polyurethane foam forms, and sandbags. Custom fitting the forms on a child who has already undergone numerous painful procedures requires skill and patience. This is especially true for children being fitted for a mask in preparation for radiation to the head. Great care should be taken to ensure that making the mask is not traumatic. This can often be accomplished by utilizing play therapy to demonstrate the procedure.

Masks are made from a lightweight, porous, mesh material. First, the technologist should explain and demonstrate the entire mask-making process to the child. The child then lies down on a table. The technologist places a sheet of the mask material in warm water to soften it. This warm mesh sheet is placed over the child's face and quickly molded to her features. The child can breathe the entire time through the mesh material, but must hold still for several minutes as the mask hardens. The mask is lifted off the child's face, and the technologist cuts holes in it for the eyes, nostrils, and mouth.

> The cancer center staff had scheduled two hours for mask making for my three-year-old daughter. I asked them to very quietly explain every step in the process. I told her that I would be holding her hand, and I promised that it would not hurt, but it would feel warm. I asked her to choose a story for me to recite as they molded the warm material to her

face to make the time go faster. She picked "Curious George Goes to the Hospital." She held perfectly still; I recited the story; the staff were gentle and quick; and the entire procedure took less than twenty minutes.

For children having radiation to areas other than the head, immobilization devices can be as simple as velcro straps to hold the body in place. Some children will have special foam or plaster molds made of their body to allow greater accuracy when directing the radiation.

Immobilization devices can be fitted on well-prepared, calm children or sedated children. The following are parent suggestions for preparing a child for the fitting of her immobilization device:

• Give the child a tour of the room where the fitting will take place.

• Explain in clear language each step in the process.

• Be honest in describing any discomfort the child may experience.

• For small children, fit the device onto a mannikin or stuffed animal to demonstrate the process.

• For older children or teenagers, show a video or read a booklet describing the procedure.

> *Seventeen-month-old Rachel was fitted with two immobilization devices. They made a mask to hold her head in position, as well as a body mold from her neck to her thighs.*

The more time spent on preparation, the less time will be spent on fitting a device. If the fitting goes well, it establishes trust and good feelings that will help make the actual radiation treatments proceed smoothly.

Sedation

All infants, most preschoolers, and some school-age children require sedation or anesthesia to ensure that they will remain perfectly still during radiation therapy. Most radiation facilities use a combination of anesthetics that are effective, yet allow the child to recover quickly.

The radiation facility should give parents written instructions concerning pediatric anesthesia. Generally, the child must not eat for eight hours prior to his appointment. Clear liquids are usually allowed four hours prior to anesthesia. Children can eat and drink immediately after treatment.

Kenny had 24 cycles of radiation under anesthesia to treat his rhab-domyosarcoma. At first it was really horrible for me to leave him in that big, dark room. I would hold his anesthesia mask over his face until he was asleep, and then I would leave. I was the last and first face he saw every time. Kenny was so brave. Towards the end of the 24 treatments, he would stand in front of the big doors yelling, "Hurry up in there! It's my turn to go night-night!" The only request he had was that a Coke and a green popsicle be waiting for him when he woke up.

Anesthesia is given through a mask, or through the child's catheter or IV while the parent is holding or comforting him. The parent must leave the room while the treatment takes place. Once the child is easily aroused, the child and parents can leave. The entire procedure takes from 30 to 60 minutes. Nausea and vomiting are occasional side effects of anesthesia.

Most of the young children at our facility were sedated, but it was not necessary for Rachel (seventeen months old). She had just spent nine weeks in the hospital and was very weak. She just laid there and didn't move. The first day she whimpered and cried a bit, but after that it didn't seem to bother her.

During a course of radiotherapy, the dose, drugs, and methods to sedate or anesthetize the child may need to be changed because some children develop a tolerance to certain drugs. Good communication between parent and members of the treatment team should prevent unnecessary anxiety about increased dosages or the use of a different drug. In some cases, less anesthesia is needed if the child is gently coached on ways to hold still.

Each time my young son came in for radiation to the orbit, part of the routine was to place the hard plastic mesh mask over his face while he was awake, just for an instant, to get him used to the idea of trying to wear it for treatments without sedation. No pressure was ever put on him about it, it was just mentioned as a possibility of something he could try, something that would let him keep eating and drinking all through the day, instead of having to fast for a few hours before each sedation, which was very hard for such a small boy who was getting sedation twice a day.

They left the mask on him for a tiny bit longer each time, until he was tolerating it for several seconds, and by the end of the third week, close to a minute. His fifth birthday was at the exact middle of treatment, and he decided that since he was such a big boy now, he would try to do it without sedation. I know he was trying to please and impress all these kind people. He worked it out quietly with a favorite technician, asked the "sleepy medicine doctor" to wait outside the treatment room, let them screw the mask down to the table and did the whole thing awake.

I've never been more proud in my life. Everyone cheered and hugged him. He finished the last three weeks of treatments without sedation, sometimes eating and drinking on his way in the door just to show off that he could!

What is a radiation treatment like?

Radiation can be a very stressful time for both children and parents. This section will describe radiation simulation and the process involved in the various types of radiation therapy.

Radiation simulation

Prior to receiving any external radiation therapy, measurements and technical x-rays are taken to map the precise area to be treated. This preparation for therapy is called the "simulation." The simulation will take longer than any other appointment, from thirty minutes to two hours. Because simulation is not a treatment with high-dose radiation, parents are often allowed to remain in the treatment room to help and comfort their child. As discussed previously, some children will need to be sedated for the simulation.

During simulation, the radiation oncologist and technologist use a specialized x-ray machine to outline the treatment area. They will adjust the table that the child lies on, the angle of the machine, and the width of the x-ray beam needed to give the exact dosage in the proper place. In addition, the oncologist or technologist will put small ink marks on the skin to pinpoint the area to be treated. These marks should not be scrubbed in the bath or shower. They do fade with time, so the technologist may need to add more ink at some point in the child's treatment.

Children who wear masks during treatment will have these ink marks put on the mask, not their skin. At some institutions, children who require spinal radiation may have tiny black dots permanently tattooed on their skin. These tattoos are made by putting a drop of India ink on the skin, then pricking with a pin. They look like tiny black freckles.

After the simulation is completed, the child can leave while the radiation oncologist carefully evaluates the developed x-ray film and measurements to design the treatment field.

External radiation treatment

To receive external radiation, children are given appointments to visit the radiation clinic for a specific number of days, the same time each day. They usually have the weekend off. At some institutions and for some protocols, children go more than once a day to receive hyperfractionated dosing. When the parent and child arrive, they must check in at the front desk. The technologist comes out to take the child into the treatment room. Often, parents accompany young children into the room. If the child requires anesthesia, it will usually take place in the treatment room.

The technologist will secure conscious children or teens in place with an immobilization device. Measurements are taken to verify that the child's body is perfectly positioned. Frequently, the technologist will shine a light on the area to be irradiated to ensure that the machine is properly aligned. The technologist and parents leave the room, closing the door behind them.

At some institutions, parents are allowed to stay and watch the TV monitor and talk to their child via the speaker system. If this is the case, the parent should be careful not to distract the technologist as he administers the radiation. At other institutions, parents must wait in the waiting room. The treatment takes only a few minutes, and can be stopped at any time if the child experiences any difficulty. When the treatment is finished, the technologist turns off the machine, removes the immobilization device, and parents and child can go home. There is no pain at all when receiving x-ray treatment.

> I desperately wanted my three-year-old to be able to receive the radiation without anesthesia. I asked the center staff what I could do to make her comfortable. They said, "Anything, as long as you leave the room during the treatment." So I explained to my daughter that we had to find ways for her to hold very still for a short time. I said, "It's such a short time, that if I played your Snow White tape, the treatment would be over before Snow White met the dwarves." Katy agreed that was a short time, and asked that I bring the tape for her to listen to. She also wanted a sticker (a different one every day) stuck on the machine for her to look at. I brought her pink blanket to wrap her in because the table was hard and the room cold. Each day, she chose a different comfort animal or doll to

hold during treatment. So we'd arrive every day with tapes, blanket, stickers, and animals. She felt safe, and all treatments went extremely well.

· · · · ·

There was something about the radiation or the anesthesia that frightened Shawn terribly. He would scream in the car all the way to the hospital. It was a scream as if he was in pain. He had nightmares while he was undergoing radiation and every night after it was over. We decided a month after radiation ended to bring a box of candy to the staff who had been so nice. Shawn asked, "Do I have to go in that room?" When I explained that it was over and he didn't need to go in the room anymore, he asked if he could go in to look at it once more. He stood for a long time and just looked and looked at the equipment. Somehow he made his peace with it, because he never had any more nightmares.

Internal radiation treatment

To receive internal radiation, children are admitted to the hospital. A hospital room is specially designed for patients undergoing this type of treatment. The walls are made from lead, and often items such as sheets and eating utensils are disposable. This is because the child and everything they touch will become radioactive during therapy.

Internal radiation may be given intravenously in the child's hospital room. If it is administered in the operating room, the child will then be transported to the special room, where he will remain until he is no longer radioactive.

When a child receives internal radiation, he poses a radiation risk to others. Children and pregnant women should not visit while the child is receiving internal radiation. Parents and nursing staff have a limited amount of time they can spend in the child's room. This may be distressing for very small children who are unable to understand why people must maintain a safe distance. It may be possible to keep the door to the child's hospital room open. In these instances, parents can sit in the hall and talk to their child to help alleviate any fears or feelings of boredom. Parents should talk with the nursing staff and the play therapist and ask if they have suggestions on how to make the child as comfortable as possible.

Our son was five years old when he was admitted for his internal radiation. The biggest issue we had to deal with was boredom. It was hard for him to understand that I wasn't allowed to spend all my time at his bedside. The door to his room was open at all times, so I moved a reclin-

ing chair into the hall, and that was where I stayed for four days. I would read him stories, stopping from time to time to hold up the book so he could see the pictures. He had a Nintendo machine and a VCR in his room, and that helped to keep him entertained. The nurses even thought of clever games to play. They would inflate rubber gloves and bat them into his room as they passed by his door. After a while they became more and more creative, taking time to draw faces and hair onto the rubber gloves.

Total body radiation (TBI) treatment

Total body radiation is given prior to bone marrow transplantation. There are numerous protocols, each with a different treatment schedule. Two examples are 200 rads given twice a day for three days, or 120 rads given three times a day for four days. The treatments are usually five to six hours apart. Prior to treatment, the child will be measured by the radiation therapist using tape measures and calipers. The therapist will give the family a tour and will show the two cobalt machines on either side of the stretcher in the middle of the room.

On the first day of treatment, the child will be brought to the room (at some institutions small kids will ride a trike or are pulled in a wagon), and may choose to watch TV or a movie, or to listen to a tape or radio. He will lay on the stretcher between the two cobolt machines, and the therapist will position him on his side or on his back. These positions will alternate each treatment, once on the back, then on the side. It doesn't matter which side, so if a child has a sore left side, he can always lie on his right. The child can move a bit—scratch his nose or cross his ankles—but cannot get off the stretcher. The therapist will remove all metal from the child and his clothing— watches, zippers, rings, clamps. Anything with tight elastic—diapers or tight socks—will be loosened or removed. Treatment time lasts from 18 to 35 minutes, depending on the size of the child or teen.

Antinausea drugs are given to prevent vomiting, and these often make the child drowsy enough to doze through the treatment. Some small or extremely active children are sedated.

> *The radiation was easy. When I wasn't sleeping, I watched TV or listened to the radio. I threw up once, but they gave me benadryl and I never was sick again from the radiation. The room was neat, it was painted lots of bright colors and had two big blue machines— one on each side of me.*

Possible short-term side effects

Generally, radiation given to children with cancer lasts a few weeks. When side effects occur, it is often hard to differentiate those caused by radiation from those caused by the high-dose chemotherapy that is sometimes being given at the same time. The severity of the side effects will be dependent upon the sensitivity and the size of the area being radiated. The radiation oncologist is familiar with these conditions and will be responsible for their treatment. Possible short-term side effects are:

- Loss of appetite

- Nausea and vomiting

- Mouth sores and/or sore throat

- Fatigue

- Slightly reddened or itchy skin

- Hair loss

- Low blood counts

- Changes in taste and smell

- Sleepiness (somnolence syndrome) from cranial radiation

- Swollen parotid (salivary) glands from TBI

- Decreased saliva

Methods of coping with most of the above side effects are contained in Chapter 16, *Common Side Effects of Chemotherapy*.

> *When Sean (age eighteen) was diagnosed with rhabdomyosarcoma, part of his treatment included 25 days of radiation therapy to the chest and shoulder area. For the first few weeks his only side effects were low white blood cell counts. However, by the sixteenth treatment, he developed bad burns under his arm and in his throat. This caused him to stop eating and drinking, which led to a hospitalization because he was dehydrated.*

> *Sean had radiation recall twice since his radiation treatments have ended. It seems that each new chemotherapy causes it to come back. The recall makes him lose his appetite, so when he feels good I make sure he eats everything his heart desires to build him back up—just in case it happens again.*

Somnolence syndrome is uniquely associated with cranial radiation and is characterized by drowsiness, prolonged periods of sleep (up to twenty hours a day), low-grade fever, headaches, nausea, vomiting, irritability, difficulty swallowing, and difficulty speaking. It can occur anywhere from three to twelve weeks after radiation treatment ends, and can last from a few days to several weeks.

> Hunter developed somnolence syndrome as a result of his total body irradiation. It caused him to sleep often during the day, sometimes for as much as twenty hours. Luckily, his doctors were just a phone call away. They reassured me that his symptoms were a result of the syndrome. His doctors really listened to me and put my mind at ease. I had been worried because he was experiencing many of the same symptoms that he'd had at diagnosis.

Possible long-term side effects

While short-term effects appear and subside, long-term side effects may not become apparent for months or years after treatment ends. The effects of radiation on cognitive functioning, bone growth, soft tissue growth, teeth and sinuses, puberty, and fertility, range from no late effects to severe, life-long impacts. Second tumors in the radiation field are also a possible long-term side effect. Detailed information about possible late effects can be found in *Childhood Cancer Survivors: A Guide to the Future* by Nancy Keene, Wendy Hobbie, and Kathy Ruccione.

> Matthew had his own calendar outside the radiation treatment room. For every treatment he received, he picked a sticker to place on his calendar. It was a wonderful way to show him how far he had come and how much farther he had to go before he were finished. Matthew loved rummaging through the sticker box for the perfect addition to his calendar. When the last treatment had been given, he was allowed to remove the calendar from the wall and bring it home as a keepsake. We still have our son's calendar. It now has a special place in his scrapbook of memories.

CHAPTER 18

Surgery

Hoping means seeing that the outcome you
want is possible and then working for it.

—Bernie S. Siegel, MD

MOST CHILDREN DIAGNOSED with solid tumors have surgery at some point in their treatment. Surgery is used to biopsy a suspicious mass at diagnosis, stage a disease, insert a central line, and remove or debulk a tumor. The surgeon is an important member of the medical team that works together to make your child well again.

This chapter explains several common types of surgery for childhood solid tumors and describes when they are necessary. Information is provided on the preoperative evaluation process and what happens in the operating room. Then caring for your child after surgery is discussed.

Types of surgery

Children with solid tumors almost always need surgery as part of their treatment. This section describes several of the more common surgeries used to treat children with solid tumors.

Biopsy

Biopsies are used to help diagnose a child with a suspected solid tumor and to determine the extent of disease during the staging process. Biopsies of possible tumors should be done at a pediatric cancer center. This is especially important if the tumor is one which requires surgery as part of the treatment, as poor biopsy technique can affect the success of future surgery.

> *Courtney's original laparotomy (abdominal surgery) was to stage her*
> *disease and hopefully remove her tumor, but that wasn't possible because*

of its size. She had four rounds of chemo to shrink it, then surgery was performed to remove the remainder of her tumor.

• • • • •

Jessica was two years old when she had her biopsy. The surgeon removed a chunk of her tumor to see what it was, and that's when the word, "neuroblastoma" first entered our lives.

Some biopsies are performed in the treatment room of the child's hospital ward under a local anesthetic. Others are done in the operating room under a general anesthetic. The type of biopsy needed depends on many factors, including the characteristics and location of the mass.

Excisional biopsy

A surgical procedure that removes an entire tumor is called an excisional biopsy. This technique is used when the surgeon feels that he can remove the entire mass safely. The surgeon will also remove the tissue around the mass. The healthy tissue removed from around the tumor is called the "margin." The pathologist carefully checks this tissue to see if any microscopic disease remains.

Incisional biopsy

A surgical procedure that removes only a portion of a tumor is called an incisional biopsy. This technique is used when removal of the entire mass is not possible or to obtain tumor samples for diagnostic purposes. It is most commonly utilized when the mass is located in an area that is difficult to reach, when the tumor is too large to remove safely, or it surrounds vital structures that can be saved if the tumor is first treated with chemotherapy.

Fine needle aspiration (FNA) biopsy

Fine needle aspiration (FNA) is another way to obtain a sample of a suspicious mass. FNA can be performed under a local anesthesia in the operating room, the treatment room of the clinic, or in the radiology department. A needle is inserted into the tumor and a small sample of cells are removed. If the amount of tissue removed is too little, a core needle biopsy will often be performed. A core needle biopsy uses the same technique, but the needle is slightly larger so that it can remove a greater sample. Sometimes the surgeon uses a CT scan or ultrasound to pinpoint the exact area to be biopsied.

Vascular access

Children with solid tumors have to endure many months of treatment. The placement of a central catheter for venous access (see Chapter 6, *Catheters*) is a surgery performed on almost all children with cancer. Direct access to a blood vessel allows the administration of chemotherapy, antibiotics, blood products, and hyperalimentation (IV nutrition), and avoids the pain of repeated needle sticks for the child.

Enteral access

Adequate nutrition plays an important role in the child's overall well-being and prognosis. For those children who are unable to eat or drink a liquid diet, enteral access may be necessary. Enteral access, which provides a method to deliver nutrients directly to the gastrointestinal tract, can be accomplished through several techniques, including the insertion of a naso-gastric tube (a tube passed down the nose to the stomach) or the surgical installation of a gastrostomy tube (a tube placed through the abdominal wall into the stomach).

Resection of a primary tumor

Surgical removal of the primary tumor offers the best chance of a cure for most children diagnosed with a solid tumor. Resection of the primary tumor may precede or follow initial chemotherapy. In a few instances, complete resection may be the only treatment required. Resection of a primary tumor usually involves major surgery performed under a general anesthesia. The surgeon will remove the affected organ or all of the mass along with a margin of tissue (the area immediately around the mass that appears normal).

Resection of metastases

Surgery is used to treat some children with metastatic disease. Oncologists use their knowledge of the typical patterns of spread for each disease to determine when this procedure will be beneficial. In the case of osteosarcoma with lung metastases, for example, surgery may be needed each time metastases appear. In other cases, surgery is not indicated for metastatic disease.

Debulking a tumor

Sometimes a tumor can be too large for the surgeon to remove safely. Debulking the mass (removing as much of the tumor as possible without removing it entirely) can have several benefits. The child is often more comfortable after the mass has been debulked and chemotherapy and radiation are sometimes more effective on a smaller tumor. In some situations, the surgeon can install special radiopaque clips used to help direct external radiation with greater accuracy while debulking the tumor.

Second-look procedures

Some children with solid tumors have a second-look procedure three to six months after the tumor is removed. Second-look procedures allow the surgeon to visually inspect the area to check for recurrence and to biopsy surrounding tissue.

Amputation and enucleation

For some children with retinoblastoma and sarcomas, surgery includes the removal of all or a portion of a body part. With the advances being made in childhood cancer treatment, amputation and enucleation (removal of the eye) are less frequently necessary. Researchers are looking for better methods to treat these diseases that will provide the best possibility of a cure while saving the affected limbs and eyes.

Palliation

Surgery can be a method for palliation to improve the child's quality of life. Surgery is sometimes used to create a bypass around an obstructed organ or to reduce pain or pressure caused by a tumor.

> *During her bone marrow transplant, Courtney needed surgery to clear a bowel obstruction being caused by an enormous hematoma (a localized collection of blood). She also needed another surgery to remove a necrotic gall bladder and an appendix that had managed to relocate itself at the top of her liver. While it was difficult for her to go through, it did make her feel better.*

Presurgical evaluation

Soon after a diagnosis of a solid tumor has been made, parents meet with the pediatric surgeon to discuss procedures included in the treatment protocol. This includes the insertion of a central catheter, which usually occurs soon after diagnosis. The consultation is important because it provides the surgeon with background information on your child, including your family medical history. The surgeon will explain the procedures to you, answer questions, and address any concerns you might have. Only an experienced, board certified pediatric surgeon is equipped to handle the special circumstances surrounding a pediatric tumor.

> *My son had several surgeries at different points in his treatment. Each time we had a long discussion with his surgeon to review the procedure and to talk about the possible complications. It made me feel scared when I thought about my little boy lying on an operating table being cut with a knife. Still, I'm glad that the surgeon was so thorough in explaining everything to us. I think that if I didn't know what was going to happen, my imagination would have really given me a hard time.*

The following is a list of questions that you can ask before signing a consent form for surgery:

- What is the purpose of the surgery? What are the expected findings?
- Is this an experimental procedure? If so, how many other children have had it?
- How long will the operation take?

> *Hunter was admitted for surgery to have his primary tumor removed on December 31, 1997. The surgery took four hours. It was the longest four hours of my life.*

- Will administration of blood be required?
- What are the common and rare complications that can occur?
- Will he have a nasogastric (NG) tube or catheter after the operation?
- Will my child need to remain on a ventilator afterwards? For how long?

> *When my child had surgery, the doctor said that there was a possibility that he would need to stay on the ventilator for a few days. Thankfully, that never happened, and he came from the recovery room breathing completely on his own.*

- Will my child need to stay in the intensive care unit after the surgery?

- How much pain will my child have after the surgery? How will it be controlled?

> *An epideral (a catheter inserted into the space just outside the spinal cord to deliver pain control medications) was in place for three days for pain control after Hunter had surgery. It helped to make him very comfortable. He also had a Foley catheter to take out the urine. This was quite uncomfortable for him, but he only needed it for a day or so.*

- When will my child be able to eat?

- How long will it take my child to recover?

> *Zachary had two surgeries to resect an abdominal tumor. He recovered from the first fairly quickly, but the second wasn't so easy. It was a horrible three week long recovery period involving painful bladder spasms, extreme diarrhea, infections, and weight loss. But the good news was that his tumor was able to be completely removed the second time around without losing any of his organs.*

- Will I need to learn how to care for her operation site after she is discharged?

- What are the possible long-term effects of this procedure?

- Will the scar be very noticeable?

> *Logan, who had hepatoblastoma at age one, has many scars. He has a two-inch scar from his port. He has a big scar from his G-tube. It's deep and quite large and it looks just like another bellybutton. He has two drainage tube scars. Logan always says that he had boo-boos in his stomach and the doctors had to cut them out. His doctors always called his scar the Mercedes cut: an upside-down V with a two-inch cut in the center going up the breast bone. Every time we were near a wishing well, we would rub money on Logan's belly and wish that his tumor would never come back. So now every time Logan's has a coin, he pulls up his shirt and rubs the money all over his scar. I tell him they're just his battle scars and he has a special tummy (since he does have two belly buttons). But I hope they'll fade out some.*

Your child may undergo myriad tests prior to the day of the operation, depending on the type of surgery and the child's medical condition. Some of the tests that may be ordered are: blood work, urinalysis, x-rays, EKG, echocardiogram, and pulmonary function tests. Your child's surgeon will explain what tests are necessary.

Some children undergo surgeries that permanently change their appearance. This includes children with sarcomas who need amputation and children with retinoblastoma who have one or both eyes removed. These children should have psychological support in place prior to the operation.

Anesthesia

The anesthesiologist is a key member of the surgical team. It is his responsibility to ensure that the child is properly anesthetized and monitored during the operation. Prior to the surgery, you will have a consultation with the anesthesiologist during which he will ask you about your child's medical history and any allergies to medications. Take this opportunity to ask the doctor any questions you have or to express concerns. For instance, if your child is very frightened, ask the anesthesiologist if he could prescribe a presurgical sedative.

The following is a list of questions you can ask the anesthesiologist before the surgery:

- Will my child be sedated prior to the operation?
- What are the names of the anesthetics you plan to use?
- What are some of the common side effects of these drugs?

> Surgery was a scary time for me. My mother and sister don't do very well under anesthesia, and we were afraid that Sean might react badly to it also. Sean did very well and came through the procedure without any complications.

- Will my child need to remain on a ventilator afterwards? For how long?

You will be asked to sign a consent form prior to the administration of any anesthesia. The anesthesiologist will answer any questions or concerns you might have before you are asked to sign.

The surgery

The surgical technique that will be used is dependent on several factors, including the type and location of disease, your child's general medical condition, and the type of procedure being performed. However, some principles apply to all operations requiring a general anesthetic. Children are usually given anesthesia through a breathing mask, an intravenous injection, or both. A breathing tube is placed in the trachea (windpipe) and connected to the ventilator that will "breathe" for the child every few seconds. Your child will be anesthetized before the breathing tube is inserted.

During the operation your child will be connected to many different monitors to ensure that there is an adequate supply of oxygen in the blood and that intravenous fluids, including blood, are being maintained at proper levels. Blood pressure, heart rate, and other functions are carefully monitored.

Operating room procedures are carried out under very sterile conditions. To minimize the risk of infection, parents are not permitted in the operating room, but are generally able to stay with their child until she is ready to be placed under a general anesthesia. After the surgery, the doctor will meet with the parents and explain how everything went.

> The surgery was handled very well. Paige was treated with kindness and prepared, so she wasn't too scared. We were informed of her progress while surgery was taking place, and the surgeon explained the outcome as soon as he could.

Once the child awakens from the anesthesia, only a liquid diet will be permitted for the next several hours. Solid foods can be given once the doctor feels that it is safe.

> Michelle had over ten major surgeries and more minor ones than I remember. She hated waking up to a liquid diet of popsicles, jello, and juice. One day she pleaded with the doctor to have something else. The doctor replied, "If you can think of anything else that's clear, you can have it." Michelle thought and thought, and she finally came up with jelly, no seeds. So on her next liquid diet tray were little packets of clear grape jelly.

Many children with abdominal tumors may not be able to eat for several days after surgery and may have an NG tube to keep the stomach empty.

Most children having a surgical procedure will not experience serious complications. The risk of complication in the pediatric patient is usually lower than that of the adult, because children tend to become ambulatory (able to move and walk) sooner. Children are remarkably resilient.

My son was anxious to start moving about a few hours after he had his surgery to remove his tumor. He really amazed me. His mobility was limited for a few days, but he didn't let the operation stop him from trying to do most activities.

· · · · ·

I think one of the hardest things about Sean's abdominal surgery was forcing him to follow the doctor's orders and be up and about. He would cry when we would try to make him walk. I felt like such a bad mom, even though I knew it would help him heal faster.

Discharge

When your child is discharged from the hospital after surgery, you are given written instructions on how to care for your child. These may include directions on dressing changes. The most important thing to remember when caring for the operation site is to use proper techniques. Hands should be thoroughly washed with soap and water prior to beginning any dressing changes. All supplies used should be sterile, including gloves and bandages.

You may also be responsible for ensuring that your child complies with daily physiotherapy exercises. Before discharge, the physiotherapist will discuss this with you, and directions to complete the exercises properly are given in writing.

Once Hunter was home from his operation to remove his primary tumor, he was back to himself in under two weeks. However, it did take his left side many months to recover its strength. Physical therapy was provided once a week.

Luke's (age two) surgery occurred four days after diagnosis, so we were still in shock when it happened. There hadn't been any indication that he had cancer except for a fever and partial leg paralysis that gave rise to the diagnosis. He looked sick, but relatively normal, which made it hard for us to accept that he had a cancerous tumor inside of him. His surgery was initially for biopsy only, but once his doctor was in, she decided to do a partial resection. A short operation turned into six hours. We were given updates throughout, which alternately buoyed (she thought

there was a single, encapsulated tumor that she could remove) and dashed our spirits (she found more).

The hard part was seeing him in the recovery room. Our baby, who looked physically perfect and cheerful going into surgery came out bruised, full of tubes, and miserable. I felt like I had inflicted this on him, even though intellectually I knew that it had to be done. I also felt the first pangs of guilt over not being able to "do something" about his illness. After the surgery, he was so hungry and he couldn't understand why I wouldn't feed him. This went against every motherly instinct in me—a mother feeds her child, right? So surgery was an emotional roller coaster ride for me.

More than a year has passed and today Lucas is a happy, energetic little boy. We do all we can to hear his laughter, and enjoy every precious minute of life.

CHAPTER 19

Bone Marrow and Stem Cell Transplantation

The courage of life is often a less dramatic spectacle than the courage of the final moment; but it is no less a magnificent mixture of triumph and tragedy.

—John Fitzgerald Kennedy
Profiles in Courage

BONE MARROW TRANSPLANTATION (BMT) and peripheral blood stem cell transplantation (PSCT) are complicated procedures used to treat childhood cancers and some blood diseases that were once considered incurable. In these procedures, the patient's bone marrow is totally destroyed by high-dose chemotherapy, with or without radiation. Normal marrow or stem cells are then infused into the patient's veins. The marrow or stem cells migrate to the cavities inside the bones where new, healthy blood cells are then produced.

Such transplants, although frequently life-saving, are expensive, technically complex, and potentially life-threatening. Understanding the procedures and their ramifications at a time of crisis can be tremendously difficult. This chapter will present the basics of bone marrow and stem cell transplantation in simple terms, as well as share the experiences of several families.

If a bone marrow or stem cell transplant has been recommended for your child, see Appendix D, *Books and Online Sites*, which lists several easy-to-read publications, as well as many technical articles which will provide more in-depth coverage of the subject.

When are transplants necessary?

At present, some types of childhood cancer cannot be cured with conventional doses of chemotherapy, radiation, surgery, or other forms of treatment.

These tumors may be sensitive to extremely high doses of chemotherapy but these doses permanently damage normal bone marrow. A bone marrow or stem cell transplant allows the delivery of such high-dose, potentially curable therapy, then bone marrow or stem cells are reinfused to rescue bone marrow function.

Many studies using high-dose chemotherapy with or without radiation therapy followed by rescue with bone marrow or peripheral blood stem cells from the patient (autologous transplants) are currently underway for high-risk solid tumors that are sensitive to chemotherapy. For instance, high-dose chemotherapy with autologous stem cell rescue is incorporated in most current cooperative group and institutional studies for treating high-risk neuroblastoma. Tandem transplants (also called serial transplants), in which high-dose chemotherapy is repeatedly followed by stem cell rescue, are also being studied. The role of transplantation is being explored for children and teens with recurrent solid tumors such as metastatic Ewing's sarcoma, and recurrent Wilms tumor, hepatoblastoma, and rhabdomyosarcoma. Preliminary data from some of these studies is encouraging.

> Hunter's high-risk neuroblastoma was treated with a double stem cell transplant. His own stem cells were harvested previously. He had enough cells collected to do three transplants. The third deposit of cells are frozen in case they're needed. The doctor told me that they could be frozen for a very long time. His protocol was very aggressive using chemotherapy, localized radiation, and total body irradiation as the last portion of his second transplant. It has been over a year and he continues to do extremely well.

If a transplant has been recommended for your child or teenager, you may want to get a second opinion before proceeding. Chapter 26, *Relapse*, and Chapter 4, *Forming a Partnership with the Medical Team*, give several methods for obtaining an educated second opinion. In addition, to fully understand the issue, you may want to ask the oncologist some or all of the following questions:

- What are all the treatment options?
- For my child's type of cancer, history, and physical condition, what chance for survival does he have with a transplant? What are his chances with other treatment?

- What are the risks? Explain the statistical chance of each risk.

- What are the benefits of this type of transplant?

- What will be my child's short-term and long-term quality of life after the transplant?

- Will she have to take medicines after the transplant? For how long?

- What are the side effects of these medicines?

- Is this transplant considered to be experimental, or is it accepted clinical practice?

Types of transplants

Under certain circumstances, a marrow or stem cell transplant is the treatment most likely to cure your child. It is important to understand the type of transplant being recommended to enable you to better evaluate what has been proposed for your child.

Autologous marrow transplant

During an autologous bone marrow transplant, the patient's own marrow is withdrawn (harvested) from the large bones of the hips. While the child is under general anesthesia, the doctor inserts a large needle into the bones and withdraws bone marrow. Marrow is withdrawn up to fifty times to draw out a total of one to two pints. The entire process takes less than one hour.

Because the amount of marrow that is removed contains less than 5 percent of the patient's developing blood cells, it takes only a few days for the body to replace the marrow. The child is usually sore for a day or two, and may feel a bit tired for several days. Recovery time varies from child to child.

> Initially, we planned an allogeneic transplant for Matthew. The entire family was HLA-typed to see who was most compatible to act as a donor. My daughter turned out to be a usable match, but the plan was later changed to try for an autologous transplant. We had both bone marrow and peripheral blood stem cells harvested in preparation for the procedure. The bone marrow harvesting was done in the operating room under a general anesthesia. Matthew was returned to the recovery room afterwards experiencing very little discomfort, sporting two bandages on his lower back area.

> *A few months later he underwent stem cell harvesting. Unlike the bone marrow harvest, it required a three day hospitalization. The first step was to have a large catheter inserted in the femoral/groin area. The catheter was used for the actual apheresis of his stem cells. After two days of collection, we had secured enough stem cells to do several transplants. His catheter was removed a few hours later and we were discharged from the hospital. The only real complaint Matthew had was that he had to remain in bed for the entire three days. We had to be sure that the catheter wasn't dislodged through unnecessary movement. It wasn't a big deal for him, though. In fact, he took the catheter home as a keepsake.*

Currently, there are ongoing studies to evaluate the risks and benefits of purged versus unpurged autologous transplants. It is clear from gene marker studies that most relapses following autologous marrow transplantation involve cancer cells infused with the marrow.

After the marrow is harvested and treated, it is cryopreserved (a type of freezing). The patient then undergoes high-dose chemotherapy (and sometimes radiation) to kill all of his existing marrow. The frozen marrow is then thawed, and reinfused into the child or teen intravenously.

> *Courtney (age eighteen months) received an autologous bone marrow transplant as part of her treatment for neuroblastoma. Her bone marrow was harvested eight days prior to day 0—transplant day. Two days after the collection she started high dose chemotherapy, including cisplatin, VM-26, Adriamycin, and melphalan. This took three days to complete and was followed by a day of rest. Two days before day 0 she began total body irradiation (TBI), given in fractions over three days. On the third and final day of TBI, Courtney was given back the bone marrow that had been harvested eight days earlier. That was nine years ago and she has been disease-free ever since.*

Peripheral blood stem cell transplant (PBSCT)

When doctors aspirate liquid bone marrow from the cavities in bones, it is full of stem cells—cells from which all other cell types evolve. Stem cells can also be found in the circulating (also called peripheral) blood, although in a much less concentrated form.

In a peripheral blood stem cell transplant (PBSCT), the cancer patient's own stem cells are harvested in a procedure called apheresis or leukapheresis.

Blood is removed through a central venous catheter or a catheter placed in a vein and circulated through a machine which extracts the stem cells. The blood is then returned to the patient. Each pheresis session lasts two to four hours, and generally four to six sessions are required to harvest enough stem cells for a PBSCT. The stem cells are frozen until the transplant is performed. As with bone marrow, these stem cells are infused intravenously after high-dose chemotherapy.

> Sean had an autologous stem cell transplant. His cells were collected in a process called apheresis. He was connected to a machine that was a lot like what is used for kidney dialysis. He had a catheter installed in his groin area that was used to connect him to the apheresis machine. His blood was removed through the catheter and run through a centrifuge which removed his stem cells and returned the remaining blood components back to his body. His stem cells were purged before they were given back to him on transplant day.

Other transplants

Allogeneic transplants use donor marrow from a family member or an unrelated person. Placental transplants use stem cells from the cord blood of a sibling or unrelated donor. Syngeneic bone marrow transplants are those in which the patient's donor is an identical twin. Since these types of transplants are only very rarely used to treat children with solid tumors (mainly children with neuroblastoma), they are not covered here. If you need information on them, see Appendix D.

> Jeremy had a syngeneic transplant from his identical twin brother as his donor to treat his secondary AML after treatment for Ewing's. He received cytoxan and radiation in his conditioning regimen. One of the worst side effects he experienced was the nausea and vomiting. He was released from the hospital on day 9, readmitted on day 11 because of an infection, and discharged again on day 12. We stayed near the hospital and then we were allowed to go home on day 30. He has done very well.

For more information on types of transplants, write or phone the *Blood and Marrow Transplant Newsletter*, 1985 Spruce Avenue, Highland Park, IL 60035, (888) 597-7674. The *BMT Newsletter* is also electronically published on the Internet at *http://www.bmtnews.org*.

Choosing a transplant center

Choosing a transplant center is a very important decision. Institutions may just be starting a marrow or stem cell program, or may have vast experience. Some may be excellent for adults, but have limited pediatric experience. Some may allow you to room in with your child, while others may isolate the patient for weeks. Protocols vary among institutions as well. The center closest to your home may not provide the best medical care available for your child, or allow the necessary quality of life (rooming in, social workers, etc.) that you need.

The Autologous Blood and Marrow Transplant Registry (ABMTR) collects patient data on autologous blood and marrow transplants performed in North and South America. More than 450 transplant centers from 48 countries are listed on their Web site at *http://www.ibmtr.org/* (click on transplant centers). You can contact them by phone at (414) 456-8325.

To help you learn about the policies of different transplant centers, here are some questions that you might ask:

- How many pediatric transplants did the institution do last year? How many of the type recommended for my child?

- How successful is your program? What are the one-, two-, and five-year survival rates? (Remember that some institutions accept very high-risk patients, and their statistics would not compare to a place that performs less risky transplants.)

- What is the nurse-to-patient ratio? Do all the staff members have pediatric training and experience?

- What are the institution's rules on parents staying in the child's hospital room?

- What are the institution's anti-infection requirements? Isolation? Gown and gloves? Washing hands?

- Describe the BMT procedure in detail. Is radiation part of the pretransplant treatment?

- Explain the risks and benefits of this procedure.

- Assuming all goes well, how soon could my child leave the hospital? Leave the area to go home?

- What will his life be like assuming all goes perfectly? If there are problems?

- What are the long-term side effects of this type of transplant?

- What long-term follow-up is available?

- Explain the waiting list requirements.

- What support staff is available (educator, social worker, child life therapist, chaplain, etc.)?

- How much will this procedure cost? How much will my insurance cover? (This is not applicable in Canada, where the cost of the procedures are covered by provincial health programs.)

Many transplant centers have videos and booklets for patients and their families that explain services and describe what to expect before, during, and after transplant. Call any transplant center that you are considering, and ask them to send you all available materials.

To explore more fully what questions to ask various transplant centers, obtain the *Candlelighters Guide to Bone Marrow Transplants in Children* (listed in Appendix D). This excellent book has an entire chapter devoted to questions to ask to find the best transplant center for your child.

To obtain additional information on how to choose the appropriate transplant center, write or phone the *BMT Newsletter* to obtain the January 1994 issue "Choosing a BMT Center."

> The head of oncology at UCLA comes to our city every two months to follow up on the kids who have been treated there. It was a big draw to us to have post-transplant follow-up at home, rather than having to travel a great distance to get back to the center. The other thing was that children are not put in laminar air flow, and families weren't required to cap and gown, only scrub their hands. Since I'm allergic to those hospital gloves, this allowed me to stay with my daughter throughout. We did, however, call around to several centers to compare facilities, costs, and insurance coverage.

Making an informed consent is a serious decision when considering a life-threatening procedure such as a bone marrow or stem cell transplant. Do not hesitate to keep asking questions until you fully understand what is being proposed. Ask the doctor to use plain English if she has lapsed into medical jargon. Bring a tape recorder or friend to help remember the information. Include your child or teen in the discussion and decision-making process if she wishes. Do not sign the consent form until you feel comfortable that you understand the procedure and have had every single question answered.

Paying for the transplant

Bone marrow and stem cell transplants are expensive. Some bone marrow transplants are considered standard of care, so insurers cover the procedure without problems. However, you will need to carefully research whether your insurance company considers the type of transplant proposed for your child to be experimental and therefore not covered. Most insurance plans have a lifetime cap, and many only pay 80 percent of the costs of the transplant up to the cap. Often, transplant centers will not perform the procedure without all of the money guaranteed. With time of the essence, this can cause great anguish for families who struggle to raise funds or mortgage all of their belongings to pay.

> Our first quote from the transplant center was $350,000, but we were able to negotiate for a lower price.

· · · · ·

> My son died soon after the transplant. I hate to talk about the money, because I don't want people to think I begrudge spending it. I know that I would feel differently if the transplant had been successful, but I honestly think that we were misled about the real chance of success for his type of disease. We spent the equity on our house, plus took out a second mortgage. We will be paying it off the rest of our lives.

If you are having difficulty getting your insurance company to pay for the transplant, contact the Childhood Cancer Ombudsman Program for help (see Appendix C, *Resource Organizations*, for contact information).

If you are not insured (or are underinsured) and must raise all or part of the necessary funds, contact the organizations that provide financial assistance listed in Appendix C. They may be able to offer financial help, and can supply advice on how to quickly and effectively raise funds. Before working with any of these organizations, ask for all printed information available, and ask questions about any fees or costs associated with their services. Make sure that when the treatment is completed or the child dies, remaining funds may be applied to outstanding medical debts. You might also call the *BMT Newsletter* and ask for the November 1993 issue, "Successful Fundraising."

In Canada, each province and territory has a provincial health plan that covers the medical costs of transplant. However, there are still expenses that will need to be covered by the family. Children will often have to travel long distances to facilities that are capable of performing a bone marrow transplant. Travel, accommodations, and related costs have to be paid for by the parents. Bone marrow or peripheral blood stem cell transplants place financial burdens on Canadian families even though the country has a standardized healthcare system.

The transplant

Prior to the actual transplant, the patient's bone marrow is destroyed using high-dose chemotherapy with or without radiation. This portion of treatment is called conditioning. The purpose of the high-doses of chemotherapy and radiation is to kill all remaining cancer cells in the body and make room in the bones for the new bone marrow or peripheral blood stem cells.

Conditioning regimens vary according to institution and protocol, and also depend on the medical condition and history of the patient. Typically, the chemotherapy is given for two to six days, and radiation (if part of conditioning) is given in multiple small doses over several days.

The transplant itself consists of simply infusing the marrow or stem cells through a central venous catheter or IV into the patient, just like a blood transfusion. The marrow or stem cells travel through the blood vessels, eventually filling the empty spaces in the long bones. Engraftment is the process in which new marrow begins to produce healthy white cells, red cells, and platelets.

> *I couldn't believe how beautiful the bone marrow was—a bag of shimmering red liquid. It just glistened. It meant life.*

Emotional responses

Bone marrow transplant can take a heavy emotional toll on the child, the parents, and the siblings. It can be a physically and mentally grueling procedure, with the possibility of months or years of after-effects. Most transplant team members are extensively trained to meet the needs of the patient and family during the transplant and long convalescence. The team usually includes physicians and nurses, as well as psychiatrists, social workers, educators, nutritionists, and child life therapists.

> Leah was feeling very good and very healthy when she went in for her transplant. We lived near the transplant center, and she had a least twenty visitors a day. I think the visits and the nonstop telephone conversations really kept her spirits up.

. . . . .

> Levi's transplant experience was like watching someone wake up from a deep sleep. For the two weeks he was flat on his back, suffering greatly from mucositis and a tummy bug that caused diarrhea for three days straight. It was a real horror. Then one evening he sat up and said, "What's all that stuff?" He was referring to all the gifts that had piled up in the corner of his room. He opened every toy, got down on the floor and drew pictures of all the foods he was craving, and never looked back. He was disgusted that all food tasted like cardboard when he was feeling so hungry. It was like an instant transformation. I think my own recovery was longer. I believe part of me froze in order to survive the transplant, and it took a long time to thaw.

Organizations that can offer emotional support to families during the transplant experience are listed in Appendix C.

> What helped me the most was the decorations and having a positive attitude. My mom decorated the area outside the transplant room with balloons, cards, and posters. It was hard to take the medicine, so my mom made a huge poster to mark off how well I did. Every time I took my medicine, I got a sticker. When I got one hundred stickers, I got some roller blades.

Complications

Some children have a smooth journey through the transplant process while others bounce from one life-threatening complication to another. Some children live, and some children die. There is no way to predict which children will develop problems, nor is there any way to anticipate whether the new development will be a mere inconvenience or a catastrophe. This section will present some of the major complications that can develop post-transplant, and the experiences of several families in facing these problems.

> *The transplant center was very clear about all of the potential problems. That was good, for it prepared me. My attitude is watch for them, hope they don't happen, if they do, then live with them. She had an easy time with the transplant, she's a happy third grader, she's alive, and we feel so, so very lucky.*

Infections

Most infections following transplant come from organisms within the body (e.g., CMV, gut bacteria). Good handwashing and adequately controlled ventilation can minimize infections with staph and fungi.

The immune system of healthy children quickly destroys any foreign invaders; this is not so for children who have undergone a bone marrow transplant. The diseased immune system of these children has been destroyed by chemotherapy and radiation to allow the healthy marrow or stem cells to grow. Until the new marrow or stem cells engraft and begin to produce large numbers of white cells (two to four weeks), post-transplant children are in danger of developing serious infections.

To prevent and combat bacterial infections, children receive large doses of several kinds of antibiotics if their temperature goes above 101°F (38.5°C) any time in the first weeks after transplant. Fungal infections can also occur. Ironically, the antibiotics used to treat bacteria allow fungi to flourish.

After the first month post-transplant, children are also susceptible to serious viral infections, most commonly herpes simplex virus, cytomegalovirus, and varicella zoster virus. Viral infections are notoriously hard to treat, although a few are sensitive to the antiviral agents acyclovir and ganciclovir. Many centers use prophylactic acyclovir or granciclovir or immunoglobulin to prevent these infections.

CMV is usually preventable if the patient and donor are both CMV negative and all transfused blood products are CMV negative or filtered to remove white blood cells.

> *Our daughter (age nine) had a peripheral blood stem cell transplant to treat her Ewing's sarcoma. It's been several months and her white blood cell count is still low, but we have come to the conclusion that we can't*

make her live in a bubble anymore. We are careful to avoid potential risks, though, such as being around large crowds of people.

Preventing infections is the best policy for those children who have had a bone marrow or stem cell transplant. The following are suggestions to minimize exposure to bacteria, viruses, and fungi:

- Medical staff and all family members must wash their hands before touching the child.

- Keep your child away from crowds and people with infections.

- Do not let your child receive live virus inoculations until the immune system has fully recovered.

- Keep your child away from anyone who has recently been inoculated with a live virus (chicken pox, polio).

- Keep your child away from barnyard animals and all animal feces.

- Avoid remodeling your home while your child is recovering.

- Call the doctor at the first sign of a fever or infection.

> *After Hunter's double stem cell transplant, we had to follow many precautions. We had to be careful when we took him out, avoiding large crowds or public places (especially those indoors). He needed to wear a mask when we took him to his doctor's visits. We would take him to plenty of outdoor places for fun. I found the precautions easy to follow.*

For more information on infections, obtain the September 1993 *BMT Newsletter*, "Infections," or read Chapter 8 of *Bone Marrow Transplants: A Book of Basics for Patients*, by Susan Stewart (listed in Appendix D).

Venoocclusive disease

Venoocclusive disease (VOD) is a complication that can occur after bone marrow or stem cell transplantation in which the flow of blood through the liver becomes obstructed. Children who have had more than one transplant or previous liver problems are more at risk to develop VOD. It can occur gradually or very quickly. Symptoms of VOD include jaundice (yellowing of the skin), an enlarged liver, pain in the upper right abdomen, fluid in the abdomen, and unexplained weight gain. Treatment includes fluid restriction, diuretics (such as furosemide), anti-clotting medications, and removal of all but the most essential amino acids from IV nutrition (hyperalimentation).

Long-term side effects

Increasing numbers of children are being cured of their disease and surviving years after a bone marrow or peripheral blood stem cell transplant. The intensity of the treatment prior to, during, and after transplant can cause major effects not apparent for months or years. This section describes a few of the major long-term side effects that sometimes develop after a transplant.

Recurrence

Despite the intensive chemotherapy and/or radiation given prior to the bone marrow or stem cell transplant, some children suffer a recurrence of the original disease. Recurrence is most likely to occur in the first two years after the transplant.

Problems with the eyes

Many children treated with total body radiation (TBI) develop cataracts. How the radiation is administered affects the child's chance of developing this complication. If the total body radiation is given in one dose, approximately 80 percent of children develop cataracts. If the TBI is given in smaller doses over several days (fractionated), the chances of developing cataracts is less than 25 percent. Most protocols use fractionated TBI.

> Naomi has had cataracts for the past six years as a result of radiation given prior to her BMT. She has approximately 50 percent cataract coverage in one eye and 66 percent in the other. She has maintained 20/20 vision in spite of the cataracts. The only thing that she does find, though, is that the contrast of light to dark is affected. For example, in school, the white chalk writing on the black board is difficult to read at times. Bright summer sun or the reflection of the sun off snow really bothers her. She wears good quality sunglasses with UV protection when she is out in bright sunlight.

Decreased tear production may also be a late effect after radiation treatment.

Growth and dental development

Irradiation can affect growth. If your child had total body radiation (TBI) as part of preparation for the transplant, she should be closely monitored for learning disabilities, dental problems (facial bone and jaw growth, delayed development of permanent teeth, incomplete root development), and growth hormone deficiency resulting in delayed or decreased growth.

Thyroid function

Children who receive chemotherapy only do not develop thyroid deficiency as a result of treatment. Those children who receive TBI do, however, have a 25 to 50 percent chance of having low thyroid function due to a decreased production of thyroid hormone. Tablets containing thyroid hormone are usually effective in treating the problem.

Puberty and sterility

Children who had only chemotherapy during the conditioning regimen usually have normal sexual development, though not always. Those who had total body irradiation, however, are particularly likely to experience delayed puberty (the incidence is lower if the radiation was given in several smaller doses). All children who had transplants should be followed closely by a pediatric endocrinologist, who can prescribe hormones (testosterone for boys, estrogen and progesterone for girls) to assist in normal pubertal development. Girls are more likely to need hormonal replacement; boys usually produce testosterone but not sperm.

Children who receive total body radiation usually, but not always, become sterile. This means that after growing up, girls will not be able to become pregnant, nor will boys be able to father children. Ability to have a normal sex life is not affected. Some children treated only with chemotherapy have remained fertile, and to date all offspring have been normal.

Secondary malignancy

Children who receive a BMT or stem cell transplant have a theoretical risk of developing a second malignancy (cancer), particularly if total body irradiation was used in the preparative regimen. Since transplants are relatively new treatments for children and teens with solid tumors, the overall impact and long-term effects are not yet clear. Your doctor can explain known risks given your child's disease and treatment.

Courtney was just eighteen months old when she was diagnosed with stage IV neuroblastoma. We lived in a small country town that was eleven hours away from the nearest oncology center. Her disease had progressed so far that her doctors were amazed that she was still able to walk and that her organs hadn't started to fail. Her treatment consisted of chemotherapy, surgery, radiation, and bone marrow transplantation, including TBI. The transplant was very hard on Courtney and her appearance changed dramatically. It was hard to believe that just days before she had been a chubby little girl who was celebrating her second birthday.

We were told that the transplant would take four to six weeks, but it ended up being a five-month hospitalization for her. It seemed everything that could possibly go wrong just about did. That was almost nine years ago and Courtney is doing well. My advice to parents is to never lose track of the fact that happy endings are possible. The transplant experience was a bad time for her—but it was worth it. Today, she's a beautiful, happy child.

CHAPTER 20

Record Keeping
and Finances

Prosperity is not without many fears and
distastes; and adversity is not without comfort
and hopes.

—Francis Bacon
On Adversity

KEEPING TRACK OF THE voluminous paper work—both medical and financial—is a trial for every parent of a child with cancer. It is a necessary evil, however, because accurate records prevent medical errors and insurance over-billings. Poor record keeping can allow changes in lab results to go unnoticed and untreated. Poor organization of bills often results in parents being hounded by collection companies.

This chapter suggests simple systems for keeping both medical and financial records. Financial record keeping is most important in countries such as the United States. In countries with standardized healthcare, such as Canada, parents never receive a bill for their child's cancer treatment.

Keeping medical records

Think of yourself as someone with two sets of books: the hospital's and yours. If the hospital loses your child's chart or misplaces lab results, you have yours. If your child's chart becomes a foot thick, you will still have your simple system to make it easy to spot trends and retrieve dosage information.

Information that you should record follows:

*   Dates and results of all lab work

*   Dates of chemotherapy, drugs given, and dose

*   All changes in dosages of medicine

- Any side effects from drugs

- Any fevers or illnesses

- Dates for all medical appointments and name of the doctor seen

- Dates for any procedures done

- Child's sleeping patterns, appetite, and emotions

Keeping daily records of your child's health for many months or years is hard work. But remember that your child will be seen by pediatricians, oncologists, residents, radiation therapists, lab technicians, nutritionists, psychologists, and social workers. Your records will keep it all straight and help pull all the information together. They will help you remember questions to ask, prevent mistakes, and notice trends. They will help busy doctors remember what happened the last time your child was given a certain drug. Your records will help the entire team provide your child with the best possible care.

There are as many good ways to record the above information as there are parents. Some of the methods used by veteran parents follow.

Journal

Keeping a notebook works extremely well for people who like to write. Parents make entries every day about all pertinent medical information and often include personal information such as their own feelings or memorable things that their child has said. Journals are easy to carry back and forth to the clinic, and can be written in while waiting for appointments. They have unlimited space. Unfortunately, however, they can be misplaced.

In *You Don't Have To Die: One Family's Guide to Surviving Childhood Cancer*, Geralyn Gaes writes of the value of keeping a journal:

> *Some days my entries consisted of only a few words: "Good day. No problems." Other times I had so many notes and questions to jot down that my handwriting spilled over into the next day's space. I must confess that I probably went overboard, documenting every minute detail of Jason's life down to what he ate for each meal. If he gets over this disease, I thought, maybe this information will be useful for cancer research.*
>
> *I'm not so sure I was wrong. Jason went two years without a blood transfusion, unusual for a child receiving such aggressive chemotherapy. Studying my journal, one of his physicians remarked, "This kid eats more oatmeal than anybody I've ever seen." Which was true. Jason wolfed it*

down for breakfast, after school, and before bedtime. The doctor specu-
lated, "Maybe that's why Jason's blood is so rich in iron and builds back
up so fast."

. . . . .

Record keeping—very important! My father came to the hospital
soon after diagnosis and brought a three-ring binder and three-hole
punch. I would punch lab reports, protocols, consent forms, drug informa-
tion sheets etc. and keep them in my binder. A mother at the clinic showed
me her weekly calendar book, and I adopted her idea for recording blood
counts and medications. Sometimes the clinic's records disagreed with
mine as to meds and where we were on the protocol. I was very glad that I
kept good records.

Calendar

Many parents report great success with the calendar system. They buy a new
calendar each year and hang it in a convenient place such as next to the telephone. Parents can record counts on the calendar while talking to the nurse
or lab technician on the phone and take it with them to all appointments.

Each year I purchase a new calendar with large spaces on it. I write
all lab results, any symptoms or side effects, colds, fevers, and anything
else that happens. I bring it with me to the clinic each visit, as it helps
immensely when trying to relate some events or watch trends. I also use it
like a mini journal, recording our activities and quotes from Meagan.
Now that she's off treatment, I'm superstitious enough to still bring it to
our monthly checkups.

. . . . .

I wrote the counts on a calendar or on little pieces of paper which got
lost. But, to be honest, I didn't keep the medical records very well. I'm
upset with myself when I think of it now.

. . . . .

For a long time I was unorganized, which is very unlike the way I
usually am. I found that my usual excellent memory just wasn't working
well. It all seemed to run together, and I began to forget if I had given her
all of her pills. Then I began using a calendar for both counts and medica-
tions. I wrote every med on the correct days, then checked them off as I
gave them.

Blood count charts

Many hospitals supply folders containing xeroxed sheets for record keeping.

> *The folder used by the hospital that my daughter went to contained four sheets with thirty lines per page. Each line had a space for the date, WBCs, ANC, Hct (hematocrit), platelets, chemotherapy given, and side effects. By the end of treatment I had to xerox more pages.*

• • • • •

> *My record-keeping system was given to me by the hospital on the first day. We were given a notebook with information about the illness and treatment. Also included were charts that we could use to keep all the information about the child's blood work, progress, reactions to drugs, etc. While we were at the hospital we were able to get the information off one of the computers on our floor each afternoon. My notebook holds records and notes for three years. Perhaps I was being compulsive with my record keeping, but it made me feel that I was part of the team working on bringing my boy back to health.*

• • • • •

> *I have several binders that contain Matthew's medical records. One binder contains a copy of every blood test he's ever received, all organized by date and test. CBCs are in the front, chemistries are in the back.*

Appendix B, *Blood Counts and What They Mean*, contains examples of actual lab sheets, and a record-keeping sheet that you can use to keep track of your child's blood counts.

Tape recorder

For parents who keep track of more information than a calendar can hold and who find writing a journal too time consuming, using a tape recorder works well. Small machines are very inexpensive, and can be carried in a pocket.

> *I started keeping a journal in the hospital, but I was just too upset and exhausted to write in it faithfully. A good friend who was a writer by profession told me to use a tape recorder. It was a great idea and saved a lot of time. I could say everything that had happened in just a few minutes every day. I kept a separate notebook just for blood counts so that I could check them at a glance.*

Computer

For the computer literate, keeping all medical records on the computer is a good option. Parents can print out bar graphs of the blood counts in relation to chemotherapy and quickly spot trends.

Keeping financial records

You will not need a calendar or journal for financial records, just a big, well-organized file cabinet. It is essential to keep track of bills and payments. Dealing with financial records is a major headache for many parents, but keeping good records can prevent financial catastrophe.

The following are ideas on how to organize financial records:

*   Set up a file cabinet just for medical records.

*   Have hanging files for hospital bills, doctor bills, all other medical bills, insurance explanations of benefits (EOB), prescription receipts, tax deductible receipts (tolls, parking, motels, meals), and correspondence.

*   Whenever you open an envelope, file the contents immediately. Don't lay it on the desk or throw it in a drawer.

*   Keep a notebook with a running log of all tax deductible medical expenses, including the service, charge, bill paid, date paid, and check number.

*   Don't pay a bill unless you have checked over each item listed to make sure that it is correct.

*   Start new files every year.

> I bought an accordion-style file folder each year to hold everything to do with Stephan. It had a slot each for hospital bill printouts, insurance explanation of benefits, receipts for all prescriptions, all Candlelighters newsletters, pediatrician bills, laboratory bills, and other information.

· · · · ·

> To be honest, the paper trail really gets me down. I can only deal with the stacks every few months. I open things and make sure that the insurance company is doing their part, and then I try to sort through and pay our part.

· · · · ·

*I started out organized, and I'm glad I did because the hospital bill-
ing was confusing and full of errors. I cleared out a file cabinet and put in
folders for each type of bill and insurance papers. I filed each bill chrono-
logically so I could always find the one I needed. I made copies of all letters sent to the insurance company and hospital billing department. I
wrote on the back of each EOB any phone calls that I had to make about
that bill. I wrote down the date of the call, the person's name that I spoke
to, and what she said. It saved me a lot of grief.*

What are deductible medical expenses?

It is estimated that families of children with cancer spend 25 percent or
more of their income on items not covered by insurance. Examples of these
expenses are gas, car repairs, motels, food away from home, health insurance deductibles, prescriptions, and dental work. Many of these items can be
deducted on federal income tax. Often parents are too fatigued to go
through stacks of bills at the end of the year to calculate their deductions. If
a monthly total is kept in a notebook, then all that needs to be done at tax
time is add up the monthly totals.

Medical expenses that could be deducted on US taxes for 1998 were: acupuncture, ambulance, artificial limb, artificial teeth, expenses to modify your
home to provide medical care for your child, crutches, dental treatment,
HMO fees, hearing aids, hospital services, insurance premiums, laboratory
fees, special school or tutor for child with learning disabilities, lodging costs
for family when child is hospitalized, meals at hospital, physician's services,
medicines, nursing care, operations, osteopath, oxygen, psychiatric care,
psychological care, therapy, transplants, transportation to obtain medical
care, wheelchair, and x-rays.

To find out what can be legally deducted for the years your child is undergoing cancer treatment, get IRS publication 502. This booklet is available at
libraries and IRS offices or by calling (800) TAX-FORM, (800) 829-3676
from 8 a.m. to 5 p.m. weekdays and 9 a.m. to 3 p.m. Saturdays.

Canadian families are able to deduct many of the same medical expenses as
those living within the US. To find out what can be legally deducted in Canada for the years your child is undergoing cancer treatment, contact Revenue Canada and ask for IT-519R2—Medical Expense and Disability Tax
Credits. Call Revenue Canada at (800) 959-8281 between the hours of 8:15
a.m. and 5 p.m. weekdays.

If you keep a calendar, an easy way to keep track of tax-deductible items is to glue an envelope inside its cover. Whenever you incur a tax-deductible expense, put the receipt in the envelope, and file it when you get home.

Dealing with hospital billing

Unfortunately, problems with billing are the norm rather than the exception for parents of children with cancer. Here are two typical experiences:

> *Insurance was an absolute nightmare. It almost gave me a nervous breakdown. After all we go through with our children to have to deal with the messed-up hospital billing was just too much—it was the worst part of the whole experience.*

> *We would stack the bills up and try to go through them every two or three months. Our insurance was supposed to pay 100 percent, but the billing was so confusing that they refused to cover some things because it wasn't clear what they were being billed for. The hospital frequently double billed, especially for prescriptions. We just stopped getting our prescriptions there.*

> *We would call them to try to get the mess straightened out, but the billing department was just as confused as we were. They kept sending our account to collections. We did everything in our power to get it straight, but we never did.*

• • • • •

> *We had two distinctly different experiences at the two institutions that we dealt with. The university hospital where my daughter received her radiation gave me a folder the first day. It included, among other things, a sheet from a financial counselor giving all the information needed for preventing and solving billing problems. I never needed to call her because the hospital billing was clear, prompt, and organized.*

> *The children's hospital where she was a frequent inpatient and clinic patient was another story altogether. They billed from three different departments, put charges from the same visit on different bills, frequently over-billed, continuously made errors, and constantly threatened to send the account to collections. I never spoke to the same billing clerk twice. It was a never-ending grind and a constant frustration.*

It is impossible to prevent billing errors, but necessary to deal with them. The following are step-by-step suggestions for solving billing problems:

- Keep all records filed in an organized fashion.

- Check every bill from the hospital to make sure there are no charges for treatments not given or errors such as double billing.

   The hospital changed billing systems halfway through Carl's treatment. For some reason, they were unable to retrieve the records for charges already billed. They lost several hundreds of dollars of charges. I kept calling to get it resolved, but they assured me that the new bills were correct. I gave up trying to pay what we owed.

- Check to see if the hospital has financial counselors. If so, make contact early in your child's hospitalization. Counselors provide services in many areas, including help with understanding the hospital's billing system, billing insurance carriers, understanding explanations of benefits, hospital/insurance correspondence, dealing with Medicaid, working out a payment plan, designing a ledger system for tracking insurance claims, and resolving disputes.

- If you find a billing error, call the hospital immediately. Write down the date, the name of the person you talk to, and the plan of action.

   I often couldn't even get through to the billing representative, I was just put on hold forever. Then I tried to discuss the problems with the director of billing, but she was never in. After about twenty phone calls, I finally said to her secretary, "You know, I have a desperately sick child here, and I have more important things to do than call your boss every day. I've been as patient and polite as I can. What else can I do?" She said, "Honey, get irate. It works every time." I told her to put me through to somebody, anybody, and I would. She connected me to the person who mediates disputes, I got irate, and we went through all the bills line by line.

- If the error is not corrected on your next bill, call and talk to the billing supervisor. Explain politely the steps you have already taken and how you would like the problem fixed.

   The hospital billing was so bad, and I had to call so often, that I developed a telephone relationship with the supervisor. I always tried to be upbeat, we laughed a lot, and it worked out. She stopped investigating every problem and would just delete the charge from the computer.

- If the problem is still not corrected, write a brief letter to the billing supervisor explaining the steps you have taken and requesting immediate action. Keep a copy of each letter that you write.

- Every time you receive an explanation of benefits (EOB) from your insurance company, compare it to the hospital bill. Track down any discrepancies.

- If you are inundated with a constant stream of bills and there are major discrepancies between the hospital charges and what is being paid for by your insurance, ask both the hospital billing department and your insurance company, in writing, to audit the account. Insist on a line-by-line explanation for each charge.

> Within five months of my daughter's diagnosis, the billing was so messed up that I despaired of ever getting it straight. When the hospital threatened to send the account to a collection agency, I took action. I wrote letters to the hospital and the insurance company demanding an audit. When both audits arrived, they were $9,000 apart. I met with our insurance representative, and she called the hospital, and we had a three-way showdown. We straightened it out that time, but every bill that I received for the duration of treatment had one or more errors, always in the hospital's favor.

· · · · ·

> Our account for last year was being audited (at my request) because there was a discrepancy in the out-of-pocket amount. My figure was way different from theirs; their records indicated that we hadn't met it, my figures say we had exceeded it by about $7,000. I had to copy all my records (more than 100 pages) and send them to the company. To make a long story short, they reprocessed the bills and sent me 43 checks—for thousands!

- If you are too tired or overwhelmed to deal with the bills, ask a family member or friend to help. He could come every other week, open and file all bills and insurance papers, make phone calls, and write all necessary letters. Some friends might even enter all your records on a computer for storage.

- Don't let billing problems accumulate. Your account may end up at a collection agency, which can quickly become a nightmare.

Our insurance was constantly months behind in paying our bills to the hospital. The hospital sent our account to collections, despite my assurances that I was doing everything I could to get the insurance to pay. We were hounded on the phone constantly by the collection people, often until we were in tears. We finally just took out a second mortgage and paid off the hospital, but now I don't know if we will be reimbursed by insurance.

Not all stories are so grim. People who are in a socialized healthcare system or on public assistance never even see bills. Many people with insurance encounter no problems throughout their child's treatment.

Our insurance paid 80 percent of everything, no questions asked and always paid us within a month. People shouldn't have to worry about finances or their insurance program at a difficult time like this.

· · · · ·

We have a low income, so we are on the state plan. They give us coupons for each child, and we just hand over a coupon at each visit. I have never seen a bill.

Coping with insurance

Finding one's way through the insurance maze can be a difficult task. Understanding the benefits and claims procedures can help parents get the bills paid without undue stress. The following sections outline steps that will help prevent problems with insurance.

Understand your policy

As soon as possible after diagnosis, read your entire insurance manual. Make a list of any questions you have on terms or benefits.

- Learn who the "participating providers" are under the plan, for, in today's managed healthcare climate, there may be a limited network of providers and hefty penalties or no benefits if the patient goes outside the network.

- Find out what your deductible is.

- Find out if there is a point where coverage increases to 100 percent.

- Determine if there is a lifetime limit on benefits.

- Find out when a second opinion is required.

- Learn when you have to notify the company about hospitalizations—many firms require pre-notification except in the case of emergency.

> *I realized that my daughter had been treated for over four months and I had never called the insurance company. When I read the manual, I was horrified to find out that I had not pre-notified them about three scheduled hospitalizations. There was a $200 penalty for each lapse. I called in tears, and they only charged me for one mistake, not all three.*

Get a copy of every form that you may need to submit—claim forms for inpatient care, outpatient care, or prescriptions. You can cut down on paperwork by filling in all the subscriber information on one of each type of form (except date and signature) and then making many copies. You will have a form ready to send in with each bill.

It may be helpful to determine whether your policy has benefits for counseling. If so, find out how many visits are covered and the level of training required (sometimes only counseling by persons with an MA or PhD degree is covered). Ask if there is a home nursing benefit and how many visits are covered.

> *We changed to a new pediatrician, and he asked me if I thought it would be easier on my son to have visiting nurses come to our home to do the chemotherapy injections and some blood work. Since he had very low counts, it made a lot of sense not to have to go out. It also lessened his fears to be able to stay at home and have the same nurse come to do the procedures. It was a pleasant surprise to find these services covered by our insurance.*

Find a contact person

As soon as possible after diagnosis, call your insurance company and ask who will be handling your claims. Explain that there will be years of bills with frequent hospitalizations, and it would be helpful to always deal with the same person. Insurers may be able to offer parents a contact person for claim review or special needs. Ask the contact person to answer any questions that you have on benefits. Try to develop a cooperative relationship with your contact person because she can really make your life easier. Also, the employer may have a benefits person who can operate as a liaison with the insurer.

My employee benefits representative was Bobbi. She was just wonderful. The hospital would send her copies of the bills at the same time as they sent mine. Since I found so many errors, she would hold the bills a week until I called to tell her that they were correct before she paid them. She was very pleasant to deal with.

Negotiate

Don't be afraid to negotiate with the insurance company over benefits. Often, your contact person may be able to redefine a service that your child needs to allow it to be covered.

My husband works for a small city that contracts out health insurance. A year into our child's treatment, the contract was being renegotiated. He brought home a copy of the proposed contract, and I was horrified to see that they had halved the benefit for transplants, from $200,000 to $100,000. I called the members of the committee negotiating the contract, the union representative, the city insurance liaison, and the city attorney. I was very polite, but I told them that if my child needed a bone marrow transplant, the new contract would bankrupt us. We would lose our home and have to sell all of our belongings to pay our part of the procedure. Then I called two transplant centers, and had them fax me the estimated cost of a routine bone marrow transplant (about $220,000). I sent copies of the fax to everyone that I could think of, and followed it up with phone calls. They changed the new contract back to $200,000. One person can make a big difference.

Challenging a claim

The key to obtaining the maximum benefit from your insurance policy is to keep accurate records and to challenge any denied claims. Some tips on good record keeping are:

- Make photocopies of everything you send to your insurance company, including claims, letters, and bills.

- Pay bills by check, and keep all of your canceled checks.

- Keep all correspondence from billing companies and insurance.

- Write down the date, name of person contacted, and conversation of all phone calls concerning insurance.

- Keep accurate records of all medical expenses and claims submitted.

Policyholders have the right to appeal a claim denial by their insurance company. The following are suggested steps to contest a claim:

- Keep original documents in your files, and send photocopies to the insurance company with a letter outlining why the claim should be covered. Make sure to get the reply in writing.

> We were making inquiries into hospice care, feeling it was time to explore that option. I found out that the only pediatric hospice provider in the state of Georgia was not on the preferred provider list. They would pay for benefits, but at a reduced rate; not a good thing since the lifetime maximum for hospice care was $7,500. With these benefits, we would get 78 days of hospice care. I felt like my only options were reduced pediatric care or full benefits using adult services. I wrote a letter of appeal stating that medically and ethically, neither of these were good choices. Well, we got a better outcome than I asked for. Not only will they cover the pediatric provider, but they have waived the lifetime maximum!

- If the insurance company is refusing coverage because they claim the procedure is "investigational" or "experimental" and therefore not covered, contact the Childhood Cancer Ombudsman Program for assistance. This organization offers a free service to help families maximize benefits or resolve disputes. See Appendix C, *Resource Organizations*, for contact information.

- Contact your elected representative to the US Congress. All Senators and members of the House of Representatives have staff who help constituents with problems.

- If all of the above steps do not resolve the dispute, take your claim to small claims court, or hire an attorney skilled in insurance matters to sue the insurance company.

Above all, don't be afraid to ask questions, and be persistent!

Sources of financial assistance

Sources of financial assistance vary from state to state and province to province. To begin to track down possible sources, ask the hospital social worker for assistance. In addition, some hospitals have community outreach nurses or case workers who may point out potential sources of assistance.

Hospital policy

If you find yourself unable to pay your hospital bills, don't sell your house or let your account go to collections. Ask the social worker to set up an appointment for you with the appropriate person to discuss the hospital policy on financial assistance. Many hospitals write off a percentage of the cost of care if the patient is uninsured or under-insured. Be proactive and talk to the hospital about setting up a monthly payment plan.

SSI (Supplemental Security Income)

SSI is a federal (US) program administered by the Social Security Administration, and is an entitlement based on family income. Recipients must be blind or disabled and have a low family income and few assets. Children with cancer qualify as disabled for this program, making some of them eligible for monthly aid if the family income and assets are low enough. To find out if your child qualifies, look in the phone book under "United States Government" for "Social Security Administration." Call the nearest field office to determine if your child is eligible for SSI.

Medicaid

Medicaid is administered by state governments in the US, with the federal government providing a portion of the entitlement. Rules on eligibility vary, but families with private insurance sometimes are eligible if huge hospital bills are only partially covered. Call your local or county social service department to obtain the number for the Medicaid office in your area. If they tell you that your child is ineligible, ask if the state has an "Aged, Blind, Disabled, Medically Needy" program.

In addition to helping pay some or all hospital bills, Medicaid sometimes also pays transportation and prescription costs. Some states cover children under the age of 21 if they are hospitalized for more than 30 days, regardless of parental income. States are supposed to have Children's Medical Services programs to pay for medical treatment of physically disabled children. These programs allow a higher income level than Medicaid. Ask for a detailed list of benefits available in your state.

Free medicine programs

Many drug companies have programs to provide free medicines (including chemotherapy) to needy patients. Eligibility requirements vary, but most are available to those not covered by private or public insurance programs. You can get a free copy of the Directory of Pharmaceutical Patient Assistance from the Pharmaceutical Manufacturers Association in Washington, DC (toll-free hot line for physicians: (800) PMA-INFO; online at *http://www.pharma.org/patients/*).

While the cost of in-hospital treatment in Canada is covered by provincial governments, families have to pay for other medications at their own expense. For those without private insurance, this usually creates an extreme financial hardship. In many instances, the Department of Social Services can help pay for medications. The qualifications vary in each province and the decision is based on financial need. Canadian parents should contact their provincial Department of Social Services for further information.

Service organizations

There are numerous service organizations that can help families in need. They provide all kinds of aid: transportation, wigs, special wheelchairs, and food. Often, all a family has to do is describe their plight, and good Samaritans appear. Some organizations that may exist in your community are: American Legion; Elks Club; fraternal organizations such as the Masons, Jaycees, Kiwanis Club, Knights of Columbus, Lions, and Rotary clubs; United Way; Veterans of Foreign Wars; and churches of all denominations. In addition, local philanthropic organizations exist in many communities. To locate them, call your local Health Department, speak to the social worker, and ask for help.

Organized fund raising

Many communities rally around a child with cancer by organizing a fund. Help is given in various ways, ranging from mason jars in local stores to an organized drive using all of the local media. There are many pitfalls to avoid in fund raising, and great care must be exercised to protect the privacy of the sick child as much as possible. If you are contemplating starting a fund, read Sheila Peterson's *A Special Way to Care,* listed in Appendix D, *Books and*

Online Sites. This guide gives detailed, step-by-step advice on determining the needs of the family, finding benefits, using publicity, generating community support, and managing the fund.

If your child is on or seeking Social Security or Medicaid eligibility, funds must be held in a special needs trust and paid directly to providers. If the family receives the money or the child's Social Security number is used to open the bank account, the child can lose both Social Security and Medicaid.

> We had excellent insurance coverage, so we never experienced any major financial difficulties during my son's treatment. However, insurance company literature can be so complicated that I felt I almost needed an advanced degree in rocket science to decipher our coverage. Our hospital has a financial counselor available for families that need help. Given the enormous stress that parents are under, I think it's an invaluable service.

CHAPTER 21

Nutrition

*Let your food be your medicine and your
medicine be your food.*

—Hippocrates (fifth century B.C.)

THE EATING HABITS of children with cancer go haywire. Parents know that eating the right types of food will help their child heal faster, feel better, and continue to grow. Moreover, cancer treatment itself increases the need for balanced nutrition. The child's body works hard to repair the damage to healthy cells caused by chemotherapy, and to break down and excrete the cancer cells killed by treatment. Just metabolizing chemotherapy drugs stresses children's systems.

Despite knowing that children need to eat nutritious meals, the reality is that sick children often do not want to eat. This chapter discusses eating problems, explains good nutrition, suggests ways to pack extra calories into small servings, and offers tips on how to make food more appealing to children.

Treatment side effects and eating

Eating is tremendously impacted by most types of chemotherapy. Listed below are several common side effects of treatment which can prevent good eating. Other common side effects, including nausea, vomiting, diarrhea, constipation, and mouth and throat sores, are covered in detail in Chapter 16, *Common Side Effects of Chemotherapy*.

Loss of appetite

Anorexia, or loss of appetite, is one of the most common problems associated with the treatment of cancer. Children suffering from nausea and vomiting, diarrhea or constipation, altered sense of smell and taste, mouth sores, and other unpleasant side effects understandably do not feel hungry. Loss of appetite is most pronounced during the most intensive periods of treatment.

> *My son looked like a skeleton several months into his protocol. I used to dress him in "camouflage" clothes—several layers thick. This kept him warm and prevented stares.*

If your child loses more than 10 to 15 percent of her body weight, she may need to be fed intravenously or by tube. Sometimes this can be avoided by parents learning how to increase calories in small amounts of food.

In addition to simple loss of appetite, your child may experience a side effect of chemotherapy called early filling. This means that the child has a sense of being full after only a few bites of food. If the child is suffering from early filling and eats only when hungry, she may begin losing weight and become malnourished. This chapter will provide dozens of creative ways to encourage your child to eat more.

Increased appetite and weight gain

When children are given high doses of steroids such as prednisone or dexamethasone, they develop voracious appetites. They are hungry all the time, develop food obsessions, and frequently wake parents up during the night begging for another meal.

> *Early in her treatment when Carrie Beth was taking dexamethasone, she would start hitting me in the face in the middle of the night demanding food. I learned to have a bag of snacks and a bottle sitting next to the bed, so I could just hand them over and go back to sleep.*

Most parents become very concerned when their child consumes huge quantities of food and gains weight. A moon face with chubby cheeks and a rotund belly are classic features of a child on high-dose steroids. Much of the extra weight is fluid which steroids cause the body to retain. Avoid foods with increased salt that can contribute to fluid retention and high blood pressure. There are two important points for parents to remember about treatment with steroids. First, when the steroids stop, the extra fluid is excreted and weight drops. Second, the child's appetite usually goes from voracious to poor.

Do not put your child on a diet when he is taking steroids. Instead, try to make the most of this brief time of good appetite to encourage consumption of a variety of nutritious foods. A well-balanced diet now will help your child withstand the rigors of treatment ahead.

If you are concerned about the weight gain, consult your child's oncologist. If the fluid retention is extreme, the doctor may have you restrict your child's salt intake, and in some cases children are given drugs called diuretics to rid the body of excess fluid.

Lactose intolerance

Lactose intolerance occurs when the body can't absorb the sugar (lactose) contained in milk and other dairy products. Both antibiotics and chemotherapy can cause lactose intolerance in some individuals. The part of children's intestines that breaks down lactose stops functioning properly resulting in gas, abdominal pain, bloating, cramping, and diarrhea. If your child develops this problem, it is important to talk to a nutritionist to learn about low-lactose diets and alternate sources of protein. The following are suggestions for parents of lactose-intolerant children:

- Add enzyme tablets or drops to dairy products to make them digestible. Some of these are over-the-counter additives, while others require a prescription. Discuss these additives with the oncologist prior to using.

- Replace milk with cheese, nonfat yogurt, buttermilk, or sour cream.

- Replace milk with acidophilus milk or soy milk, which are easier to digest.

- Remember that milk is a common ingredient in other foods, even bread. Read ingredient lists carefully.

- If no dairy products are tolerated, supply calcium by serving canned salmon, sardines, or calcium-fortified fruit juices. Consult your child's oncologist and nutritionist about calcium supplements.

- Always be sure that products are pasteurized, not raw.

Diet and Nutrition and *Eating Hints* are free booklets available from the National Cancer Institute, (800) 4-CANCER. They both contain recipes and suggestions for lactose-restricted diets.

Altered taste and smell

One common reason why children do not eat is because food has no taste or tastes bad. If the problem is food having no taste, try serving highly seasoned food (e.g., Italian, Mexican, or curried foods). If foods taste bitter or metallic, avoid using metal pots, pans, and utensils. Serve the child's food with plastic knives, forks, and spoons. Replace red meat with tofu, chicken or turkey, eggs, and dairy products.

Some children's taste returns to normal a few months into treatment, some after treatment ends, and for a few children, it takes years before some foods taste pleasant again.

What is a balanced diet?

A good diet includes sufficient calories to ensure a normal rate of growth, fuel the body's efforts to repair and replace damaged normal cells, and provide the energy the body needs to break down the various chemotherapy drugs and excrete their by-products. Research has shown that a well-nourished body will:

- Tolerate more treatment

- Tend to have fewer side effects

- Maintain weight

- Recover faster from treatment

When the body becomes malnourished, body fat and muscle decrease. This leads to:

- Weakness, lack of energy, weight loss

- Decreased ability to digest food

- Limited ability to heal and fight infection

To keep your child's body well-nourished, foods from all of the five basic food groups are needed. The five groups are breads and cereals, fruits, vegetables, dairy products, and meats and meat substitutes. The groups and recommended daily servings are shown in Figure 21-1.

Examples of foods contained in each group are listed next, with a small child's serving size in parentheses beside each food. Consult a nutritionist to determine the serving size appropriate for your child.

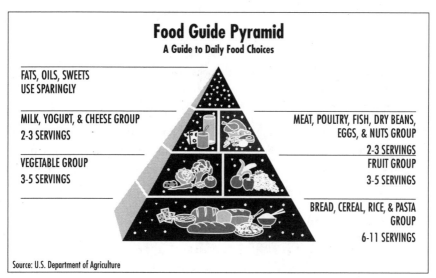

Figure 21-1 Food guide pyramid.

Meat and Meat Substitutes (2 or 3 servings per day)

Meat (1 ounce)

Fish (1 ounce)

Poultry (1 ounce)

Cheese (1 ounce)

Eggs (1)

Peanut butter (2 Tbsp.)

Dried beans, cooked (1/2 cup)

Dried peas, cooked (1/2 cup)

These foods provide protein, which helps build and maintain body tissues, supplies energy, and forms enzymes, hormones, and antibodies. Some typical one-ounce servings of meat and meat substitutes are: a meatball one inch in diameter, a one-inch cube of meat, one slice of bologna, a one-inch cube of cheese or one slice of processed cheese. As you can see, two to three meatballs a day provide all the protein needed by a school-aged child.

Dairy Products (2 or 3 servings per day)

Milk (1/2 cup)

Cheese (1 ounce)

Ice cream (1/2 cup)

Tofu (1/2 cup)

Custard (1/2 cup)

Yogurt (1/2 cup)

These foods provide calcium, vitamin D, and protein.

Breads and Cereals (6 to 11 servings per day)

Bread (1/2 slice)	Dry cereal (1/2 cup)
Oatmeal (1/2 cup)	Granola (1/2 cup)
Cream of wheat (1/2 cup)	Cooked pasta (1/2 cup)
Graham crackers (1 square)	Saltines (3 squares)
Rice (1/2 cup)	Potatoes (1 baked)

These foods supply vitamins, minerals, fiber, and carbohydrates. Try to use only products made with whole wheat flour and limited sugar to get more nutrients per serving. One sandwich made with two slices of bread provides 4 servings of this food group.

Fruits (2 to 4 servings per day)

Fresh fruit (1 medium piece)	Dried fruits (1/4 cup)
Canned fruit (1/4 cup)	Fruit juice (1/4 cup)

Fruits provide vitamins, minerals, and fiber. Fruits can be camouflaged by pureeing them with ice cream in the blender to make a tasty milk shake, or by adding them to cookie and muffin recipes.

Vegetables (3 to 5 servings per day)

Raw vegetables (1/4 cup)	Cooked vegetables (1/4 cup)

Vegetables, like fruit, are excellent sources of vitamins, minerals, and fiber. If your child does not want vegetables, they can be grated or pureed and added to soups or spaghetti sauce. If you own a juicer, add a vegetable to fruits being juiced.

Fats (several servings a day)

Butter or margarine	Cheese
Mayonnaise	Whipped cream
Peanut butter (or nuts)	Avocado
Meat fat (in gravy)	Olives
Ice cream	Chocolate

Although the food pyramid calls for fats to be used sparingly, higher consumption of fats is needed for children being treated for cancer. Experiment to find the fats that your child enjoys eating and serve them frequently.

Vitamin supplements

Vitamin supplements are usually necessary. The nutritional needs of kids with cancer are higher than other children's, yet kids on treatment eat less food. Most children and teens with cancer are unable or unwilling to eat the variety of foods necessary for good health. In addition, damage to children's digestive systems from chemotherapy alters the body's ability to absorb the nutrients contained in the food they do manage to eat.

Vitamin supplementation should be done only after consultation with your child's oncologist. Oversupplementation of some vitamins, folic acid for example, can make your child's chemotherapy less effective. But providing other vitamins can make the difference between a child with dull hair, no energy, and dry peeling skin to one with stronger hair, clear skin, and a better attitude. Vitamin supplements should be individually tailored for your child in consultation with the oncologist and nutritionist.

> I gave my teenaged daughter supplements of vitamins and some minerals. I also increased her vitamin intake by using the juicer every day. She always drank a big glass of fruit or vegetable juice, and I really think it helped her do as well as she has.

Making eating fun and nutritious

In some homes, mealtimes turn into battlegrounds, with worried parents resorting to threats or bribery to get their child to eat. After such scenes, parents, the ill child, and siblings are exhausted, and nutritious food still has not been consumed. The next several sections are full of methods used successfully by many veteran parents to make mealtimes fun and nutritious.

How to make food more appealing

Many children are finicky eaters at the best of times. Cancer and its treatment can make eating especially difficult. The following are general suggestions to make eating more enjoyable for your child:

- Give small portions throughout the day rather than three large meals. Feed your child whenever she is hungry.

- Remember that your child knows best which foods he can tolerate.

In the beginning of treatment, we decided that my son had to eat what the rest of the family was having. If he didn't eat that, he got no more food. He usually just didn't eat. Some mornings, I had trouble waking him up. He was limp, and would have his eyes rolled back in his head. He was tested, and diagnosed with hypoglycemia (low blood sugar). The doctor told us to make sure he ate something right before bed, even if it was ice cream or cookies and milk. Since he has been off chemo, he has not had any problems.

- Explain clearly to your child the importance of eating a balanced diet.

- Make mealtimes pleasant and leisurely.

- Rearrange eating schedules to serve the main meal at the time of day when your child feels best. If she wakes up feeling well most days, make a high-protein, high-calorie breakfast.

- Praise and encourage eating well.

- Don't punish the child for not eating.

- Set a good example by eating a large variety of nutritious foods.

- Have nutritious snacks available at all times. Carry them in the car, to all appointments, and packed in knapsacks for school.

- Serve fluids between meals rather than with meals to keep your child from feeling full after only a few bites of food.

- Limit the amount of less desirable foods in the house. Potato chips, corn chips, soda pop, and sweets with large amounts of sugar will fill your child up with empty calories.

- If your child is interested, include him when making a grocery list, shopping for favorite foods, and preparing food.

Make mealtime fun

The following are suggestions on how to make mealtime more fun:

- Try to take the emphasis off eating food because it's good for you and focus instead on setting a mood of enjoying each other's company while sharing a meal. Encourage good conversation, tell stories and jokes, perhaps light some candles.

- Make one night a week restaurant night. Use a nice tablecloth, candles, allow the children to order from a menu, and pretend the family is out for a night on the town.

- Since any change in setting can encourage eating, consider having a picnic on the floor occasionally. Order pizza or other takeout, spread a tablecloth on the floor, and have an in-home picnic. Some parents even send lunch out to the treehouse for a lark.

> My son enjoyed eating in different places around the house and seemed to eat more when he was having fun. I sometimes fed the kids on their own picnic table outdoors in good weather, and at the same picnic table in the garage during the winter. They were thrilled to wear their coats and hats to eat. Occasionally I would let them eat off TV trays while watching a favorite program or tape.

- Some families have theme meals, such as Mexican, Hawaiian, or Chinese. They use decorations, wear costumes, and cook foods with exotic spices.

- Some children seem to eat better if food is attractively arranged on the plate or is decorated in humorous ways. Preschoolers enjoy putting a smiling face on a casserole using strips of cheese, nuts, or raisins. Sandwiches can be cut into funny shapes using knives or cookie cutters.

> My daughter liked to have food decorated. For example, we would make pancakes look like a clown face by using blueberries for eyes, strawberry for a nose, orange slices for ears, etc. She also enjoyed eating brightly colored food, so we would add a drop of food coloring to applesauce, yogurt, or whatever appealed to her.

How to serve more protein

Since many children and teens cannot tolerate eating meat while on chemotherapy, the following are suggestions for increasing protein consumption:

- Add one cup of dried milk powder to a quart of whole milk, then blend and chill. Use this extra-strength milk for drinking and cooking.

- Use extra-strength milk (above), whole milk, evaporated milk, or cream instead of water to make hot cereal, cocoa, soup, gravy, custards, or puddings.

- Add powdered milk to casseroles, meat loaf, cream soups, custards, and puddings.

- Add chopped meat to scrambled eggs, soups, and vegetables.

- Add chopped, hard-cooked eggs to soups, salads, sauces, and casseroles.

- Add grated cheese to pizza, vegetables, salads, sauces, omelets, mashed potatoes, meat loaf, and casseroles.

- Serve bagels, English muffins, hamburgers, or hot dogs with a slice of cheese melted on top.

- Spread peanut butter on toast, crackers, and sandwiches. Dip fruit or raw vegetables into peanut butter for a quick snack.

- Spread peanut butter or cream cheese onto celery sticks or carrots.

- Serve nuts for snacks, and mix nuts into salads and soups.

- Serve yogurt and granola bars for extra protein. Top pie, Jell-O, pudding, and fruit with ice cream or whipped cream.

- Use dried beans and peas to make soups, dips, and casseroles.

- Use tofu (bean curd) in stir-fried vegetable dishes.

- Add wheat germ to hamburgers, meat loaf, breads, muffins, pancakes, waffles, vegetables, and as a topping for casseroles.

Guidelines for boosting calories

Parents need to alter their perceptions of what constitutes healthy food when they are struggling to feed a child on chemotherapy. Many parents have ingrained habits of low-fat cooking and food preparation. That habit must be replaced by methods that add calories to their child's food:

- Add butter or margarine to hot cereal, eggs, pasta, rice, cooked vegetables, mashed potatoes, and soups.

- Use melted butter as a dip for raw vegetables and cooked seafood such as shrimp, crab, and lobster.

- Use sour cream to top meats, baked potatoes, and soups.

- Use mayonnaise instead of salad dressing on salads, sandwiches, and hard-cooked eggs.

- Add mayonnaise or sour cream when making hamburgers or meat loaf.

- Use cream instead of milk over cereal, puddings, Jell-O, and fruit.

- Make milkshakes, puddings, and custards with cream instead of milk.
- Serve your child whole milk instead of 2 percent milk to drink.
- Saute vegetables in butter.
- Serve bread hot so it will absorb more butter.
- Spread bagels, muffins, or crackers with cream cheese and jelly or honey.
- Make hot chocolate with cream, and add marshmallows.
- Add granola to cookie, bread and muffin batters. Sprinkle granola on ice cream, pudding, and yogurt.
- Serve meat and vegetables with sauces made with cream and pan drippings.
- Combine cooked vegetables with dried fruit.
- Add dried fruits to recipes for cookies, breads, muffins.

Nutritious snacks

Try to get into the habit of always bringing a bag of nutritious snacks whenever you leave home with your child. This allows you to feed her whenever she is hungry and avoids stopping for non-nutritious junk food. The following are some examples of healthful snacks:

- Apples or applesauce
- Baby foods
- Burritos made from beans or meat
- Buttered popcorn
- Celery sticks stuffed with cheese or peanut butter
- Cookies made with wheat germ, oat meal, granola, fruits, or nuts
- Cereal
- Cheese
- Cheesecake
- Chocolate milk
- Cottage cheese
- Crackers with cheese, peanut butter, tuna salad

- Custards made with extra eggs and cream
- Dips made with cheese, avocado, butter, beans, or sour cream
- Dried fruit such as apples, raisins, apricots, or prunes
- Fresh fruit
- Granola mixed with dried fruit and nuts
- Hard-cooked and deviled eggs
- Ice cream (made with real cream)
- Juice (made from 100 percent fruit)
- Milkshakes (made with whole milk or cream)
- Muffins
- Nuts
- Peanut butter on crackers or whole wheat bread
- Pizza
- Puddings
- Sandwiches (with real mayonnaise or butter)
- Vegetables like carrot sticks or broccoli florets
- Yogurt, regular or frozen

Ask for help

It is very helpful to consult the hospital nutritionist to obtain more information and ideas on how to add more protein and calories to your child's diet.

> I had two quite different experiences with hospital nutritionists. At the children's hospital, I couldn't get the doctors concerned about my daughter's dramatic weight loss. She was so weak she couldn't stand, and her muscles seemed to be wasting away. I finally asked the receptionist to please send in a nutritionist. A very young woman came in and talked to me about the major food groups. I felt my cheeks begin to flush, and my eyes glistened as I said, "I know what she is SUPPOSED to eat, I need to know how I can make her want to eat." I must have sounded a bit crazy, because she just handed me a booklet and backed out the door.
>
> The next week when my daughter began her radiation, the radiation nurse took one look at her and called the nutritionist right down. This

nutritionist was very warm and caring. She helped me to understand that I needed to think fat, protein, and calories, and she gave me lots of practical suggestions on how to boost calories. I think that she probably saved my daughter from tube feedings.

Another resource is the American Institute for Cancer Research Nutrition Hotline, (800) 843-8114, Monday through Friday, 9 a.m. to 5 p.m. EST. A registered nutritionist will answer your questions about your child's nutrition.

What kids really eat

The previous part of the chapter listed ideas for increasing calories and making food more appealing. What follows are accounts of what several kids really ate while on chemotherapy. You'll notice how varied the list is, so experiment to see what your child finds palatable. Remember also that children's tastes and aversions change as time passes while on treatment.

Judd craved chicken chow mein and fried rice take out from a Chinese restaurant. He also loved spaghettiOs and hot dogs.

· · · · ·

I let Preston eat whatever tasted good to him which was usually lots of potatoes and eggs. He liked spicy food (especially Mexican).

· · · · ·

Katy typically only ate one food for days or weeks at a stretch. One time, she ate pesto sauce (made from olive oil, garlic, Parmesan cheese, and basil leaves) on pasta every meal for weeks. She also went through a spicy barbecue sauce phase, in which she wouldn't eat any food unless it was completely immersed in sauce. She ate no fruits, vegetables (except potatoes), or meat for the entire period of treatment. She ate mostly cereal and beans when she was feeling well, and mostly pureed baby food when she was really sick.

· · · · ·

In the beginning when Meagan lost so much weight, we snuck Polycose (a powdered nutritional supplement) into everything. She finally got stuck on cans of mixed nuts. They are high calorie, and were instrumen-

tal in putting back on the weight. She also craved capers, and would eat them by the tablespoonful.

· · · · ·

All Brent asks for are "peanut butter and jelly sandwiches, cut in fours, no crusts, with Fritos." The only fruit he has eaten for three years is an occasional banana, and he eats no vegetables. He always ate everything before his diagnosis at age six.

· · · · ·

The doctor told me to keep Kim on a low-salt, low-folic-acid diet. She wouldn't eat anything, so he eventually said he didn't care what she ate, as long as she ate. She liked spaghettiOs, Chick-fil-A nuggets, Chick-fil-A soup, and McDonald's sausage and pancakes.

· · · · ·

All that Carl ate was dry cereal, dry waffles, oatmeal, and bacon. He ate no other meat or vegetables throughout treatment, but did drink milk. I thought that he would never be healthy, but he's fifteen now (diagnosed when two), eats little junk food, never gets sick, and looks great.

· · · · ·

John (fourteen months old) craved creamed corn and pork and beans. I would just sit him on a potty chair at the table and let him eat, and it would go in one end and out the other. When on prednisone, he would sit at the table almost all day. He also drank a gallon of apple juice a day. He rarely eats meat to this day (two years off treatment).

· · · · ·

I guess Carrie Beth is the exception that proves the rule, because she has an excellent appetite. She eats fruits, vegetables, and lots of meat.

Parent advice

Parents whose children have completed therapy offer the following suggestions on how to handle the inevitable eating problems children have during treatment.

Doctors sometimes reassure parents by saying, "His appetite will return to normal." Don't be surprised if this does not happen after the most intensive parts of treatment are completed.

· · · · ·

Let the child control what type of food and how much he wants. In the beginning, any food is good food.

· · · · ·

Buy a juicer, and use it every day. This was the only way we got any fruits or vegetables into our daughter. Make apple juice and sneak in a carrot. Sometimes we would make the juice, then blend it in the blender with ice cubes to make an iced drink, which we would serve with a straw.

· · · · ·

I solved my daughter's salt cravings by buying sea salt and letting her dip french fries in it once a week. For some reason, that satisfied her and stopped her from begging for regular table salt at every meal.

· · · · ·

Try not to worry about your child's future eating habits. During treatment, you just have to let go of normal requirements and feed him whatever he wants, whenever he is hungry.

· · · · ·

Try to work around their taste problems. For example, my son wouldn't drink milk, so I made his oatmeal and cream of wheat with milk instead of water.

· · · · ·

If you only keep good food in the house, and don't buy junk food, your child will eat more nutritious food

· · · · ·.

Take good care of yourself by eating well. We are all under tremendous stress and need good nutrition. I gave my daughter healthy foods and glasses of juiced fresh fruits and vegetables while I was living on lattés (a coffee drink). I now have breast cancer and wish that I had eaten well during my daughter's treatment.

· · · · ·

There is reason for hope. My daughter ate almost nothing while on treatment. After treatment ended, she ate more food but still no variety. She didn't turn the corner until a year off treatment, but now she is gradually trying new foods, including fruits and vegetables again. I'm glad I never made an issue of it.

Commercial nutritional supplements

Many children cannot tolerate solid food or can eat only small amounts each day. Liquid supplements can help provide the necessary calories. The following is a sampling of the variety of supplements that can be purchased at pharmacies or grocery stores. If you are unable to locate a particular brand, your pharmacist may be able to order it for you:

- **Sustacal.** Lactose-free liquid. Flavors are chocolate, vanilla, eggnog, and strawberry. Also comes in a high-protein or extra-fiber formula. 240 calories and 15 grams of protein per 8 oz. can (Mead Johnson).

- **Sustacal Pudding.** Sustacal in pudding form. Flavors are chocolate, vanilla, and butterscotch. 240 calories and 6.8 grams of protein per 5 oz. can (Mead Johnson).

- **Sustacal HC.** Concentrated liquid. Flavors are vanilla, chocolate, strawberry, and eggnog. 360 calories and 14 grams of protein per 8 oz. can (Mead Johnson).

- **Ensure.** Lactose-free liquid. Flavors are chocolate, vanilla, black walnut, coffee, butter pecan, banana, and strawberry. Other formulas are high protein or extra fiber. 250 calories and 9 grams of protein per 8 oz. can (Ross Laboratories).

- **Ensure Plus.** Concentrated liquid. 355 calories and 13 grams of protein per 8 oz. can (Ross Laboratories).

- **Isocal.** Lactose-free liquid. Vanilla. 250 calories and 8 grams of protein per 8 oz. can (Mead Johnson).

- **Enrich.** Liquid with fiber. Lactose free. 260 calories and 9 grams of protein per 8 oz. can (Ross Laboratories).

- **Instant Breakfast.** Powder, which is added to milk. Variety of flavors. When mixed with 8 oz. whole milk, it provides 280 calories and 15 grams of protein (Carnation Co.).

- **Citrotein.** Powder, which is added to water or juice. Orange flavor. 127 calories and 8 grams of protein per 1/4 cup (Doyle Pharmaceutical).

- **Polycose.** Liquid or powder. Powder is added to milk, juice, gravy, or soups. Adds carbohydrates for extra calories. One tablespoon adds 30 calories.

Feeding by tube and IV

Tube feedings or TPN are a necessity for some children with cancer. These types of feedings do not represent a failure on the part of parents or children to "eat properly." Although feeding by tube and IV may require additional hospitalization, parents should understand the benefits clearly. If a child with cancer becomes malnourished, events are set in motion that can have grim consequences. As appetite and weight decrease, the child's ability to repair cellular damage caused by treatment is impaired. The child becomes progressively weaker and resistance to infection decreases. Infections and weakness may require interruptions in treatment. This scenario needs to be prevented. Most protocols require tube or IV feeding after a certain percentage of body weight is lost. There are two types of supplemental feeding.

Total parenteral nutrition (TPN)

Total parenteral nutrition, also known as hyperalimentation, is a form of intravenous feeding used to prevent malnutrition in children who cannot eat enough to meet basic nutritional needs. Some of the many reasons why your child may require TPN are: severe mouth and throat sores which prevent swallowing, severe nausea, vomiting, and diarrhea, and a loss of more than 10 percent of body weight. TPN ensures that the child receives all of the protein, carbohydrates, fats, vitamins, and minerals she needs. The TPN is administered through the central or IV line, but children receiving TPN can also eat solids and drink fluids.

Enteral nutrition

If a child requires supplemental feeding and the bowel and intestines are still functioning well, enteral nutrition may be recommended. Enteral feedings are better than IV when possible. Enteral nutrition is feeding via a tube placed through the nose, mouth, or directly into the stomach through the abdominal wall. See "Gastronomy" in Chapter 2, *Coping with Procedures*. Nutritionally complete liquid formulas are fed through the tube. The appropriate formula will be decided by the oncologist and nutritionist. Infrequent side effects of enteral nutrition are irritated throat, nausea, and constipation.

One parent shared her thoughts on her son's chemotherapy-induced eating problems with these words:

> I feel good nutrition is very important to good health, but the reality of the situation with our child was that he hated anything nutritious when he was on chemotherapy. I could doctor it up, add the best toppings, make it look terrific, season it just right, and it would still be rejected. So I decided since my son wasn't allowed to make any decisions in regards to the pills, treatments, tests, or hospital stays, he wouldn't be forced to eat everything nutritious if he didn't want to. Whether this was a right or wrong decision, I don't know. I just know that I served him a lot of processed foods during those years and he's a healthy and happy teen ten years later. After he was finished with chemotherapy, however, we did require that he eat healthier foods.

CHAPTER 22

School

Most of us had two feelings at the same time:
wanting to go back to school and
being scared of going back.

—Eleven children with cancer
There Is a Rainbow
Behind Every Dark Cloud

CHILDREN WITH CANCER often experience disruptions in their education due to repeated hospitalizations, side effects from chemotherapy, or generally not feeling well enough to fully participate in daily school life. As their health improves and treatment allows, returning to school can be either a relief or a challenge for children with cancer.

For many children, school is a refuge from the world of hospitals and procedures—a place for fun, friendship, and learning. Because school is the defining structure of every child's daily life, returning to school signals normalcy; indeed, expectations of school attendance impart a clear and reassuring message that there is a future. Other children, especially teens, may dread returning to school because of temporary or permanent changes to their appearance or concerns that prolonged absences may have changed their social standing with their friends. Additionally, school can become a major source of frustration for children who develop learning disabilities as a result of treatment. These learning differences, if handled in an insensitive or uninformed manner, can affect a child's confidence and self-esteem.

The issues of educating children with cancer are complex, but most can be successfully managed through planning and good communication. In this chapter, many veteran parents share advice and experiences to help you meet the educational needs of your child.

Keeping the school informed about treatment

Communicating with the school often does not enter a parent's mind during the nightmarish days after diagnosis. Keeping the school informed, however, lays the foundation for the months or years of collaboration as the child goes through the rigors of treatment for cancer. Parents need to forge a strong alliance with the school professionals to ensure that their child, who may be emotionally and/or physically fragile, continues to be welcomed and nurtured at school.

As soon as your child is diagnosed, notify the principal in writing of the child's diagnosis and hospitalization. The next step in ensuring a good relationship is choosing an advocate to be the liaison among hospital, family, and school. The advocate will work to keep information flowing between the hospital and school, and will help pave the way for a successful school re-entry for the sick child. Often the advocate is the hospital social worker, but it may also be a hospital or school nurse, psychologist, principal, or other motivated individual. The most important qualifications for this role are good communication skills, knowledge of educational programs and procedures, comfort in dealing with school issues, and organizational skills. It must be someone you trust to act fairly on your child's behalf.

You will need to sign a release form authorizing the school and hospital to exchange information. Schools have these forms.

The advocate should locate a contact person at the school (or hospital) and should provide frequent updates about the child's medical condition, treatment, emotional state, and tentative re-entry date. The advocate should encourage questions, and address staff concerns about having a seriously ill child in school.

> We had absolutely no problem keeping the school informed as we lived directly behind it. The teacher would frequently stop by on her way home to drop off homework assignments and cards or messages from Stephan's classmates. The school nurse, psychologist, and teacher were at my beck and call. Whenever I felt that we needed to talk, I'd call and they would set up a meeting within 24 hours. I gave them the Candlelighters' book "Educating the Child with Cancer" and they even attended a Candlelighters meeting. They have been wonderful.

Keeping teacher and classmates involved

While your child is hospitalized, it is vital to his well-being to stay connected with his teacher and classmates. Children attend school not only for instruction, but also to develop communication and social skills.

The teacher should be getting updates through the advocate, but the parent can help by calling the teacher periodically, and bringing notes or taped messages to the classroom. The following are suggestions for keeping the teacher and classmates involved:

- Give the teacher copies of *Educating the Child with Cancer* and *Back to School: A Handbook for Teachers of Children with Cancer* (listed in Appendix D, *Books and Online Sites*).

- Have the pediatric oncology nurse or social worker come to class to give a presentation about what is happening to their classmate and how he will look and feel when he returns. This should include a question and answer session to clear up misconceptions and allay fears. Teenagers should be involved in deciding what information should be given to classmates.

- Send pictures of your child on treatment to the school. Some families fill photo albums with pictures that are shared with the classmates.

- Encourage classmates to keep in touch by sending notes, calling on the phone, sending class pictures, or making a banner.

Call the American Cancer Society, (800) ACS-2345, and ask for a comprehensive list of the printed materials and outreach programs available for teachers and parents. Canadians can find information through the Canadian Cancer Society's Cancer Information Service at (888) 939-3333.

Keeping up with schoolwork

Whenever your child is able, keeping up with schoolwork should be a priority. Learning can continue despite school absences. Parents should communicate with the teacher to keep abreast of the subjects being covered in school. Often, the teacher will send assignments and materials home with siblings, or arrangements can be made for pick-up.

To help your child keep up in school, you need to request special education eligibility. Then the child can qualify for an itinerant teacher. Without an IEP or 504 plan, the child is legally entitled to nothing except what the school voluntarily provides, and this is not enforceable.

Joanne Holt, a high school Director of Special Education, suggests:

> *If children are having difficulty remaining interested in school work due to fatigue and not feeling well, it may be useful to consider alternative learning activities. In such circumstances, a parent and child might identify an area of special interest or curiosity (e.g., dinosaurs, space, animals, nature, the Wild West, etc.). Children may find it more interesting to develop reading skills, learn math concepts, develop writing skills, and learn research and study principles in the context of a high-interest area while still learning and maintaining the concepts being introduced in school. Play is a significant part of such activities and can often spark imaginative activities. It is important that the school be aware of and supportive of such an approach; most often they are and, in fact, may be valuable resources for ideas and activities. The goal is to encourage confidence and prepare the child for the least disruptive re-entry to school routines.*

Siblings need help, too

The diagnosis of cancer catastrophically affects all members of the family. Siblings can be overlooked in the early months when the parents are spending most of their time caring for the ill child at the hospital, clinic, or in the home. Many siblings keep their feelings bottled up inside to prevent placing additional burdens on their distraught parents. Often, the place where siblings act out the most is at school. It is very common for siblings to withdraw or become disruptive in the classroom, cry easily, become frustrated, fall behind in classwork, bring home failing grades, cut classes, become rebellious towards authority, or have fistfights with classmates. Siblings, like parents, are overwhelmed by feelings, and generally have fewer coping skills.

You should send a letter to the school principal of each sibling, asking the principal to alert teachers, counselors, and nurses about the cancer diagnosis in the family and ask for their help and support for the siblings.

> *Lindsey was in kindergarten when Jesse was first diagnosed. Because we heard nothing from the kindergarten teacher, we assumed that things*

were going well. At the end of the year, the teacher told us that Lindsey frequently spent part of each day hiding under her desk. When I asked why we had never been told, the teacher said she thought that we already had enough to worry about dealing with Jesse's illness and treatment. She was wrong to make decisions for us, but I wish we had been more attentive. Lindsey needed help.

Remember to include the siblings' teachers in all conferences at school. If the siblings' teachers are in different schools or they have several teachers (e.g., in middle school and high school), ask the principal to send a school representative. They need to be aware of the stresses facing the family, and understand that feelings may bubble to the surface in their classroom. It is essential that parents advocate for the healthy child's emotional and educational needs as well as their sick child's. Chapter 23, *Siblings*, deals exclusively with problems, feelings, and burdens, and contains suggestions for coping.

Returning to school

Although it is normal that parents don't think about school during the early efforts to save their child's life, hospital personnel should reinforce the importance of an early return to school. Going to school helps children regain a sense of normalcy and provides a lifeline of hope for the future.

Preparation is the key to a successful re-entry to school. The parent should ask the physician or primary nurse to prepare a letter for the school staff containing the following information:

- The student's health status and its probable affect on attendance.

- Whether she will attend full or half days.

- Whether he can attend unrestricted general physical education classes, general phyical education with restrictions (e.g., no running), or Adaptive Physical Education for disabled children.

- How much recess is allowed, if any.

- A description of any changes in her physical appearance (e.g., will she bring a wig?).

- Her feelings about returning to school.

- Any anticipated behavioral changes resulting from medication or treatment.

- The possible effect of medications on her academic performance.

- When any medications or other health services need to be given at school.

- A reminder to never give any medication, especially aspirin, which can cause uncontrollable bleeding, without parental permission.

- Any special considerations such as extra snacks, rest periods, extra time to get from class to class, use of the nearest restroom (even if its the teacher's), and the need to leave for the restroom without permission.

- Dietary restrictions, if any.

- Concerns about exposure to communicable disease.

- A list of signs and symptoms requiring parent notification—e.g., fever, nausea, pain, swelling, bruising, or nosebleeds. If parents are divorced, which parent to notify or which to notify first.

- A reminder that the teacher's job is to teach, and the parent and nurse will take care of all medical issues.

Once the faculty has a chance to read the letter, request an IEP meeting that includes faculty, administrators, school nurse, school counselor and psychologist, and special education personnel. At this meeting, answer any questions about the information contained in the letter, pass out booklets on children with cancer in the classroom, formulate a communicable disease notification strategy (if necessary), discuss the ongoing need for appropriate discipline, and do your best to establish a rapport with the entire staff. Take this opportunity to express appreciation for the school's help and your hopes for close collaboration in the future to create a supportive climate for your child.

> I still feel unbelievable gratitude when I think of the school principal and my daughter's kindergarten teacher that first year. The principal's eyes filled with tears when I told her what was happening, and she said, "You tell us what you need and I'll move the earth to get it for you." She hand-picked a wonderful teacher for her, made sure that a chicken pox notification plan was in place, and kept in touch with me for feedback. She recently retired, and I sent her a glowing letter which I copied to the school superintendent and school board. Words can't express how wonderful they were.

· · · · ·

Shoshana (sixteen years old) did incredibly well psychologically while being treated for osteosarcoma. She kept up with school (tutors at home and hospital for tenth and eleventh grade). She also took the SATs and went for a college interview (bald and on crutches). She wrote a research paper using a college library (she was the brains and I was her legs) that blew them over at the interview. She also helped to create a multimedia project for patient information at the hospital.

Shoshana was back in school for her senior year. It was a big adjustment socially. Some kids didn't remember her, some thought she was a transfer student. She was still recovering from the side effects of chemo (lower counts, weight loss, low energy). Shosh was determined to put it all behind her and made college plans. She interned in a research lab and won an award from our community called Courage to Come Back. She won a full-scholarship to our local university (Distinguished Honor Scholar) and moved into the dorm in the fall of '97.

The following are additional parent suggestions on how to prevent problems through preparation and communication:

- Keep the school informed and involved from the beginning. This fosters a feeling that "we're all in this together."

- Reassure the staff that even if the child looks frail, he really needs to be in school.

  The school librarian had a bed set up in the library for ailing students to use. I found out that sometimes Preston would spend the whole day there, because he was just too exhausted to attend class. It was very important to him and his sense of well-being to be at school. He would just drag himself in there in order to be with the other kids. Fortunately, all of his classmates were always nice to him.

  • • • • •

  There was a beanbag chair in the back of Brent's class, and he just curled up in it and went to sleep when he needed to.

- Reassure other children that your child poses no health threat to anyone.

- Bring the pediatric oncology nurse back into the class to talk about cancer and answer questions whenever necessary. This should also be done at the beginning of each new year to prepare the new classmates.

Adam was not comfortable going back to school (kindergarten) when his hair fell out. His blood counts were down most of the time and he caught every cold that came around. When people asked what happened to his hair, he would simply reply, "Cancer," but he wouldn't go into detail. After five years, he still doesn't go into details. I think that he tries to put it behind him and go on with life. He's done a very good job with that.

• Ask the school to bend some rules and policies if you think it will help your youngster. For example, wearing a hat can sometimes eliminate teasing and leaving a three-ring binder with notes, papers, tests, etc., in the classroom can prevent the need to carry a heavy backpack.

My sixteen-year-old son was allowed to leave each textbook in his various classrooms. This prevented him from having to carry a heavy backpack all day. They also let him out of class a few minutes early because he was slower moving from room to room.

• For elementary school children, enlist the aid of the hospital advocate or school counselor to help select the teacher for the upcoming year. Although this violates the policy at some schools, it can go a long way toward preventing problems. Although you have no legal right to this, you can ask nicely to have the policy modified for your child.

Because my son has had such a hard third-grade year, I have really researched the fourth-grade teachers. I sat in and observed three teachers. I sent a letter to the principal, outlining the issues, and requested a specific teacher. The principal called me and was very upset. He said, "You can't just request who you want. What would happen if all the parents did that? You'll have to give me three choices just like everybody else." I said, "My son has had three years of chemotherapy, has a seizure disorder, behavior problems, and learning disabilities. Can you think of a child who has greater need for special consideration?" My husband and I then requested a meeting with him, and at the meeting he finally agreed to honor our teacher request.

• Prepare both teacher(s) and student for the upcoming year.

I asked for a spring conference with the teacher selected for the next fall and explained what my child was going through, what his learning style was, and what type of classroom situation seemed to work best. Then I brought my son in to meet the teacher several times, and let him

*explore the classroom where he would be the next year. This helped my
son and the future teacher adjust to one another.*

- Get professional help. The school counselor can talk with your child
  about problems with grades or classes. A mental health professional can
  help your child express emotions about what is happening in school and
  other areas in your child's life.

  *My daughter went to a psychotherapist for the years of treatment. It
  provided a safe haven for frank discussions of what was happening, and
  also provided a place to practice social skills, which was a big problem for
  her at school.*

- Realize that teachers and other school staff can be frightened, biased,
  overwhelmed, and discouraged by a child with a life-threatening illness
  in their classroom. Accurate information and words of appreciation can
  provide much needed support.

Avoiding communicable diseases

The dangers of communicable diseases to immunosuppressed children were
discussed in Chapter 16, *Common Side Effects of Chemotherapy.* To prevent
exposure, parents need to work closely with the school to develop a chicken
pox, shingles, and measles outbreak plan. Check to see if your child's school
already has an organized disease notification plan. Parents need to be notified immediately if their child has been exposed to chicken pox so that the
child can receive the varicella zoster immune globulin (VZIG) injection
within 72 hours of exposure.

There are several methods used to ensure prompt reporting of outbreaks.
Some parents notify all the classmates' parents by letter to ask for help. If the
parent has a good rapport with the teacher, she can have the teacher report
any cases.

*My daughter's preschool was very concerned and organized about the
chicken pox reporting. They noted on each child's folder whether he or she
had already contracted chicken pox. They told each parent individually
about the dangers to Katy, and then frequently reminded everyone in the
monthly newsletters. The parents were absolutely great, and we always
had time to keep her out of school until there were no new cases. With the
help of these parents, teachers, our neighbors, and friends, Katy dodged*

exposure for almost three years. She caught chicken pox seven months after treatment ended and had a perfectly normal case.

Other parents enlist the help of the office workers who answer the phone calls from parents of absent children.

> *We asked the two ladies in the office to write down the illness of any child in Mrs. Williams' class. That way the teacher could check daily and call me if any of the kids in her class came down with chicken pox.*

What about preschoolers?

A large proportion of children diagnosed with cancer are preschoolers. Parents face the dilemma of continuing preschool through treatment, risking exposure to all the usual childhood viruses and diseases, or holding their child out, which denies them the opportunity for social growth and development. The decision is a purely personal one made after considering the following issues:

- Has the child already had chicken pox?
- Is the child already enrolled and comfortable in a preschool program?
- Are social needs being met by siblings and/or neighbors?
- Is preschool an option given medical considerations?

> *Elizabeth was in preschool at the time of her diagnosis. The manager did a wonderful job of integrating her back into the fold. All of the other children at the school were taught what was happening to Elizabeth and what would be happening (such as hair loss). They learned that they had to be gentle with her when playing. The manager was a former home health nurse, so I was very confident that she would be able to take care of my daughter in the event of an emergency. She was already familiar with central lines and side effects from chemotherapy. She was a gem!*

The terminally ill child and school

In the sad event that the child's health continues to deteriorate and all possible treatments have been exhausted, it is time for the students and staff to discuss ways to be supportive during his final days. Classmates need timely information about their ill classmate, so that they can deal with his declining health and prepare for his death. The possibility of death from cancer should have been sensitively raised in the initial class presentation prior to the student's return to school, but additional information is needed if the student's health declines. The following are suggestions on how to prepare for the death of a classmate:

- The entire school staff needs to be in continuous communication with parents and hospital. They need to be reassured that death will not suddenly occur at school, that the child will either die at home or in the hospital.

- Staff needs to be aware that participation at school is vital to a sick child's well-being. They should welcome and support the child's need to attend school as long as possible.

- Staff can design flexible programs for the ill student—for example, part-time school attendance and/or part-time home tutoring (if appropriate) for a child too weak to attend school all day.

> Jody was lucky because he went to a private school, and there were only sixteen children in his class. Whenever he could come to school, they made him welcome. Because children worked at their own pace, he never had the feeling that he was getting behind in his classwork. He really felt like he belonged there. Sometimes he could only manage to stay an hour, but he loved to go. Toward the end when he was in a wheelchair, the kids would fight over whose turn it was to push him. The teacher was wonderful, and the kids really helped him and supported him until the end.

- Staff can designate a "safe person" and "safe haven" in the school building so that the student can retreat if physically or emotionally overwhelmed.

- The hospital advocate should meet with school personnel and the student's class to answer questions about the student's health status and to address fears and misconceptions about death.

- It is helpful to provide reading materials on death and dying for the ill child's classmates, siblings' classmates, teachers, and staff.

- Extraordinary efforts should be made to keep in touch once the child can no longer attend school. Cards, banners, tapes, telephone calls, or conference calls (on the principal's speaker phone) from the entire class are good ways to share thoughts and best wishes.

- Visits to the hospital or child's home should be made, if appropriate. If the child is too sick to entertain visitors, the class could come wave at the front window and drop off cards or gifts.

- The class can send a book of jokes, a Walkman and tapes, or a basket of small gifts to the hospital.

- The class can decorate the family's front door, mailbox, and yard when the child is returning home from the hospital.

All of the above activities encourage empathy and concern in classmates, as well as help them adjust to the decline and imminent death of their friend.

When the child dies, a memorial service at school gives students a chance to grieve. School counselors or psychologists should talk to the classmates to allow them to express their feelings.

Parents appreciate receiving stories or poems about their departed child from classmates, and attending the funeral also supports the grieving family.

Identifying cognitive late effects

State-of-the-art treatment for childhood cancer has increasingly resulted in greater numbers of long-term survivors, but not without cost. Some survivors suffer neurotoxic effects, which cause changes in their learning style as well as social behavior. These differences may be treatment related, may have been pre-existing and aggravated by treatment, or may be caused by prolonged absences from school and friends.

It is important that parents and educators remain vigilant for potential learning problems to allow for quick intervention. The signs of possible learning disabilities are problems with:

- Handwriting.
- Spelling.
- Reading or reading comprehension, especially compound sentences.
- Understanding math concepts, remembering math facts, comprehending math symbols, sequencing, and working with columns and graphs; difficulty using calculators or computers.
- Auditory or visual language processing, which cause trouble with vocabulary, blending sounds, and syntax.

- Attention deficits. Some children become either inattentive or hyperactive or both. These behaviors are indicative of neurologically based deficits in attention, which can cause children to be more impulsive and distractible than their peers.

- Short-term memory and information retrieval.

- Planning and organizational skills.

- Social maturity and social skills.

You should also suspect learning difficulties if:

- Your child was an A student prior to cancer, and she is working just as hard and getting Cs.

- Your child takes three hours to do homework that used to take one hour.

- Your child reads a story and then has trouble explaining the plot.

- Your child frequently comes home frustrated from school, saying he just doesn't understand things as well as the other kids.

- Your child's teacher complains that she "just doesn't pay attention" or "just needs to work harder."

- Your child complains that he can't hear the teacher.

If any of the above situations are occurring, take action to begin the evaluation process before your child's self-esteem plummets. It is often hard to take this first step because children affected by radiation and/or chemotherapy can reason well and think clearly and may be above average academically in several areas. They may fall behind their classmates, however, on tasks that require fast processing skills, short-term memory, sequential operations, and organizational ability, especially visual. Once identified, these differences can be addressed by strategies such as utilizing resource services in memory enhancement, eliminating timed tests, improving organizational skills, and acquiring extra help in mathematics, spelling, reading, and speech.

> When she entered adolescence, my daughter became very angry
> about her learning disabilities. She used to be gifted, and now does very
> well, but it is a struggle for her. We honestly explained that the choices
> were life with the possibility of some academic problems versus death, and
> we chose life.

Your legal rights (United States)

The cornerstone of all federal special education legislation in the United States is Public Law 94-142, the Individuals with Disabilities Education Act (IDEA). The major provisions of this legislation are the following:

- All children, regardless of disability, are entitled to a free and appropriate public education and necessary related services.

- Children will receive fair testing to determine if they need special education services.

- Schools are required to provide a free and appropriate public education through an individually designed instructional program for every eligible child. An amendment to 94-142, called Public Law 99-457, requires early intervention programs for infants and toddlers at risk.

- Children with disabilities will be educated in the least restrictive environment, usually with children who are not disabled.

- The decisions of the school system can be challenged by parents, with disputes being resolved by an impartial third party.

- Parents of children with disabilities participate in the planning and decision making for their child's special education.

Of course, each school district has different interpretations of the requirements of the law, and implementation varies, so you should contact the school superintendent, director of special education, or special education advisory committee to obtain a copy of the school system's procedures for special education ("Notice of Parents' Rights"). Depending on the district, this document may range from two to several hundred pages. Also write to your state Superintendent of Public Instruction to obtain a copy of the state rules governing special education. To get the address, ask the school principal or a reference librarian.

Children off treatment may also be eligible for services and accommodations under the federal Rehabilitation Act, "Section 504."

> *Destiny (age eleven) has some long-term effects from her treatment for stage IV neuroblastoma nine years ago. Her treatment included high-dose chemotherapy, radiation to the head and brain, and bone marrow transplantation. Her learning ability (in particular, comprehension and short-term memory) has been affected. The special ed department at the*

school told us she was entitled to extra help because of her "other health-impaired" status. This is a label given to children who have undergone specialized treatments that have been proven to result in learning problems. Destiny is in a normal classroom setting, but a special education teacher comes into the room several times daily to give extra help to the kids who need it. Examples of services are: helping with problem solving (especially math), giving her extra time to do work, as well as allowing her to repeat tests that she didn't perform well on. We have found this to be a great help in Destiny's education. She is now making As and Bs as well as exhibiting a more positive attitude toward school in general.

Your legal rights (Canada)

The Canadian special education process is very similar to that used in the US. Provincial guidelines are set down by the national Ministry of Education and governed by the Education Act, but most decisions are made at the regional, district, or school level. Evaluations are done by a team that may include a school district psychologist, a behavioral specialist, a special education teacher, other school or district personnel, and in some cases a parent, although the latter is not required by law as it is in the US.

Children between the ages of six and twenty-two may qualify for special education assistance under the Designated Disabled Program (DDP), the Special Needs Program (SNP), or the Targeted Behavior Program (TBP), depending on the evaluation.

A full range of placement options is available for Canadian students, from home-based instruction to full inclusion. Students from rural or poorly served areas may receive funding to attend a day program outside of their home area.

Referral for services

You will need to be an advocate for your child as he goes through the several steps necessary to determine the best possible education available to him. The steps that will be taken are referral, evaluation, eligibility, developing an individual education plan (IEP), annual review, and triennial assessment.

My son had problems as soon as he entered kindergarten while on treatment. He couldn't hold a pencil, and he developed difficulties with math and reading. By second grade, I was asking the school for extra help, and they tested him. They did an IEP, and gave him special attention in small remedial groups. The school system also provided weekly physical therapy, which really helped him.

Parents or teachers can make a referral by writing the school principal and requesting special education testing. Some school districts will automatically set up an IEP for any child who has had cranial radiation as part of his therapy, while other school districts are extremely reluctant to even evaluate struggling children for possible learning disabilities. Therefore, it is best for the parent or physician to send a written request to the principal stating that the child is "health impaired" due to treatment for cancer, list his problems, and request assessments and an IEP meeting.

Once the referral is made, an evaluation is necessary to find out if the school district agrees that the child needs additional help, and if so, what types of help would be most beneficial. Usually, a multidisciplinary team consisting of at least the teacher, school nurse, district psychologist, speech and language therapist, resource specialist, medical advocate (whoever is serving as the hospital liaison with the school), and social worker meet to administer and evaluate the testing. Areas usually included in the evaluation process are educational, medical, social, psychological, and others.

Some survivors of childhood cancer require neuropsychological testing, which is best administered by psychologists experienced in testing pediatric patients. Most large children's hospitals have such personnel, but it sometimes takes very assertive parents to get the school system to use these experts. Your written consent is required prior to your child's evaluation, and you have the right to obtain an independent evaluation if you believe that the school's evaluation is biased or flawed in any way. However, you are responsible for this cost unless the district agrees or you follow the notice procedures.

After the evaluation, a conference is held to discuss the results and reach conclusions about what actions will be necessary in the future. Make sure that in all written correspondence with the school, you clearly express a wish to be present at all meetings and discussions concerning your child's special education needs. You know him best, and you and your spouse have the right to be there.

Parents need to be aware that children of very high intelligence can, unfortunately, fall into a gap where services will not be offered. This is because they may continue to perform "adequately," according to the school district standards (e.g., achievement scores within two grade levels of the child's age). Gifted children may receive good enough grades (As, Bs, and Cs), even though their potential is that of an A+ student. These assertions may be unlawful if the child meets other eligibility requirements. This discrepancy can frustrate them significantly. In this case, parents should be strong advocates, and continue to seek special services through the school. If you decide to pay for any services out of pocket, give prior written notice to the school and seek professional help to determine if you qualify for reimbursement.

Individual Education Plan (IEP)

The Individual Education Plan describes the special education program and any other related services specifically designed to meet the individual needs of your child with learning differences. It is developed as a collaboration between parents and professional educators to determine what the student will be taught, and how and when the school will teach it. Students with disabilities need to learn the same things as other students: reading, writing, mathematics, history, and other subjects in preparation for college or vocational training. The difference is that, with an IEP in place, many specialized services, such as small classes, home schooling (usually five hours per week), speech therapy, physical therapy, counseling, and instruction by special education teachers, are used.

The IEP has five parts:

1. **A description of the child.** Includes present level of social, behavioral, and physical functioning, academic performance, learning style, and medical history.

2. **Goals and objectives.** Lists skills and behaviors that your child can be expected to master in a specific period of time. These should not be vague like "John will learn to cooperate," but rather, "John will prepare and present an oral book report with two regular education students by May 1." Each goal should answer the following questions: Who? What? How? Where? When? How often? When will the service start and end?

3. **Related services.** There are many specialized services that might be mandated by the IEP which will be provided at no cost to the family.

These can include hearing or speech therapy, health services, occupational therapy, parent counseling and training, physical therapy, and transportation. For these services, the IEP should list the frequency and duration, e.g., "Jane will receive physical therapy from 9 to 10 a.m. on Tuesday and Thursday from September until December, when her needs will be re-evaluated."

4. **Placement.** Describes the least restrictive setting in which the above goals and objectives can be met. For example, one student would be in the regular classroom all day with an aide present, while another might leave the classroom for part of each day to receive specialized instruction in the resource room or physical therapy. The IEP should state the percent of time the child will be in the regular education program and the frequency and duration of any related services.

5. **Evaluating the IEP.** At least once a year, and more frequently if requested by a parent or teacher, a meeting is held to review the progress towards meeting the short- and long-term goals and objectives of the IEP. Some states have limits on the number of IEP meetings per year.

It is best to create a positive relationship with the school so that you are able to work together to promote your child's well-being. If, for whatever reason, communication deteriorates and you feel that your child's IEP is inadequate or not being followed, there are several facts you need to know:

• Changes to the IEP cannot be made without parental consent.

• If parents disagree about the content of the IEP, they can withdraw consent and request (in writing) a meeting to draft a new IEP, or they can consent only to portions of the IEP with which they agree.

• Parents can request to have the disagreement settled by an independent mediator and hearing officer.

The IEP in Canada is almost identical to those used in the US. In Canada, the IEP is updated yearly, or more frequently if needed. A formal review is required every three years. In Canada, if disputes arise between the school or the district and the parents, there is a School Division Decision Review process available to resolve them. The concept known as due process in the US is usually referred to as fundamental justice in Canada.

This year (third grade) has been a nightmare. My son has an IEP that focuses on problems with short-term memory, concentration, writing, and reading comprehension. The teacher, even though she is special ed qualified, has been rigid and used lots of timed tests. She told me in one conference that she thought my son's behavior problems were because he was "spoiled." We asked her at the beginning of the year to please send a note home with my son if he has a seizure, and she has never done it. She even questions him when he tells her that he had a seizure at recess. I began communicating directly with the principal, and I finally received a written notice that he had a seizure. I learned that the IEP is only as valuable as the teacher who is applying it.

· · · · ·

Initially, the school was reluctant to test Gina because they thought she was too young (six years old). But she had been getting occupational therapy at the hospital for two years, and I wanted the school to take over. I brought in articles from Candlelighters Childhood Cancer Foundation, and spoke to the teacher, principal, nurse, and counselor. She had a dynamite teacher who really listened, and she helped get permission to have Gina tested. Her tests showed her to be very strong in some areas, and very weak in others. Together, we put together an IEP which we have updated every spring. Originally, she received weekly occupational therapy and daily help from the special ed teacher. She's now in fourth grade and is doing so well that she no longer needs occupational therapy, and she only gets extra help during study hall. They even recommended her for the student council, which has been a tremendous boost for her self-confidence.

Services for infants and preschoolers

US federal law also mandates early intervention services for disabled infants and toddlers, and in some cases, children at risk of having developmental delays. Infants, toddlers, or preschoolers with cancer may be eligible for these services in order to avoid developmental delays caused by cancer treatments. These services are administered either by the school system or the state health department. You can find out which agency to contact by asking the hospital social worker or by calling the special education director for your school district.

The law requires services not only for the infant or preschooler, but for the family as well. Therefore, instead of an IEP, an Individualized Family Service Plan (IFSP) is developed. This plan includes:

- A description of the child's physical, cognitive, language, speech, psychosocial, and other developmental levels.

- Goals and objectives for family and child.

- The description, frequency, and delivery of services needed, such as:
  - Speech, occupational, and physical therapy.
  - Health and medical services.
  - Family training and counseling.

- A caseworker who locates and coordinates all necessary services.

- Steps to support transition to other programs and services.

> *We have had an excellent experience with the school district throughout preschool and now in kindergarten. We went to them with the first neuropsych results, which were dismal. They retested him, and suggested a special developmental preschool and occupational therapy. Both helped him enormously. He had an IEP done, and now has a full-time aide in kindergarten. He is getting the help he needs.*

Record keeping

Other than medical record keeping, no records are more important to keep than those concerning your child's special education. Many parents recommend that you keep a yearly file that includes the name of the teacher, principal, and district psychologist, a copy of the IEP and all test results, all correspondence, a current copy of the local and state regulations, and all of your child's report cards. You should also include in the file a list of the medications taken by your child during the year. The thought of this may seem overwhelming, but try to think of it this way: appropriate schooling is what will enable your child to overcome the cancer experience and become a productive adult. Your child needs your help to secure that future.

Do not throw these records out—give them to your child when she reaches eighteen. These records can be crucial for college testing and college accommodations.

On accepting disabilities

Many of the disabilities of survivors of childhood cancer are invisible. To help children and teens reach their true potential, changes in intellectual functioning and social skills must be diagnosed early and addressed. Students whose style of learning has changed as a result of treatment need their parents and teachers to explore the many excellent methods to enhance their ability to learn.

It is also important to remember that higher cognitive functioning often remains intact, it is just getting the information in ("processing") that is impaired. Children who were gifted usually remain so; children with average abilities retain them. Their performance may be slower; they may require extra instruction in memory enhancement and organizational skills, but they can still achieve to their potential. There are thousands of survivors in their late teens and twenties who are successfully attending college, or who have graduated and are pursuing professional careers. A disabled survivor of Wilms tumor who is now an expert on disability law wrote:

> These children are not going to have their rights protected, or be eligible (presuming they are eligible) for various services, benefits, programs, and affirmative action unless they say they are disabled. As far as the civil rights laws are concerned, they will be considered disabled from diagnosis till death, even if they are as healthy as the average person. Furthermore, the limited civil rights protection that applies to their parents, siblings, spouses, and partners won't apply unless they say they are disabled.

> I do not think that there is anything shameful or stigmatizing about saying you are disabled. I think the efforts some parents have gone to so they can avoid this word are similar to the old days, when black children wore their hair like white children, and other families changed their last names and stopped speaking their native tongues for fear of "not fitting in." I think if disability is correctly explained to children, they will understand and accept. When I was a child, I was told I wasn't disabled (that was for people who were deaf, retarded, or in a wheelchair), I was merely "very sick" most of the time. It is better to make the effort to teach and have the children enjoy friendships with both nondisabled and disabled children. Otherwise, you end up with adults who feel isolated from even their own siblings.

Armed with the information from this chapter, and material from Appendix D, you will be prepared to effectively work with the school to ensure the very best education possible for your child, the survivor.

My son Zachary has been out of school for over a year. Zachary received a stem cell transplant for his neuroblastoma, and school has not been an option for him in the months afterwards. He is taught by a teacher provided by our county for "homebound" students. She's great, and Zach is ahead of the regular second grade curriculum.

Zach is so comfortable with his teacher that he doesn't want to return to school in the fall. He feels everyone will think he's weird and will tease him. So I tell him we're all weird in our own way and everyone gets teased over something! Actually, I'm not that glib about it. I realize this is an important issue for him, so he is seeing a therapist in preparation for return to school. I feel that will help him a great deal.

CHAPTER 23

Siblings

There's no place like home.

—Dorothy in *The Wizard of Oz*

CHILDHOOD CANCER touches all members of the family, with especially long-lasting effects on siblings. The diagnosis creates an array of conflicting emotions in siblings; not only are the siblings concerned about their ill brother or sister, but they usually resent the turmoil that the family has been thrown into. They feel jealous of the gifts and attention showered on the sick child, yet feel guilty for having these emotions. The days, months, and years after diagnosis can be difficult indeed, for the sibling of a child with cancer.

Of all the topics covered in this book, parents expressed the most regret and guilt over how they handled the pain and worry of their "healthy" children. They share their experiences, in the hope that they will help you to find the time to listen to and love the frequently overlooked brothers and sisters.

Emotional responses of the siblings

Brothers and sisters are shaken to the very core by cancer in the family. Their parents, the leaders of the family clan, are immobile for a while. There is no time, and little energy, to focus on the siblings. During this major crisis for the siblings—this time when their beings are flooded with anger and concern, jealousy and love, when they are in conflict as never before—they often have no one to turn to for help. They may feel utterly alone, abandoned, desolate in their pain. If you recognize these strong emotions of siblings as normal, not pathological, you will be better able to help your child talk about and cope with his overpowering feelings.

Although the time after diagnosis is emotionally potent, stress levels associated with life-threatening illnesses tend to decrease over time. Siblings also tend to have good psychological outcomes. In many cases, siblings report the experience as life changing in many positive ways.

Concern for sick brother or sister

Children really worry about their sick brother or sister. It is hard for them to watch someone they love be hurt by needles, sickened by medicines, lose weight, and be bald. It is hard to feel so healthy and full of energy when the brother or sister has to stay indoors because of weakness or low blood counts. The siblings may also be old enough to understand that death is a possibility. There are plenty of reasons for concern.

> Christine's younger sister has really developed the nurturing side of her personality as a result of the disease. She frequently puts her arm around her sister, comforts her with soothing words or touches, and seems to feel her pain.

Fear

It is very common for young siblings of children with cancer to think that the disease is contagious, that they can "catch it." Many also worry that one or both parents may get cancer. The diagnosis of cancer changes children's views that the world is a safe place. They feel vulnerable, and they are afraid. Depending on their age, siblings worry that their brother or sister may get sicker, or may die. Some siblings develop symptoms of illness in an attempt to regain attention from the parents.

Fears of things other than cancer may emerge: fear of being hit by a car, fear of dogs, fear of strangers. Many fears can be quieted by accurate and age-appropriate explanations from the parents or medical staff.

> My three-year-old daughter vacillated between fear of catching cancer ("I don't ever want those pokes") to wishing she was ill so that she would get the gifts and attention ("I want to get sick and go to the hospital with mommy"). She developed many fears and had frequent nightmares. We did lots of medical play which seemed to help her. I let her direct the action, using puppets or dolls, and I discovered that she thought there was lots of violence during her sister's treatments. She continues to ask questions, and we are still explaining things to her, four years later.

Jealousy

Despite feeling concern for the ill brother or sister, almost all siblings also feel jealous. Presents and cards flood in for the sick child, mom and dad stay at the hospital with the sick child, and most conversations revolve around the sick child. When the siblings go out to play, the neighbors ask about the sick child. At school, teachers are concerned about the sick child. Is it any wonder that they feel jealous?

The siblings' lives are in turmoil, and, being human, they feel a need to blame someone. It's natural for them to think that if their brother didn't get sick, life would be back to normal.

> Our nine-year-old son seemed to be dealing with things so well until one evening as I was tucking him in he confided that he had tried to break his leg at school by jumping out of the swing. He began to cry and told me he doesn't want his brother to be sick anymore; that he needs some attention, too. I was always so concerned with our sick child that I didn't realize how much our healthy child was suffering.

Guilt

Young children are egocentric; they feel that the world revolves around them. It is logical to them to feel that since their sister has cancer, they caused it. They may have said in anger, "I hope you get sick and die," and then their sister got sick.

This notion should be dispelled right after diagnosis. Children really need to be told, many times, that cancer just happens, and no one in the family caused it. They need to understand that just because you think something or say something, it doesn't make it happen.

Beyond feeling guilt for causing the cancer, most siblings feel shame for their normal emotional responses to cancer like anger and jealousy. They think, "How can I feel this way about my brother when he's so sick?" Assure them that the many conflicting feelings they are experiencing are normal and expected. As a parent, share some of your conflicting feelings (anger at the behavior of a child on prednisone, guilt about being angry).

Some children even feel guilt for being healthy! They think, "Why should I feel great when he's so frail and sick?"

Abandonment

When parental attention revolves around the sick child, siblings may feel isolated and resentful. Even when parents make a conscious effort not to be so preoccupied with the ill child, siblings still perceive that they are not getting their fair share of attention, and may feel rejected.

> One day when my four-year-old son was in day care, we had to unexpectedly bring Erica in for emergency surgery on a septic hip. (It turned out to be a life-threatening surgery, and she ended up staying in for weeks.) I called the day care and said that I couldn't pick up Daniel by closing time and the teacher said, "No problem, I live right across the street and I'll take him home for dinner." We went to get Daniel that evening, and he was very withdrawn. Later, he exclaimed, "All the mommies came. Then teacher turned out the lights, and you didn't come to get me." Then he burst into tears. In hindsight, one of us should have gone to bring him to the hospital to just sit with us. It was tense there, but at least he would have been with us, included as part of the family.

Sadness

Siblings have many very good reasons to be sad. They miss their parents and the time they used to spend together. They miss the life they used to have, the one they were comfortable with. They worry that their brother or sister may die. Some children show their sadness by crying often; others withdraw and become depressed. Often children confide in relatives or friends that they think their parents don't love them anymore.

> When Jeremy was very sick and hospitalized, we sent his older brother Jason to his grandparents for long periods of time. We thought that he understood the reasons, but a year after Jeremy finished treatment, Jason (nine years old) said, "Of course, I know that you love Jeremy more than me anyway. You were always sending me away so that you could spend time with him." It just broke my heart that every time he made that long drive over the mountains with his grandparents, he was thinking that he was being sent away.

Anger

Children's lives are disrupted by a brother or sister's diagnosis of cancer, and it can make siblings very angry. Questions such as "Why did this happen to us?" or "Why can't things be the way they used to be?" are common. Children's anger may be directed at their sick brother, their parents, relatives, friends, or doctor. Children's anger may have a variety of causes, for instance, being left with babysitters so often, unequal application of family rules, or additional responsibilities at home. Because each member of the family may have frayed nerves, explosions of temper can occur.

> As we were driving home from school one day, Annie was talking, and I was only half listening. All of a sudden I realized that she was yelling at me. She screamed, "See, this is what I mean. You never listen, your mind is always on Preston." I pulled the car over, stopped, and said, "You're right. I was thinking about Preston." I told her that from now on I would try to give her my full attention. I realized that I would really have to make an effort to focus on what she was saying and not be so distracted. This conversation helped to clear the air for a while. I tried to take her out frequently for coffee or ice cream to just sit, listen, and concentrate on what she was saying.

Worrying about what happens at the hospital

Children have vivid imaginations, and when they are fueled by disrupted households and whispered conversations between teary parents, children can imagine truly horrible things. Seeing how their ill sister looks upon returning from a hospital stay can reinforce their fears that awful things happen at the clinic or hospital. Age-appropriate, verbal explanations can help children understand what happens at the hospital, but nothing is as powerful as a visit. Of course the effectiveness of a visit depends on your child's age and temperament, but many parents said bringing the siblings along helps everyone. The sibling gains an accurate understanding of hospital procedures, the sick child is comforted by the presence of the sibling, and the parent gets to spend time with both (or more) children.

Another method that minimizes worry is reading age-appropriate books together. Many children's hospitals have coloring books for preschoolers that explain hospital procedures with pictures and clear language. Adolescents might be helped by seeing videos on the subject or joining a sibling support group.

Veteran parents suggest that another way to reduce siblings' worries is to allow even the youngest children to help the family in some way. As long as children have clear explanations of the situation and concrete jobs to do that will benefit the family, they tend to rise to the occasion. Make them feel they are a necessary and integral part of the family's effort to face cancer together.

Concern about parents

Exhausted parents often are not aware of the strong feelings of their healthy children. They sometimes assume that children understand that they are loved, and would be getting the same attention if they were the one who had cancer. But siblings frequently do not share their powerful feelings of anger, jealousy, or worry because they love their parents and do not want to place additional burdens on them. It is all too common to hear siblings say, "I have to be the strong one. I don't want to cause my parents any more pain." But burdens are lighter if shared, and parents need to try to encourage all of their children to talk about how they are feeling.

Sibling experiences

Simply understanding the depth of the pain and fears of your "healthy" children eases their path. Being available to listen, to say, "I hear how painful this is for you," or "You sound scared. I am, too," makes siblings feel that they are still valued members of the family, that even though their brother or sister is absorbing the lion's share of parents' time and care, they are still cherished. Even if parents do not have large amounts of time to spend with them, siblings need to hear that what they feel matters. If parents understand that these overwhelming emotions are normal, expected, and healthy, they can provide solace.

Brothers and sisters of children with cancer shared the following stories to illuminate the difficulties they face.

First, Alana Friedman (eleven years old) remembers how family life changed when her sister, Laura, had cancer:

> My sister was in fifth grade, and had been sick for the last week or so. Laura always seemed to be my hero, although we got into arguments, all siblings get into fights, so I didn't worry. I didn't know what was about to happen, but neither did anyone else.
>
> I don't quite remember how my parents told me she had cancer, but I do remember a lot of tears.
>
> As time progressed my life changed. I lived with my best friend and her parents, Catherine and Bill, but that changed too. Kelsie (my friend) and I got into a lot of arguments, but we still do. I don't know if that is

why my grandmother and grandfather moved up to live in our house so that they could take care of me. Living with them was different. My grandmother had different expectations of me than my mother did.

My parents would each take turns staying at the hospital. Some nights I would live with my mom, grammy, and grandpy; and the next it would be with my dad and them.

Of course, going through this dilemma I felt left out. Here I was living with my grandparents, and my sister got to live with our parents. She got lots of flowers, cards, and gifts and all I got was the feeling of love from my relatives. I know that love is better than material things, but when you are six years old, you don't think so.

Things stayed the same for a long time. Then my sister went into remission and started living at home. I had to get used to my parents again and missed my grandparents.

My sister was spoiled at home too. They bought her a water bed, so she wouldn't get cold. What did I get? A heating blanket—a used heating blanket.

A few months after she came home, her remission ended. She went back to live in the hospital, and my grandparents moved up to live with me.

Things went downhill from there. My life was turned around again. My sister went into a coma, and didn't really have much of a chance of coming out of it. Soon it would be her best friend's birthday, and Laura had to miss it. She was taken to heaven that day. Taken out of her misery and leaving us with a feeling of shock.

The day my sister died I had no idea what was happening. Kelsie's mom took care of me and everything was going great. To me, that is. But when her mom took me back home, I remember my dad at the door talking to her. I headed in the other direction, but my father stopped me. My dad went into my parents' bedroom with me, and there I found my mom, lying on the bed helplessly, and to this day I still remember what she said to me, "It's over." Those words didn't make a lot of sense to me—I didn't know if the earth was going to explode. And then those two words sunk into my heart and I knew; my sister had died.

Alison Leake gives a six year old's perspective:

> I think having a sister with cancer is not fun. My mom paid more attention to Kathryn, my sister. I had to stay with daddy! Mommy picked Kathryn up and not me! I wanted my sister's PJs. Guess what? I did not get them! Although my mommy wanted to stay with me she did not want to leave my sister alone. Sometimes I felt like I was going to throw up. Now she has stopped having medicine and she is completely better. To celebrate that my sister and I were such good sports when my sister had cancer, we are going to Disneyland!

Allison Ellis (twenty years old), now a graduate of Smith College and counselor at a camp for victims of childhood cancer and their siblings, says siblings can become "forgotten children":

> I remember walking into my sister's room one morning and seeing large clumps of blond hair on her pillow. "Mommy, why is Lisa's hair falling out?" I asked.
>
> "She's sick," was the only reply possible from my mother; she had no time for lengthy explanations to a three year old. So I was left to solve the mystery for myself. I went with Lisa and my mother several times a week to the hospital where Lisa would get finger "pokies" and sometimes "bone marrows" (which I thought of as "bone arrows" because the procedure entailed being punctured in the back by a large needle). Lisa would always cry afterward—the kind of childhood cry that seems to go on for hours at a deafening pitch. She lost all of her hair, so she wore bonnets that my grandmother made for her until her hair grew back. Sometimes she would get sick and throw up, and sometimes she stayed overnight at the hospital. I remember not understanding at all what was happening to my sister and not receiving any explanations. I remember the toys, gifts, and candy that were given in surplus to Lisa in a futile attempt to ease her pain. I felt jealous, neglected, and isolated because of Lisa's illness and the subsequent attention that was given to her and taken from me. I spent a lot of time with babysitters and television and less with my parents and the relatives who visited only to see Lisa. It seemed as though she was the only one people cared about. In this, I was the typical sibling of a victim of childhood cancer.
>
> Lisa was diagnosed with cancer in 1973 when she was just two years old and I was three. It was not expected that Lisa would live; in fact, all diagnoses of cancer before 1970 were terminal. My parents were told not

to talk about the disease with anyone; a child dying of cancer was just too frightening. Lisa underwent radiation therapy as well as chemotherapy to rid her body of the cancer-causing cells.

Yet, the result of this trauma was that I, as a sibling, received no attention relative to the rest of my family, and I felt extremely left out. I remember having a babysitter who stayed with me and my newborn baby sister during Lisa's treatment who seemed to understand how I was feeling. She would say, "Allison, I bet you're feeling a little bit left out with all the fuss over your sisters." (The youngest was given a lot of attention because everyone pays attention to newborn babies.)

I would always utter a modest, "Yeah, I guess so," while really thinking, "Yes, nobody pays attention to me. All I do is watch Sesame Street and watch Lisa play with her new toys that she got because she is sick and she won't share them with me. You bet I feel left out!"

I remember going places with my mother and being totally ignored by the people we would meet. People would say to my mother, "How is your daughter?" I would always say, "Fine," but they were never referring to me. "Not you," they would say, "the other one," rendering my health and condition completely unimportant. I felt like a nonentity.

I began to taunt my sister, and we would fight frequently over sharing toys or clothes, which for the most part could be attributed to normal sibling rivalries, yet a lot of my hostilities ran deeper than a few pulled hairs. Lisa was the favored member of the family, and she received deferential and preferential treatment. When she came home crying after school, which was frequently the case in the first few years after her treatment was completed, she was always met with solace and understanding, whereas if I was ever upset, I was left to work things out for myself.

Today I understand better why I had the feelings that I did regarding my sister's cancer. For many years I resented her for something she had no control over and was angry at my parents for treating her differently than me. I now realize that no parent is superhuman and that they were doing what they thought was best under the unfortunate circumstances. Yet I know there are certain things I cannot change, such as being the first born. Whereas cancer made my sister vulnerable and my parents more protective, being the sibling of a cancer patient made me more independent. I was forced to find other sources of comfort at an early age, which usually meant that it had to come from within myself. Being at camp made me realize that I wasn't the only one who had experienced such a difficult role, however, and that there are many others who have been affected by childhood cancer much more deeply than me.

In conclusion, I wish to offer some advice. Siblings: please tell your parents in any way you can how you are feeling. Remember that you are not alone and you need not be forgotten, but try to understand where your parents are coming from. Parents: listen to your children. Recognize that siblings have different needs from cancer patients and try to even out attention-giving. Don't be surprised if your sibling child is angry at you. Professionals and neighbors: sometimes you are the only hope for a neglected sibling, yet you also have the potential to make things worse. Don't forget the sibling.

Erin Hall (eighteen years old), considers his brother "a legend" for surviving childhood cancer:

I'm really proud of my brother Judson for handling everything so well. During those years there were times when I was jealous of him, not only for the attention he received, but for his courage as well. This little boy was going through so much and I still cowered at getting my finger pricked. As I look back, I wonder if I would have been able to make it through, not only physically, but emotionally as well.

According to some people a person needs to be dead in order to be a legend, or to have been famous or well liked. A legend to me, though, is someone who has accomplished something incredible, enduring many hardships and pains, and still comes out of it smiling.

Judd is a legend to me because he didn't give up in a time that he might have. He is a legend because he survived an illness that many do not. Now I look at him after being in remission for almost five years, and I hope that someday if I am ever faced with a challenge like his, I will have the same strength and courage he had.

Eight-year-old Amanda Moodie explains the ups and downs of having a brother with cancer:

Sometimes having a brother with cancer is fun, like when my family goes on the Fantasy Flight to the North Pole, and going to the special summer camp, and getting special privileges at Disney World.

But other times, it can be really hard, especially when William gets put in the hospital. Right now, he can't leave his room in the hospital, and the doctors wear masks when they come in. I HATE seeing that. And he stays in for very long periods of time. The first time, he was there for almost three weeks! It comes so suddenly. He has stayed out for five months, then BAM! He's back in. And the worst of it is, people are always pitying us. "Poor little boy." "Poor William." I guess they like pitying us.

So cancer has ups and downs like everything else, but to me it's mostly downs.

Annie Walls (fifteen years old) relates a positive outcome to her and her brother's battle with childhood cancer:

One experience in my life that was in no way comfortable for my family or myself and caused me a lot of confusion and grief was when my brother had cancer. Along with the disruption of this event, it also caused me to grow tremendously as a person. The Thanksgiving of my third-grade year, Preston, my brother, became very ill and was diagnosed a few weeks later with having cancer.

This event helped me to grow to become a better person in many ways. When my brother had very little hair or was puffed out from certain drugs I learned to respect people's differences and to stick up for them when they're made fun of. Also, when Preston was in the hospital I was taught to deal with a great amount of jealousy that I had. He received many gifts, cards, flowers, candy, games, and so many other material things that I envied. Most of all though, he received all the attention and care of my mother, father, relatives, and friends. This is what I was jealous of the most. As I look back now, I can't believe that I was that insensitive and self-centered to be mad at my brother at a time like that.

The thing that made this a graced experience was the fact that it enabled me to be very close to my brother as we grew up. My brother and I are now good friends and are able to talk and share our experiences with each other. I don't think that we would have this same relationship if he never had cancer and I think that has been a very positive outcome. Another thing that has been a positive outcome of this event is the people I've been able to meet. Through all the support groups, camps, and events for children with cancer and their siblings, I have met some people with more courage and more heart than anyone could imagine. In no way am I saying that I'm glad my brother had cancer, but I will say I'm very glad with some of the outcomes from it.

Eleven-year-old Jeff Pasowicz explains what happened when "My Sister Had Cancer." (Reprinted from CCCF Canada CONTACT newsletter Vol. XVI No. 2 Spring 1994.)

My sister Jamie got cancer when she was 23 months old. I was eight, and my two other sisters were six and four.

My sisters and I were scared that my sister was going to die. We weren't able to go to public places and also weren't allowed to have friends in my house. We missed a lot of school when there was chicken pox in our school. I got teased in school sometimes because my sister had no hair. Once an older kid called my sister a freak. My mom was sad most of the time. It was very hard.

We are all pleased that Jamie is doing well, and our lives are getting back to normal. It was an experience I'll never forget, and I hope it has made me a stronger person.

Fifteen-year-old Sara McDonnall won first prize in the 1995 Candlelighters Creative Arts Contest with her essay, "From a Sibling":

Childhood cancer—a topic most teens don't think much about. I know I didn't until it invaded our home.

Childhood cancer totally disrupts lives, not only of the patient, but also of those closest to him/her, including the siblings. First, I was numbed with unbelieving shock. "This can't be happening to me and my family." Along with this came a whole dictionary full of incomprehensible words and a total restructuring of our (up to that time) fairly normal lifestyle.

One day in July 1988, I was waiting for my parents to pick me up from summer camp and anticipating the start of our family vacation to Canada. When they arrived, they informed me that my older brother Danny was very sick, and we wouldn't be taking that trip after all. The following day the call came that confirmed the diagnosis. Instead of packing for vacation, we packed our bags and headed for Children's Hospital in Denver, 200 miles away, where Danny was scheduled for surgery and chemotherapy.

I developed my own disease (perhaps from fear I would "catch" what Danny had), with symptoms similar to my brother's:

- Sympathy pains. I asked, "Why him?" when he came home from the hospital, exhausted from throwing up a life-saving drug for three days.

- Fear. "How much sicker is Danny going to get before he gets well? He is going to get well, isn't he?"

- Resentment. My parents seemed so worried about him all the time. They didn't seem to have time for me anymore.

- Confusion. Why couldn't Danny and I wrestle around like we used to? Why couldn't I slug him when he made me mad?

- Jealousy. I felt insignificant when I was holding down the fort at home.

The parts I hated the most were: not understanding what was being done to him; answering endless worried phone calls; and hearing the answers to my own questions when my parents talked to other people.

I was helped to sort out these feelings and identify with other siblings when I attended a program held just for teens who had siblings with cancer. We got together, tried to learn how to cross-country ski, and talked about our siblings and ourselves.

Perhaps you remember this story: "US [speed skating] star Dan Jansen, 22, carrying a winning time into the back straightaway of the 1000 meter race, inexplicably fell. Two days earlier, after receiving word that his older sister, Jane, had died of cancer, Dan crashed in the 500 meter" (Life magazine). Having a sibling with cancer can immobilize even an Olympic athlete. Dan was expected to bring home two gold medals, but cancer in a sibling intervened. He became, instead, the most famous cancer sibling of all time. He shared his grief before a television audience of two billion people. Dan later went on to win the World Cup in Norway and Germany, and capture the gold at the Olympics. He is the first to tell you the real champions can be found in the oncology wards of children's hospitals across our nation, and the siblings who are fighting the battle right along beside them.

Naomi Chesler gives advice to parents and siblings of those with childhood cancer:

> Twelve young people aged 7 to 29 met at the 25th Anniversary Candlelighters Conference to talk about what it is like having a sibling with cancer in the family. We talked about our families, our anger, jealousy, worries, and fears, and thought about what we wanted to tell others about our experiences. In fact, we made lists of things we wanted other people to know: one for parents, one for other children or young adults in our position, and one for the child who has been diagnosed with cancer.
>
> Some parts of these lists reflect anger and bitterness, but that was not the overriding feeling in the session. I hope it isn't the only message you take away. If nothing else, the issues raised here may provide you with a good starting point for discussions in your own family.
>
> To parents:
>
> - We know you are burdened and trying to be fair. But try harder.
> - Give us equal time.
> - Be tough on disciplining the child with cancer. No free rides.
> - Put yourself in our shoes once in a while.
> - If you are away from home a lot, at least call and tell us, "I love you."
> - Tell us what is going on. Don't just sit us in front of a video (about cancer); talk with us about it.
> - Keep special time with us like lunch once a week or something. Time for just us. And if you can't be with us, find someone who can.
> - When you talk to family members, say how everyone is doing— what we are doing is important, too.
> - Ask how we are feeling. Don't assume you know.
>
> To siblings of newly diagnosed kids:
>
> - Keep a diary if you don't want to talk to your parents.
> - Expect to not get as much attention.

- *Expect that your parents are going to be extra cautious about what your brother/sister does, who he/she hangs out with, etc.*

- *Hang in there. You're all you've got for now.*

- *Don't feel like you have to think about the illness all the time.*

- *Be understanding of your parents and stay involved.*

- *Tell someone how you are feeling—don't bottle it up.*

- *Go to the hospital to visit when you can.*

- *Make as many friends as possible at school.*

To our siblings who struggled or are struggling with cancer:

- *The world does not revolve around you.*

- *Stop feeling sorry for yourself.*

- *Not everything is related to cancer. Stop using that as an excuse for everything.*

- *I'm jealous of you sometimes, but I'm not mad. I know it sometimes seems like I'm mad, but I'm not.*

- *Don't take advantage of all the extra attention you get.*

- *Tell mom and dad to pay attention to me sometimes, too.*

- *Now that you are feeling better, where's the gratitude for all those chores that I did?*

- *I really admire your strength and courage. I wouldn't have gotten through your illness without you.*

Helping siblings cope

The following are the experiences and advice from several families on ways to help the brothers and sisters cope:

- Make sure that you explain cancer and its treatment to the siblings in terms that they understand. Create a climate of openness, so that they can ask questions and know that they will get answers. If you don't know the answer to a question, write it on your list to ask the doctor at the next appointment, or ask your child if he would like to go to the appointment with you and ask the question himself.

We always, always explained everything that was happening to Brent's older brother Zac (eight years old). He never asked questions, but always listened intently. He would say, "Okay, I understand. Everything's all right." We tried to get him to talk about it, but through all these years, he just never has. So we just kept explaining things at a level that he could understand, and he has done very well through the whole ordeal. The times that he seemed sad, we would take him out of school, and let him stay at the Ronald McDonald House for a few days, and that seemed to help him.

- Make sure that all the children clearly understand that cancer is not contagious. They cannot catch it, nor can their ill brother give it to anyone else. Impress upon them that nothing the parents or brothers and sisters did caused the cancer.

- Bring home a picture of the brother or sister in the hospital, and carry a tape recorder back and forth to relay songs and messages.

- It is very hard for mothers and babies or toddlers to be separated. Some families leave out family photo albums for the caregiver to show the toddler whenever she gets sad.

My daughter was eighteen months old when her three-year-old sister was diagnosed. Each member of the family flew in to stay at the house for two-week shifts, so she had a lot of caregivers. A friend of mine gave her a big key chain which held eight pictures. We put a picture of each member of the family (including pets) on her key chain, and she carried it around whenever we were away. It seemed to comfort her.

- Try to spend time alone with each sibling.

We began a tradition during chemotherapy that really helped each member of our family. Every Saturday each parent would take one child for a two-hour special time. We scheduled it ahead of time to allow excitement and anticipation to grow. Each child picked what to do on their special day—such as going to the park, eating lunch at a restaurant, riding bikes. We tried to put aside our worries, have fun, and really listen.

- If people only comment on the sick child, try to bring the conversation back to include the sibling. For example, if someone exclaims, "Oh look how good Lisa looks," you could say, "Yes, and Martha has an attractive new haircut, too. Don't you like it?"

- Share your feelings about the illness and its impact on the family. Say, "I'm sad that I have to bring your sister to the hospital a lot. I miss you when I'm gone." This allows the sibling an opportunity to tell you how she is feeling. Try to make the illness a family project by expressing how the family will stick together to beat it.

> *I never kept my feelings secret from Shawn's two older brothers (five and seven years old). If I was scared, I talked about it. Once when we thought he was relapsing, my stomach was so knotted up that I could barely walk. Kevin said, "Mom, I'm really worried about Shawn." I told him that I was, too, and then we both just hugged and cried together. They really opened up when we didn't hide our feelings.*

- Include siblings in decision making on matters such as how chores will be done, or devise a schedule for parent time with the healthy children.

> *We always gave the boys choices about where they would stay when Shawn had to be in the hospital. I felt like it gave them a sense of control to choose babysitters. They usually stayed at a close neighbor's house where there were younger children. It allowed them to ride the same bus to school and play with their neighborhood friends. Their lives were not too disrupted. They also really pitched in and helped with the younger kids. I think it helped them to help others.*

- Allow siblings to be involved in the medical aspects of their sister or brother's illness, if they wish it. Often the reality of clinic visits and overnight stays are easier than what siblings imagine. Many siblings are a true comfort when they hold their sister or brother's hand during spinal taps or bone marrows.
- Give lots of hugs and kisses.

> *We assumed everything was fine with Erin because she had her grandma, who adored her, staying with her. We made a conscious decision to spend lots of time with her and include her in everything. But we realized later that she felt very left out. My advice is to give triple the affection that you think they need, including lots of physical affection such as hugs and kisses. For years, Erin felt jealous. She thought her brother got more of everything: material things, time with parents, opportunities to do things she was not allowed to do. She finally worked it out while she was in college.*

- Be sure to alert teachers of siblings about the tremendous stress at home. Many children respond to the worries about cancer by developing behavior or academic problems at school. Teachers should be vigilant for the warning signals, and provide extra support or tutoring for the stressed child or teen. Continue to communicate frequently with the teachers of the siblings to make sure you are aware of any developing problems.

- Expect your other children to have some behavior problems as part of living with cancer in the family. This is a normal, not pathological, response.

> When my four-year-old "healthy" child screams and sobs over a minor skinned knee, she gets as much sympathy as my child with cancer does during a bone marrow aspiration. I put a bandage on the knee, rock her, sing a song, and get her an ice pack. The injuries are not equal, but the needs of each child are. They both need to be loved and cared for; they both need to know that mom will help, regardless of the severity of the problem. I even let the sib use EMLA for routine shots. My pediatrician laughs at me, but I just tell him, "Sibs need perks, too."

- The child with cancer receives many toys and gifts resulting in hurt feelings or jealousy in the siblings. Provide gifts and tokens of appreciation to the siblings for helping out during hard times, and encourage your sick child to share.

> Matthew received many new toys during the course of his disease. We finally told family members that we would prefer it if they could bring a toy for Matthew and his brother and sister, or to bring nothing at all. We told them that Matthew was happy to see them whether they came bearing gifts or not. His siblings couldn't understand why he was getting so many new things while they didn't get anything. Matthew always shared his presents, though. He would come home from the hospital and dump his suitcase onto the living room floor for David and Kristina to pick their new toy. Those were happy days for all three of them. Not only did they have new toys to play with, but they were all together in their own home.

- Encourage a close relationship between an adult relative or neighbor and your other children. Having a "someone special" when the parents are frequently absent can help prevent problems and help your child to feel cared for and loved.

- Take advantage of any workshops, support groups, or camps for siblings. These can be of tremendous value for siblings, providing fun and friendships with others who truly understand their feelings.

Positive outcomes for the siblings

After stating all of the above potential troubles that your children might experience, it is important to note that many siblings exhibit great warmth and active caretaking while their brother or sister is being treated for cancer. Their empathy and compassion seem to grow with the crisis. Some brothers and sisters of children with cancer feel that they have benefited from the stressful experience in many ways, such as increased knowledge about disease, increased empathy for the sick or disabled, increased sense of responsibility, enhanced self-esteem, greater maturity and coping ability, and increased family closeness. Many of these siblings mature into adults interested in the caring professions, such as medicine, social work, or teaching. Character can grow from confronting personal crisis, and many parents speak of the siblings with admiration and pride.

I don't think it matters how old the siblings are—it's a reality that the healthy ones will not get their fair share for a while. From what I've been able to observe in my own and other families, the siblings do eventually take it in stride and even seem to benefit from the opportunity to learn compassion, selflessness, and responsibility. As they get older, they even take comfort in the realization that, had they been the sick one, THEY would have received all the necessary attention and that their parent(s) can cope (somehow) with whatever comes around. Libby added to her observations that she noted carefully how I reacted to Casey's illness at first (fell apart!), but that the next day I could gather my strength and do what had to be done. She likes to think she would also react similarly should the occasion arise (although, at her age, every blip in her universe is a catastrophe).

CHAPTER 24

Feelings, Communication, and Behavior

When I approach a child, he inspires in me
two sentiments: tenderness for what he is,
and respect for what he may become.

—Louis Pasteur

UNDER THE BEST OF CIRCUMSTANCES, child rearing is a daunting task. When parenting is complicated by an overwhelming crisis such as cancer, communication within the family may suffer. Prior to the diagnosis, children know the family rules and understand the limits for their behavior. Afterward, normal family life is disrupted, and all sorts of confusing and distressing feelings appear. Parenting must change in response to the frequently shifting needs of the ill child and affected siblings. This chapter examines some emotional and behavioral changes in both children and parents, and presents suggestions on how to maintain effective communication and appropriate behavior within the family.

Feelings

Chapter 1, *Diagnosis*, contains an extensive list of feelings that parents may experience after their child's cancer diagnosis. It is important to remember that children—both siblings and the ill child—are also overwhelmed by strong feelings, and they generally have fewer coping skills than do adults. At varying times and to varying degrees, children and teens may feel fearful, angry, resentful, powerless, violated, lonely, weird, inferior, incompetent, or betrayed. Children have to learn strategies to deal with these strong feelings to prevent "acting out" behaviors (behavioral problems) or "acting in" behaviors (depression, withdrawal).

> *I had cancer when I was fifteen. I tried so hard as a freshman in college to put it all behind me and get on with my life. It just didn't work.*

Next to treatment, that was the worst year of my life. It showed me that if I didn't deal with it consciously, I was going to deal with it subconsciously. I had nightmares every night. I'd wake up feeling that I had needles in my arms. I decided to start taking better care of myself in a different kind of way. I do something fun every day. I try to see the positive side of situations. I read more and write a lot. I unplug from the cancer community whenever I feel overwhelmed. I try to explore my feelings rather than shove them in the back corner. Once I started dealing with these feelings, things really improved.

For some children with cancer, the emotional impact of the disease is intensified by permanent changes to the body. This is especially true for children with sarcomas who require amputation, or those with retinoblastoma who require enucleation.

I was 26 months old when I was diagnosed with bilateral retinoblastoma. My blindness sometimes intrudes on my ability and confidence in establishing relationships. However, I value everyone and everything around me and I try to live my life to the fullest.

The majority of sarcomas in children requiring amputation occur during the teenage years. This is a time when appearance is particularly important. The adolescent has lost a part of his body, so feelings of sadness, anger, bewilderment, helplessness, and fear are normal. Depression is common after amputation. Losing a limb can cause emotions that are similar to what the child would feel when experiencing the death of someone close to them. He will go through a period of grieving. It is crucial that the teen receive support and counseling for his psychological well-being.

I was sixteen years old and on the national championship hockey cheerleading team when I was diagnosed with osteosarcoma. I never went back to high school, and I'll never cheerlead again. I had an allograph and a total knee replacement. I can't kneel, sit cross-legged, or bend my knee all the way. I lost every friend I had.

Good communication is the first step toward helping your family identify how child behavior and family functioning is being impacted and how family members may work with each other and with professionals to restore order and a nurturing climate.

Communication

Communicating with your child or teen is the foundation for trust. He needs to know from the beginning that you will be truthful in response to his questions about his disease. Taking the time talk about feelings is crucial to his emotional well-being.

Honesty

Above all else, children need to be able to trust their parents. They can face almost anything, as long as they know that their parents will be at their side. Trust requires honesty. For your ill child and his brothers and sisters to feel secure, they must always know that they can depend on you to tell them the truth, be it good news or bad. This reduces isolation and a sense of disconnection within the family.

> We were always very honest. We felt that she needed to know that she could trust us to tell her the truth, however scary that would be. I saw a few incidents in the clinic of people with totally different styles who didn't tell their kids the truth. I have run into the bathroom at the clinic crying after overhearing a mother who had deceived her child into coming to the clinic. Then he found out he needed a back poke and completely lost it. It makes me cringe. Children just have to be prepared. If they can't trust their parents, who can they trust?

· · · · ·

> We felt we had to tell Jessica the truth from the very beginning. She needed to know that she could trust us and it helped her understand why the treatments were necessary. We told her that her hair would fall out, but that it didn't matter. She would still be beautiful to us, with or without hair. It would grow back. We told her when something would hurt and when it wouldn't.

· · · · ·

> I explained everything to Zachary every step of the way. I answered all his questions and never withheld or misrepresented anything to him.

Listening

Just trying to get through each day consumes most parents' time, attention, and energy. Consequently, one of the greatest gifts we can give our children is our time: a special time when we really focus on what they are saying, when we listen to not only the words, but the feelings that generate them; a time we stop to think before we speak. Many behavior problems can be prevented if our children think that we understand—if they feel that no matter how leaky the boat is, we are all in it together.

> After my relapse at age thirteen, the chemotherapy was much more difficult to tolerate. My appearance changed dramatically due to hair loss and rapid weight gain from prednisone. After a two-month absence, when I returned to school, the treatment I received from the other students was unbearable. I finally refused to go to school. I felt so strongly about not going to school that once, on the way there, I jumped out of the car at an intersection. This helped mom and dad make the decision to send me to a private school. The kids and staff at the new school knew my situation and were very compassionate. The decision to change schools was one of the best things my parents ever did for me.

· · · · ·

> When my daughter was seven, three years after her treatment ended, I realized how important it was to keep listening. She was complaining about a hangnail and I told her that I would cut it for her. She started to yell that I would hurt her. I asked her, "When have I ever hurt you?" and she said, "In the hospital." I sat down with her in my arms, rocked her, and explained what had happened in the hospital during her treatment, why we had to bring her, and how we felt about it. I told her that I cried along with her when she was hurt by procedures. I asked her to tell me her feelings about being there. We cleared the air that day, and I expect we will need to talk about it many more times in the future. Then she held out her hand so that I could cut off her hangnail.

Talking

If you are not in the habit of talking to your children about how you are feeling, it is hard to start in a crisis. But now, more than ever, it's important to try. Parents can provide an opening for discussion by simply stating how much they miss their other children—for example, "I really miss you when I have to take your sister to the hospital. I'll call you every night just so I can hear your voice," or "Sometimes I really get mad at the cancer. I wish the family didn't have to be separated so much." It is also helpful to tell your child with cancer how the illness is affecting her siblings—for example, "It is very hard for Jim to stay at home with a babysitter when I bring you to the hospital. Let's try to think of something nice to do for him." These statements not only reassure children of your continued love for them and distress about being separated from them, but creates an opportunity for them to share with you how they feel about what is happening to the family.

> My daughter, diagnosed when one year old and now entering fifth grade, has three older siblings, so we have been through many developmental stages as far as communication goes. I try to answer their questions honestly, but only tell them what I think they can understand without overwhelming them with information. I remember one of my boys, soon after her diagnosis, asked me if she was going to die, and I said "no" emphatically. I regretted it immediately, and realized that I would have to deal with my fears about the possibility of her dying, then go back and tell him the truth. So, later, I told him that I hadn't given an accurate answer because I was scared; that we didn't know if she was going to die, we hoped not, but we would have to wait and see.

> I have found that as their understanding deepens, they come back with more questions, needing more detailed answers. So, my motto is, be honest but don't scare them. If you say everything is okay but you are crying, they know something is wrong, and they can't trust you for the truth.

Common behavioral changes of children

Discipline under the best of circumstances can be difficult. But when one child has cancer, parents are stressed, siblings are angry, and the situation may become unmanageable. First, you need to decide whether the ill child is going to be treated as if she only has a few months to live, or as if she will survive and needs to learn strategies for how to self-regulate difficult emotions. Then examine your own behavior to see if you are modeling the conduct that you expect from your children. Also, is to develop a consistent response to the angry or destructive child, then help the child develop social and emotional competence.

Barbara Sourkes, an experienced child psychologist, wrote the following in her book *Armfuls of Time: The Psychological Experience of the Child with a Life-Threatening Illness*:

While loss of control extends over emotional issues, and ultimately over life itself, its emergence is most vivid in the child's day-to-day experience of the illness, in the barrage of intrusive, uncomfortable or painful procedures that he or she must endure. The child strives desperately to regain a measure of control, often expressed through resistant, noncompliant behavior or aggressive outbursts. Too often, the source of the anger —the loss of control—goes unrecognized by parents and caregivers. However, once its meaning is acknowledged, an explicit distinction may be drawn for the child between what he or she can or cannot dictate. In order to maximize the child's sense of control, the environment can be structured to allow for as much choice as is feasible. Even options that appear small or inconsequential serve as an antidote to loss, and their impact is often reflected in dramatic improvements in behavior.

In the following sections, parents share how they handled various behaviors of their ill child.

Anger

Parents respond to the diagnosis of cancer with anger, and so do children. Not only is the child angry at the disease, but also at the parents for bringing her in to be hurt, at having to take medicine that makes her feel terrible, at losing her hair, at losing her friends, and on and on. Children with cancer have good reasons to be angry.

I was initially excited when my son finished treatment for Ewing's sarcoma in 1995. I really expected to have a normal life again. In reality, the whole family had a hard time adjusting. He has a twin brother, and both boys had a very rough transition to junior high school. They were frequently in trouble and began failing most of their subjects. It added a lot of stress to our home life to have the principal calling us two to five times a week. Although we started counseling, we still had major "blow-ups" at home.

· · · · ·

We have a case of the halo or the horns. Our son is either very defiant or an absolute angel. He argues about every single thing. I really think that it is because he has had so little control in his life. I have very clear rules, am very firm, and put my foot down. But I also try to choose my battles wisely, so that we can have good times, too. My husband reminds me when I get aggravated, that if he wasn't this type of tough kid, he wouldn't have made it through so many setbacks. Then I am just glad to still have him with us.

Tantrums

Healthy children have tantrums when they are overwhelmed by strong feelings, and so do children with cancer. In some cases, tantrums can be predicted by parents paying close attention to what triggers the outburst. This knowledge helps parents prevent tantrums by avoiding situations that create overload for their child. In other cases, there is no warning of the impending tantrum.

> *We never knew what would set off three-year-old Rachel, and to tell the truth, she didn't know what the problem was herself. She was very verbal and aware in many ways, but she had no idea what was bothering her and causing the anger. I would just hold her with her blanket, hug her, and rock until she calmed down. Later she would say, "I was out of control," but she still didn't know why.*

Of course, if the child begins to be destructive, he needs help learning other ways to vent his anger. For a child who is frequently destructive, professional counseling is necessary. *The Misunderstood Child* by Larry Silver, listed in Appendix D, *Books and Online Sites*, has a chapter that explains in detail how parents can initiate a behavior modification program at home.

> *My son had frequent, violent rages which sometimes caused damage (toys thrown at the walls, books ripped up). He was small, but strong. I talked to him when he was calm about how the tantrums would be handled. Tantrums with no damage would be ignored; afterwards we would cuddle and talk about what prompted the anger and others ways for him to handle the anger. If he began to break things or hurt people, I would wrap him in a blanket and rock him until he relaxed. I would tell him, "I need to hold you because you are out of control. Soon you will learn how to control yourself." All of the tantrums ended after he went off treatment, but, dealing with his destructive anger was one of the hardest things that I have ever experienced.*

Withdrawal

Some children withdraw rather than blow up in anger. Like denial, withdrawal can be temporarily helpful as a way to come to grips with strong feelings. However, too much withdrawal is not good for children. It can also be a sign of the kind of depression which some children suffer. Parents or counselors need to find ways to allow withdrawn children to gently express how they are feeling.

Comfort objects

Many parents worry when, after diagnosis, young children regress to using a special comfort object. Many young children ask to return to using a bottle, or cling to a favorite toy or blanket. It is reasonable to allow your child to use whatever he can to find comfort against the terrible realities of treatment. The behaviors usually stop either when the child starts feeling better or when treatment ends.

> My daughter was a hair twirler. Whenever she was nervous, she would twirl a bit of her hair around her finger. As her hair fell out, she kept grabbing at her head to find a wisp to curl. I told her that she could twirl mine until hers grew back. She spent a lot of time next to me or in my lap with her hand in my hair. It was annoying for me sometimes, but it had a great calming effect on her. When hers grew back, I would gently remind her that she had her own hair to twirl. She also went back to a bottle although we did limit the bottle use to home or hospital. Both behaviors, hair twirling and drinking from a bottle, disappeared within six months of the end of treatment, when she was six years old.

· · · · ·

> Matthew had a special teddy bear that a friend had bought for him while visiting Germany. Mr. Bear, as he was called, went through everything Matthew went through. When he received cranial radiation, Mr. Bear had his skull irradiated, too. If Matthew needed oxygen, they both got a mask. That little teddy bear even had surgery a few times. Each time my son was admitted to the hospital, Mr. Bear went along and got his own hospital identification bracelet. They went through a lot together. It's amazing how much comfort he received from a stuffed toy.

Talking about death

Part of effective parenting is allowing children to talk about topics that cause discomfort. In many cultures, the subject of death has become taboo. A diagnosis of cancer forces both parents and children to acknowledge that death is a very real possibility. Even children as young as three years old think about death and what it means.

> *Eighteen months into treatment, five-year-old Katy said, "Mommy, sometimes I think about my spirit leaving my body. I think my spirit is here (gesturing to the back of her head) and my body is here (pointing to her bellybutton). I just wanted you to know that I think about it sometimes."*

· · · · ·

> *Courtney's diagnosis was very difficult on her two older brothers. Especially Jay, who at the age of ten understood the concept of death far better than Vaughn at age six. Both boys had to deal with our sudden departure late at night, taking with us their baby brother, Jared (age nine weeks) and Courtney, who was eighteen months old at the time. One of the hardest things I've ever done in my entire life was to answer a question Jay asked me one night. He asked me if his sister was going to die. I ached to lie to him and tell him that everything would be all right. I wanted to say, "Of course she isn't," but I couldn't do it. I had always been honest with the children, and felt that, difficult as it was, now more than ever he needed to know that he could trust that what I was saying was true. I told him his sister might die, but that we were going to do everything we could to make sure that didn't happen.*

Trusting your child

Sometimes, if parents listen to their children, they will say what they need to do to persevere. It may not be the way the parents cope; it may make them nervous. But, it is the child or teen's way to make peace with the day-to-day reality of cancer.

> *Early one summer morning, twelve-year-old Preston and I left the hospital after a week-long stay. He had been heavily sedated, and was groggy and shaky on his feet. My husband and daughter were getting ready to go on a boat trip, and I felt Preston was too sick to go. We sadly*

saw them off, then returned to the car. Preston said, "Mom, I really need to go fishing. I know you don't understand, but I really need to do this."

It made me very uncomfortable, but we went home to get his equipment. We then drove up to the mountains to a very deserted spot on the river, and Preston said that he needed to be out of my sight. So, I watched him put on his waders, walk into the swift river and disappear around a bend upstream. I went out into the river and sat on a rock. I waited for two hours before Preston came back. He said, "That's what I needed; I feel much better now."

There is a fine line between providing adequate protection for our children or teens and becoming overly controlling due to worry about the disease. You might ask yourself, "If she didn't have cancer, would I let her do this?"

Coping well

Some children, due to both temperament and the environments in which they have lived, are blessed with good coping abilities. They understand what is required, and they do it. Many more develop emotional competence from facing and coping with the difficulties of cancer. Many parents expressed great admiration for their child's strength and grace in the face of adversity.

Stephan has not had any behavior problems while being treated for his initial diagnosis (age five) or his relapse (age seven). He has never complained about going to the hospital and views the medical staff as his friends. He has never argued or fought about painful treatments. Unlike many of the parents in the support group, we've never had to deal with any emotional issues. We are fortunate that he has that confident personality. He just says, "We've got to do it, so let's just get it done."

· · · · ·

Leeann has often told me that if she could have had a life without cancer or her life with osteosarcoma, she wouldn't change a thing. I see that as a very healthy viewpoint. Being comfortable with who we are is one of the most challenging parts of our lives. She accomplished that at the young age of ten.

Common behavioral changes of parents

It's impossible to talk about children's behavior without discussing parental behavior. Children's development does not occur in a vacuum, but rather in the context of their family. At different times during their child's treatment, parents may be under physical, emotional, financial, and existential stress. Their worries are endless. The crisis can cause them to behave in ways of which they are not always proud.

Some of the problem behaviors mentioned by veteran parents follow.

Dishonesty

Children feel safe when their parents are honest with them. If the parents start to keep secrets from the child or "protect" her from bad news, the child feels isolated and fearful. She thinks, "If mom and dad won't tell me, it must be really bad," or "Mom won't talk about it. I guess there's nobody that I can tell about how scared I am."

Denial is a type of "unconscious" dishonesty. This occurs when parents say things to children, such as, "Everything will be just fine" or "It won't hurt a bit." This type of pretending just increases the distance between child and parent, leaving children with no support. However horrible the truth, it seldom is as terrifying to a child as a half truth upon which his imagination builds.

Depression

Feelings of sadness or depression may occur in parents of children with cancer. If you are consistently experiencing any of the following symptoms, get professional help: changes in sleeping patterns (sleeping too much, waking up frequently during the night, awakening in the early morning), appetite disturbances (eating too little or too much), decreased sex drive, fatigue, panic attacks, inability to experience pleasure, feelings of sadness and despair, poor concentration, social withdrawal, feelings of worthlessness, suicidal thoughts, and drug or alcohol abuse. If a parent becomes depressed, children may be neglected. Depression is very common, very treatable, and should be dealt with early.

Find a counselor you "click with." Stick with that person until you truly feel some peace about your experiences and strength for dealing with the ongoing stress of treatment or whatever else might come up. I regret that I toughed it out and didn't recognize the depression I was experiencing for such a long time. I think finding sources of support in a variety of ways at the earliest moment possible can greatly mitigate long-term difficulties in coping, such as depression.

· · · · ·

It was two years after my son finished treatment that my depression became severe enough that I recognized it. I actually had a lot of suicidal thoughts and my husband urged me to see a doctor. He started me on Zoloft and it has helped me tremendously.

Losing your temper excessively

All parents lose their temper sometimes. They lose their tempers with spouses, healthy children, pets, and even strangers. But it is especially painful when the target of the anger is a very sick child. Abuse of spouses and children increases at times when either or both spouses feel incompetent and powerless. If you find yourself unable to control your temper, seek professional counseling.

I had my share of temper tantrums. The worst was when he was having his radiation. I tried to make him eat because it would be so many hours before he could have any more food. He always threw up all over himself and me, several times, every morning. It seemed like we changed clothing at least three times before we even got out of the house each day. I remember one day just screaming at him, "Can't you even learn how to throw up? Can't you just bend over to barf?" I really flunked mother of the year that day. I can't believe that I was screaming at this sick little kid, who I love so much.

· · · · ·

In the beginning, my two-year-old daughter was incredibly angry. She would have massive temper tantrums, and I would just hold her and tell her that I wouldn't let her hurt anybody. I would continue to hold her until she changed from angry to sad. When she was on the dexamethasone, she would either be hugging me or pinching, biting, or sucking my neck. It drove me crazy. Now she's not having as many fits, but she still pushes her sisters off swings or the trampoline. She has a general lack of control. Sometimes, when I can't stand it anymore, I swat her on the bottom, and then I feel really bad.

· · · · ·

I had always taught my children that feeling anger was okay, but we had to make good choices about what to do with it. Hitting other people or breaking things was a bad choice; hitting pillows, running around outside, or listening to music were good choices. But, as with everything else, they learned the most from watching how I handled my anger, and during the hard months of treatment my temper was short. When I found myself thinking of hitting them, I'd say, in a very loud voice, "I'm afraid I'm going to hurt somebody so I'm going in my room for a time-out." If my husband was home, I'd take a warm shower to calm down; if he wasn't, I'd just sit on the bed and take as many deep breaths as it took to calm down.

Unequal application of household rules

You will guarantee family problems if the ill child enjoys favored status while the siblings must do extra chores. Granted, it is hard to know the right time to insist that your ill child must resume making his bed or setting the table, but it must be done. Siblings need to know from the very beginning that any child in the family, if sick, will be excused from chores, but will have do them again as soon as he is physically able.

I spoiled my sick daughter and tried to enforce the rules for my son. That didn't work, so I gave up on him and spoiled them both. He was really acting out at school. What he needed was structure and more attention, but what he got was more and more things. They both ended up thinking the whole world revolved around them, and it was my fault.

Overindulgence of the ill child

Overindulgence is a very common behavior of parents toward their child with cancer.

I bought my daughter everything that I saw that was pretty and lovely. I kept thinking that if she died she would die happy because she'd be surrounded by all these beautiful things. Even when I couldn't really afford it, I kept buying. I realize now that I was doing it to make me feel better, not her. She needed cuddling and loving, not clothes and dolls.

. . . . .

Someone asked me once if I didn't want to spoil him rotten or baby him because he might not survive. I said, "No, because what would I do if he does survive? I'd have a raging brat." So we just try to be normal and discipline like we would if he didn't have cancer. We don't let him get away with murder. We don't believe in hitting, but we do use time-outs, loss of privileges, and loss of opportunities to do things he enjoys.

One aspect of overindulgence that is quite common is the parent's reluctance to teach the sick child life skills. After years of dealing with a physically weak and sometimes emotionally demanding child, parents may forget to expect age-appropriate skills.

I realized that I had formed a habit of treating my child as if she was still young and sick. I was still treating her like a three-year-old, and she was seven. One day, when I was pouring her juice, I thought, "Why am I doing this? She's seven. She needs to learn to make her own sandwiches and pour her own drinks. She needs to be encouraged to grow up." Boy, it has been hard. But I've stuck to my guns, and made other extended family members do it, too. I want her to grow up to be an independent adult, not a demanding, overgrown kid.

Overprotection of sick child

For a child to feel normal, he needs to be treated as if he is normal. Ask the doctor what changes in physical activity are necessary for safety, and do not impose any additional restrictions that go beyond this on your child. Let the child be involved in sports or neighborhood play, and even though it is hard, stop yourself from issuing constant reminders to "be careful."

Our son Adam was born with neuroblastoma. He was in remission until age five when he relapsed with ganglioneuroma. He had chemotherapy because it was growing. Adam has never been officially in remission because he still has inactive tumors in his abdomen. The tumors are impossible to remove surgically because of their location. For a long time, the doctors wouldn't let him play contact sports.

However, at a recent check up, he was finally given the all-clear to play whatever sports he wanted. I wasn't sure if that was what I wanted to hear, because it makes me nervous. Luckily for me, he is totally disinterested in football! It took some time, but we realized we needed to allow him to do these things if we were to ever feel normal again. Adam is now twelve and quite active.

Not spending enough time with the sibling(s)

While acknowledging that there are only so many hours in a day, the parents interviewed for this book felt the most guilt about the effect of the cancer on the siblings. They wished that they had asked family and friends to stay with the sick child more often, allowing them to use more of their precious time with the siblings. Many expressed pain that they didn't know how severely affected the siblings had been.

We didn't have problems with our child with cancer, but his brother (six years old) really suffered. He would get the flu and sob all night. He would scream that he would have to go to the hospital and that he would die. He also had behavior problems at school. I ended up quitting work because my son with cancer was having trouble making it through the entire school day, and his brother needed some loving attention. Many of the sibling problems cleared up with lots of one-on-one attention.

Using substance abuse to cope

Some parents find themselves turning to alcohol or drugs to help them cope. Not only illegal drugs are abused; overuse of over-the-counter sleeping pills or other medications also occurs. If you find yourself drinking so that your behavior is affected, or using drugs to get through the day or night, seek professional help.

Coping

Some parents have no major problems adjusting to the diagnosis and treatment of their child with cancer. They find unexpected reserves of strength and are able to ask for help from their friends and family when they need it. They realize that different needs arise when there is a great stress to the family, and they alter their expectations and parenting accordingly. These families usually had strong and effective communication prior to the illness, and pull together as a unit to deal with it.

The majority of families, however, have periods of calmness and other times when nerves are frayed and tempers short. But usually families survive intact and are often strengthened by the years of dealing with cancer.

Improving communication and discipline

Parents suggest the following ways to keep the family on a more even keel:

- Make sure that the family rules are clearly understood by all of the children. Stressed children feel safe in homes that are very structured with regular, predictable routines.

   After yet another rage by my daughter with cancer, we held a family meeting to clarify the rules and consequences for breaking them. We asked the kids (both preschoolers) to dictate a list of what they thought the rules were. The following was the result, and we posted copies of the list all over the house (which created much merriment among our friends):

   1. No peeing on rug

   2. No jumping on bed

   3. No hitting or pinching

   4. No name calling

   5. No breaking things

   6. No writing on walls

   7. No being alone in room

   If they broke a rule, we would gently lead them to the list and remind them of the house rules. It really helped.

- Have all caretakers consistently enforce the family rules.

   We kept the same household rules. I was determined that we needed to start with the expectation that Rachel was going to survive. I never wanted her to be treated like a "poor little sick kid" because I was afraid she would become one. We had to be careful about babysitters because we didn't want anyone to feel sorry for her or treat her differently. I do feel that we avoided many long-term behavior problems by adopting this attitude early.

- Give all the kids some power by offering choices and letting them completely control some aspects of their lives, as appropriate.

    For a few months we ignored Shawn's two brothers as we struggled to get a handle on the situation. We just shuttled them around with no consideration for their feelings. When we realized how unfair we were being, we made a list of places to stay, and let them choose each time we had to go off to the hospital. We worked it out together, and things went much smoother.

· · · · ·

My bald, angry, four-year-old daughter asked me for some scissors one day. I asked what she was going to do, and she said cut off all her Barbies' hair. I told her those were her dolls and she could cut off their hair if she chose. I asked her to consider leaving one or two with hair, because when she had long hair again, she might want dolls that looked like her then, too. But I said it was up to her. She cut most completely off, and left some intact. It really seemed to make her feel better.

- Take control of the incoming gifts. Too many gifts make the ill child worry excessively ("If I'm getting all of these great presents, things must be really bad") and makes the siblings jealous. Be specific if you want people not to bring gifts, or if you want gifts for each child, not just the sick one.

    Paige has a sister, Chelsea, who was five at diagnosis, and a brother, Dan, who was four months old. Chelsea had a very difficult time. She didn't like it that Paige was getting so many presents and she often felt left out. When I would try to do something special for her, she would get mad—she just wanted normalcy.

- Recognize that some problems are caused solely by the drugs. It helps to remember that these children are not naturally defiant or destructive. They are feeling sick, powerless, and altered by massive doses of toxic drugs, and they need both sympathy and clear limits. Remember, when they get off the drugs, their real personalities will return.

- If your child likes to draw, paint, knit, or do collages or other artwork, encourage it. Art is both soothing and therapeutic and it allows the child a positive outlet for feelings and creativity. Making something beautiful really helps raise children's spirits.

  When Jody was in the laminar airflow (isolation) room for weeks after his bone marrow transplant, he passed the time by doing many collages. I kept him well-supplied with all sorts of materials, and he created beautiful things.

- If your child writes or does artwork, recognize that powerful emotions may surface for both child and parents.

  At my daughter's preschool, once a week each child would tell the teacher a story, which the teacher wrote down for the child to take home. Most of my daughter's stories were like this: "There was a rhinoceros. He lived in the jungle. Then he went in the pool. Then he decided to take a walk. And then he ate some strawberries. Then he visited his friend." But the week before or after a painful procedure, she would dictate frightening stories (and this from a kid who wasn't allowed to watch TV). Two examples are: "Once there were some bees and they stung someone and this someone was allergic to them and then they got hurt by some monkeybars and the monkeybars had needles on them and the lightning came and hit the bees," and, "Once upon a time there were six stars and they twinkled at night and then the sun started to come up. And then they had a serious problem. They shot their heads and they had blood dripping down."

- Allow your child to be totally in charge of his art. Do not make suggestions or criticize (e.g., "stay inside the lines" or "skies need to be blue not orange"). Rather, encourage them and praise their efforts. Display the artwork in your home. Listen carefully if your child offers an explanation of the art, but do not pry if it is private. Above all, do not interpret it yourself or disagree with your child on what the art represents. Being supportive will allow your child to explore ways to soothe himself and clarify strong feelings.

  Jody was continually making "projects." We kept him supplied with a fishing box full of materials, and he glued and taped and constructed all sorts of sculptures. He did beautiful drawings full of color, and every per-

son he drew always had hands shaped like hearts. If we asked him what he was making, he always answered, "I'll show you when I'm done."

- Come up with acceptable ways for your child to physically release anger. Some options are: ride a bike, run around the house, swing, play basketball or soccer, pound nails into wood, mold clay, punch pillows, yell, take a shower or bath, or draw angry pictures. In addition, teach your child to use words to express his anger—for example, "It makes me furious when you do that," or "I am so mad I feel like hitting you." Releasing anger physically and expressing anger verbally are both valuable life skills to master.

Shawn was very, very angry many times. We had clear rules that it was okay to be angry, but he couldn't hit people. We bought a punching bag which he really pounded sometimes. Play dough helped, too. We had a machine to make play dough shapes which took a lot of effort. He would hit it, pound it, push it, roll it. Then he would press it through the machine and keep turning that handle. It seemed to really help him with his aggression.

· · · · ·

Our therapist recommended that we have our five-year-old daughter make an "angry sheet." She should be encouraged to draw or write what she felt like doing when she was angry, and encouraged to get it all out. It was pretty scary, because she drew pictures of stamping people, gouging their eyes out, shooting them, etc. It was amazing how much better she felt afterwards. Then we went through the pictures together and discussed which ones she could really do, and which ones she could only think about doing because really doing it would hurt someone.

- Treat the ill child as normally as possible.

When Justin was in the hospital, I could never stand to see him in those little hospital gowns. I asked if we could dress him in his own outfits, and they said yes. So even when he was in the ICU with all the tubes coming out of his body, we dressed him every day in something cute. It just felt better to see him in his clothes. Several months later my mother said that she had really admired us for doing that because we were sending the message to Justin that everything was going to be okay. That even though he couldn't breathe on his own, he was still going to get up every day and get dressed. Now I think it probably did communicate to him that things were going to be normal again.

- Get professional help whenever you are concerned or run out of ideas on how to handle emotional problems. Mental health care professionals (see Chapter 14, *Sources of Support*) have spent years learning how to help resolve these kinds of problems, so let them help you.

My daughter and I both went to a wonderful therapist throughout most of her treatment for cancer. My daughter was a very sensitive, easily overwhelmed child, who withdrew more and more into a world of fantasy as cancer treatment progressed. The therapist was skilled at drawing out her feelings through artwork and play. She also helped me with very specific suggestions on parenting. For instance, when I told the therapist that my daughter thought that treatment would never end (a reasonable assumption for a preschooler), she suggested that I put two jars on my daughter's desk. One was labeled "All Done," and the other was labeled "To Do." We put a rock for every procedure and treatment already completed in the all-done jar, and one rock for every one yet to do in the to-do jar (only recommended if the child is more than halfway through treatment). Then, each time that we came home, my daughter would move a rock into the all-done jar. It gave her a concrete way to visualize the approach of the end of treatment. She could see the dwindling number of pebbles left. On the last day of treatment, when she moved the last pebble over and the to-do jar was empty, I cried, but she danced.

- Most emotional problems that children develop as a result of treatment for cancer can be resolved by professional counseling. However, some children may also need medications to get them through particularly rough times.

My daughter was doing really well throughout treatment until a combination of events occurred that was more than she could handle. Her grandmother died from cancer during the summer, one of her friends with cancer died on December 27, then another friend relapsed for the second time. She was fine during the day, but at night she constantly woke up stressed and upset. She had dreams about trapdoors, witches brewing potions to give to little children, and saw people coming into her room to take her away. She would wake up smelling smoke. She was awake three or four hours in the middle of the night, every night. Her doctor put her

on sleeping pills and antianxiety medications, and the social worker came
out to the house twice a month.

- Teach children relaxation or visualization skills to help them cope better with strong feelings.

- Have reasonable expectations. If you are expecting a sick four-year-old to act like a healthy six-year-old, or a teenager to act like an adult, you are setting your child up to fail.

> *It seemed like we spent most of the years of treatment waiting to see a doctor who was running hours behind schedule. Since my child had trouble sitting still and was always hungry, I came well prepared. I always carried a large bag containing an assortment of things to eat and drink, toys to play with, coloring books and markers, books to read aloud, and play dough. He stayed occupied and we avoided many problems. I saw too many parents in the waiting room expecting their bored children to sit still and be quiet for long periods of time.*

- As often as possible, try to end the day on a positive note. If your child is being disruptive, or if your feelings toward your child are very negative, the following is an exercise that can end the day in a pleasant way. At bedtime, parent and child each tell one another something they did that day that made them proud of themselves, something they like about themselves, and something they are looking forward to the next day. Then a hug and a sincere "I love you" bring the day to a calm and loving close.

Checklist for parenting stressed children

A group of veteran parents compiled the following checklist to help you parent your stressed child:

- Model the type of behavior you desire. If you talk respectfully and take time-outs when angry, you are teaching your children to do so. If you scream and hit, that is how your children will handle their anger.

- Seek professional help for any behaviors that trouble you.

- Teach your children to talk about their feelings.

- Listen to your children with understanding and empathy.

- Be honest and admit your mistakes.

- Help your children to examine why they are behaving as they are.

- Distinguish between feelings (always okay) and acting on strong feelings in destructive or hurtful ways (not okay).

- Have clear rules and consequences for violations.

- Teach children to recognize when they are losing control.

- Discuss acceptable outlets for anger.

- Give frequent reassurances of your love.

- Provide plenty of hugs and physical affection.

- Notice and compliment your child for good behavior.

- Recognize that the disturbing behaviors result from stress, pain, and drugs.

- Remember that with lots of structure, love, and time the problems will become more manageable.

Our children look to us to learn how to handle adversity. They learn how to cope from us. Although it is extremely difficult to live through your child's diagnosis and treatment for cancer, it must be done. So we each need to reach deep into our hearts and minds to help our children endure and grow.

Children Learn What They Live

If a child lives with criticism, he learns to condemn.
If a child lives with hostility, he learns to fight.
If a child lives with ridicule, he learns to be shy.
If a child lives with shame, he learns to feel guilty.
If a child lives with tolerance, he learns to be patient.
If a child lives with encouragement, he learns confidence.
If a child lives with praise, he learns to appreciate.
If a child lives with fairness, he learns justice.
If a child lives with security, he learns to have faith.
If a child lives with approval, he learns to like himself.
If a child lives with acceptance and friendship,
He learns to find love in the world.

—Dorothy Law Nolte

CHAPTER 25

End of Treatment and Beyond

The best formula for longevity: have a
chronic disease, and cure it.

—Oliver Wendell Holmes

THE LAST DAY OF TREATMENT is a time for both celebration and fear. Most families are thrilled that the days of hospital stays and procedures have ended, but fear a future without drugs to keep the disease away. Concerns about relapse are an almost universal parental response, but for the majority of families, the months and years roll by without recurrence of cancer. Some children and teens quickly return to excellent physical and mental health, while others have lingering or permanent effects from the treatment.

This chapter covers the emotional and physical aspects of ending treatment. Effective medical follow-up, employment issues, and problems with insurance are then discussed.

Emotional issues

Many parents describe ending treatment as almost as wrenching an experience as diagnosis. Families begin to experience the gamut of emotions—from elation to terror—months before the final day.

Parents should anticipate that after many months or years spent watching their child go through the rigors of treatment, they will have lost the feeling of a "normal" life. They may experience relapse scares, and they may need to call the doctor to describe the symptoms and be reassured.

> *Every time Sean sneezed, I was there with a thermometer. I was constantly on the look-out for "bad germs." It took about a year before I was finally able to relax and stop feeling so paranoid.*

With diagnosis came the awareness that life can be cruel and unpredictable. Many parents feel safe during treatment and feel that therapy is keeping the cancer away. The end of treatment leaves many parents and children feeling exposed and vulnerable. When treatment ends, parents must find a way to live with uncertainty, to find a balance between hope and reasonable worry.

When treatment was finally over, we felt like we had been cut adrift at sea. Suddenly, our hospital safety net was gone. This was the day that we had been waiting for—and now we were terrified.

Last day of treatment

The last day of treatment usually includes a physical examination, blood-work, scans or x-rays (depending upon the type of cancer), and a discussion with the oncologist. The oncologist should review the treatment, outline the schedule for blood tests and exams for the future, and sensitively inform the family of the potential for long-term side effects. One group of parents presented to physicians at a major children's hospital the following list of suggestions for the last day of treatment:

- Schedule enough time to have a conversation.
- Bring a sense of closure to the active phase of treatment.
- Express happiness that all has gone well.
- Be realistic but hopeful about the future.
- Praise the child for handling a very difficult time in her life with grace (or courage, or whatever word is appropriate).
- Praise the parents for all of their hard work.
- Allow time for the parents to give the physician feedback and thanks.
- Give a certificate of accomplishment to the child.
- Be aware that families are relieved but fearful of the future.

Catheter removal

Children and teens usually cannot wait for the catheter to be removed, as it symbolizes that treatment has truly ended. Physicians have very different opinions on the best time to remove the catheter. Some remove it on the last day of treatment, while others want to wait until several weeks or months have passed. If your doctor recommends a delay, and you or your child have strong feelings about waiting, take the time to discuss it fully.

> Our son kept his catheter for several months after he finished his protocol. His oncologist felt it was necessary and we agreed. There was a high likelihood that he would relapse, so we kept the catheter in place, just in case he would still need it.

· · · · ·

> During Elizabeth's last treatment, her doctor told me he was going to schedule her for surgery to remove her central line. I was so ecstatic! To me, Elizabeth wasn't really in remission as long as the central line was still there. I know it was irrational, but part of me felt as if there were cancer cells dangling at the end of that central line. If we didn't get it out right away, Elizabeth would still have cancer. I wanted it out "right now."

Removal of the external catheter (Hickman or Broviac) is usually an outpatient procedure. The child is given a mild sedative, then the oncologist pulls the catheter out of the child's body by hand. This may also be done under general anesthesia by the surgeon or radiologist who inserted it.

> Kristin's Broviac removal wasn't too bad. They gave her fentanyl ahead of time, so she was fairly relaxed. I wished that they had offered me a sedative as well. One of the nurses had her hand on Kristin's shoulder and quietly talked to her to try to keep her focused elsewhere. I held her legs, and my wife held her hand. The doctor put one hand on her chest, and pulled on the tubing with the other. It only took about two seconds to come out. There was little blood; they just put a Band-Aid on the site and sent us home.

Implanted catheters such as the Port-a-cath are removed surgically in the operating room. Children are usually given general anesthesia, and the operation takes less than half an hour. Only one incision is made, usually just above the port at the same place as the scar from the implantation surgery. The sutures holding the port to the underlying muscle are cut, and the port with tubing is pulled out. The small incision is then stitched and bandaged. When the child begins to awaken, he is brought out to the parents. The family then waits until the surgeon has approved their departure. Often, the wait is short, for as soon as the child is awake enough to take a small drink or eat a popsicle, he is released. If your child becomes nauseated from the anesthesia, the wait can be several hours until he is feeling better.

Brent had a very easy time with his port removal surgery. We scheduled him to be the first patient early in the morning, so there was no delay getting in. Then the anesthesiologist asked him what flavor gas he wanted, which he liked. They brought him out to us while he was still groggy, and he woke up feeling goofy and happy. We went home soon thereafter. It felt more like the ending then than on the last day of treatment.

Ceremonies

Some families greatly benefit from having ceremonies to celebrate the end of cancer treatment. Especially for younger children who have spent much of their lives receiving treatment and having procedures, ceremonies can help them grasp that it is truly over. Here are ideas from many families on how to commemorate this important occasion:

- Take "good-bye" pictures of the hospital and staff.
- Take a picture of your child receiving his last treatment.
- Give trophies to your child and his siblings.

We had a big party during which my husband Scott stood up and called for everyone's attention. He gave a talk about how proud we were of Jeremy and handed him a big trophy. It had a victory angel on top and was engraved with "Jeremy, we are so proud of you and your victory. Love, Mom and Dad." We gave a plaque to his brother Jason for being the world's most supportive brother.

- Ask the clinic to present your child with a certificate.
- Let your child flush all of the leftover oral medications down the toilet.
- Let your child tear or cut up the calendar used to record dates for procedures (not a good idea if any records are on it).
- Throw a big party.
- If your child has been seeing a counselor, schedule a visit to talk about the accomplishment.

- Have friends and family send congratulations cards.

- Ask the surgeon to give your child her port or Hickman line.

> *I know that this may sound odd, but my six-year-old daughter hated her port and talked incessantly about getting it out. She even told me that she was going to slice it out herself with a knife. I told her it would be better to wait until the doctors put her to sleep, but I promised her that she could have it after the operation to do with as she wished. That idea brought a smile to her face. She came out of the recovery room clutching a baggie with the port inside. Once we were home, she carried it around for weeks, jumped on it, hit it with a hammer, and finally cut it to pieces. That port really symbolized all of the painful things that had happened to her, and it made her feel better to hurt it back.*

- If consistent with your beliefs, have a religious ceremony of thanksgiving.

- Go on a trip or vacation to celebrate.

Some parents do not feel comfortable celebrating the end of treatment. One mother described her feelings this way:

> *Finishing treatment was very difficult. I thought that I would feel like celebrating and cheering—but all I felt was fear. Treatment was over, but cancer was still a part of our lives. I think we will always live with the fear of relapse. It has taken me some time to come to grips with that reality.*

As you have read so often in this book, every child, parent, and relative reacts differently to every phase of treatment; what is important is not the differences, but the fact that each family member feels free to express and act on their own feelings, whatever they may be. You may be joyful, relieved, fearful or terrified, but end of treatment is emotionally charged for every member of the family.

What is normal?

After the trauma of cancer, families grapple with the idea of returning to normal. Unfortunately, most parents don't really know what "normal" is any longer. Parents realize that returning to the carefree days before cancer is unrealistic—life has changed. The constant interaction with medical personnel is ending, and support from family and friends recedes. While it is true that the blissful ignorance of the days prior to cancer are gone forever, families do enter a period of calm in which routines do not revolve around caring for a sick child, hospital stays, and clinic appointments. Each family needs to carve out a new definition of "normal."

> We're a year off treatment, and I really don't think about relapse very often. I do occasionally find myself studying her to see if she looks pale, or I worry when she seems tired or her behavior is bad. Usually, I'm feeling safer. But honestly, I don't think any of us will ever go back to the days when we just assumed that our kids would grow up, that the parents would die first; that sense of security is probably gone forever.

• • • • •

> Shawn's six months off treatment, and he's just like a flower beginning to bloom. He's so happy and I try to be happy with him. I try very hard to put worries about the future out of my mind, because I feel that those thoughts will rob me of just being able to enjoy Shawn.

• • • • •

> My mother still calls my daughter "the fragile child" and says other things, such as, "She's been affected, she will never be the same. She'll be lucky to live to adulthood." However, I have left cancer thoughts behind me and feel that life is normal for us again.

• • • • •

> For the month after treatment ended, Christine (six years old) drank water constantly. It was amazing how much she drank. I guess it was her body's way of flushing itself. She also threw some grand-scale temper tantrums for a month or two.

• • • • •

> For two months after ending treatment, Meagan was worried about everything that went in her mouth. She'd say, "Is this okay to eat? Will this hurt me? Am I safe? Am I going to get hurt doing this?" This paranoid phase just faded away.

• • • • •

> These first two months off treatment, I've noticed Kristin steadily gaining in self-confidence and composure.

Many parents and children resolve their complicated feelings by giving back to the cancer community in some way. Helping others, for many people, is a satisfying way to reach out or bring closure to the active phase of cancer treatment. Helping others can create something enormously meaningful out of personal tragedy. Here is what some families say they have done:

- We started a Boy Scout project to keep the toy box full at the clinic.

- My children are counselors at the camp for kids with cancer.

- After my son died, I gave up my parish to be a hospice chaplain.

- We organized a walk to raise funds for the Ronald McDonald House.

- We (a group of parents of children with cancer) requested and were granted a conference with the oncology staff to share our thoughts on ways to improve pain management and communication between parents and staff. It was very well-received.

- We circulated a petition among parents to request increased hospital funding for psychosocial support staff. We presented it to the director of the hematology/oncology service.

- I started a Candlelighters group and organized meetings, conferences, and picnics, and I write a quarterly newsletter.

- I requested that the clinic and local pediatricians refer newly diagnosed families to me if the parents wanted someone with a child who experienced the same disease to talk to. I remembered how impossible it was to go to meetings in the first few months, and how desperately I needed to talk to someone who had already traveled the same road.

- We held a bone marrow donor drive.

- I give platelets and blood regularly.

- I took all of our leftover Hickman line supplies to camp and gave them to a family who needed them.

The possibilities are endless. Parents use whatever talents they have to help others, from designing head coverings, to writing newsletters, to going online on their computer to talk with newly diagnosed families.

> I am the administrator of several online support group for parents of children with cancer. We have over 600 participants from sixteen countries all over the world. Some of the members' children have been cured for years, some are newly diagnosed, and some of the children have died. We've become a family. It's important to me to remain involved in the fight against childhood cancer. There are so many others that are follow-

ing behind in our footsteps. Perhaps showing that we've been there, too, yet we're still standing, might help another mom or dad.

An equally healthy response to ending treatment for cancer is to put it behind you. Many families, after years of struggles, just want to enjoy a new-found sense of normalcy. They don't want constant reminders of cancer, and feel that it's not good for children to be continually reminded of those hard times.

> *I realized that it was time to put it behind us when I watched my two children playing house one day. There was only one adult and one child in the family. I asked what happened to the rest of the family and they both said, "Cancer, they died." I didn't want them to have any more cancer in their lives. They had had enough. I know people who worry all the time about the cancer returning, and it is not healthy for them or their children. I decided to get out of the cancer mode, and back to being my usual upbeat self. I feel that we are finally back to normal, and it's a good place to be.*

Parents and children need to talk to one another, examine their emotions, decide what course they want to chart, and work together toward a healthy life after cancer.

Follow-up care

In the past, most survivors of cancer were on their own after treatment ended. With increasing numbers of long-term survivors, it became apparent that these young men and women often faced complex medical and psycho-social effects from their years of treatment. As a result, many institutions began late-effects clinics to provide a multidisciplinary team to monitor and support survivors. The nucleus of the team is usually comprised of a nursing coordinator, pediatric oncologist, pediatric nurse practitioner, radiation oncologist, endocrinologist, school liaison, social worker, and psychologist.

The follow-up programs usually include a review of treatments received, counseling regarding potential health risks (or lack thereof), and case-specific diagnostic tests such as cardiac evaluations, hormonal studies, or testing for learning disabilities. These follow-up clinics not only provide comprehensive care for long-term survivors, but participate in research projects that track the effectiveness and side effects from various clinical trials. In addition, the follow-up clinic acts as an advocate for survivors at schools, insurance agencies, and employers.

As Grace Powers Monaco, one of the founders of Candlelighters Childhood Cancer Foundation, said:

> Life is a hollow gift unless cancer survivors emerge from treatment as competent and worthy individuals, able to obtain insurance, equipped to earn a living, and prepared to participate in a medical surveillance program to "keep" the life they have won.

If your institution does not provide long-term follow-up care, the following issues should be addressed at the end of treatment.

Follow-up schedule

Protocols for clinical trials require specific follow-up schedules. For instance, your child may require monthly physical exams and a monthly CBC for the first year off treatment, and a less frequent schedule for the following years. Find out from the oncologist what the required schedule will be, and where the appointments will take place. Make sure that your child understands that after treatment ends doctor appointments and blood draws will still be an occasional necessity.

Possible late effects

At diagnosis, parents do not know the price their child will ultimately pay for reprieve from cancer. Short-term effects are discomfort, a bald head, and school absences. Long-term effects range from none to severe. These can include an impaired endocrine system, altered bone growth, subtle or pronounced learning disabilities, hepatitis C infection from blood transfusions or growth hormone, infertility, hearing loss, lung or heart problems, and an increased risk of secondary malignancies. It is important to know the possible risks based on the treatment your child received. You can then store this knowledge in the back of your mind. As one mother said, "I hope for the best and I deal with the rest." For detailed information on possible late-effects from childhood cancer, read *Childhood Cancer Survivors: A Practical Guide to the Future*, by Nancy Keene, Wendy Hobbie, and Kathy Ruccione.

An essential aspect of survivorship is making healthy choices. Good health habits and regular medical care help protect survivors' health as well as

reduce the likelihood of late effects from cancer treatment. A siza^l
of adult cancers are linked to lifestyle choices. Eating a healthy .
physically active, using sun screen, avoiding excessive alcohol consum_ᵣ
maintaining a healthy weight, and not smoking all help to keep survivors
healthy and cancer-free. Wearing bike or motorcycle helmets, using seat
belts, and calling a cab if the person driving you home has had too much to
drink protect survivors from injury. Survivors have little or no control over
genetic make-up or the environment in which they live. But making healthy
choices on how to live the rest of their lives gives them control over some of
their own destiny.

Immunizations

If your child was diagnosed prior to receiving all of her immunizations, ask
the oncologist when you should resume the regular schedule for vaccinations.

> My doctor said to wait a year before beginning to catch up on shots.
> It was nice for her to get a long break before any more pokes.

Risks of smoking

Teens need continuing counseling on problems associated with smoking
(cigarettes or marijuana) or other high-risk behaviors. Any child or teen who
received anthracycline therapy (adriamycin, daunomycin, or idarubicin) is at
risk for damage to the muscle of the heart. Smoking not only impacts the
lungs, but it makes blood vessels hard, further decreasing the heart's ability
to pump. The combination of heart damage from chemotherapy and smoking vastly increases the chance of heart disease, heart attack, congestive heart
failure, stroke, and cancer of the mouth, throat and lungs, or death from
sudden cardiac failure. An article on survivors and smoking contained in the
Candlelighters Winter 1994 youth newsletter ends with these words:

> If you've had cancer and your friends haven't, they don't face the
> same risks from smoking that you do. You've fought hard for your life.
> Don't put it out in an ashtray.

Safe sex

Every teen and young adult who has survived cancer should be counseled
about safe sexual practices. Despite the prevalence of sexual messages in
our culture, most teens are woefully underinformed about the facts. Many

survivors think, erroneously, that if they are infertile, they do not have to be concerned about the use of condoms or other forms of birth control. Many female survivors have found themselves unexpectedly pregnant after not using birth control. In addition, all sorts of diseases, some potentially fatal (hepatitis C, HIV/ARC/AIDS) and some not (genital herpes, genital warts, gonorrhea), can be transmitted through sexual intercourse.

One nurse practitioner at a large follow-up clinic stated:

> I tell every teenager who comes through the door, regardless of their medical background, that I think that he or she is too young to have sex, and I explain why. But then I say, in the event that you do choose to become sexually active, you ALWAYS need to use a condom, and not just any condom. I tell them to only use a latex condom with a spermicide, which is the most protective barrier. I explain that no sex is the only guarantee to avoid the many diseases out there, but a latex condom with spermicide offers the next best protection. And I really stress that this should be done whoever the partner is, and for whatever type of sex. So many teenagers think that diseases only happen to other kinds of kids.

Keeping the doctor informed

For a variety of reasons, many children and young adults are no longer cared for by pediatric oncologists who are familiar with their history. Additionally, when treatment ends, many patients and parents are not adequately informed of the risks of developing physical difficulties months, years, or decades after treatment ends. The risks of such delayed effects are real. Moreover, many primary care physicians—pediatricians, family practice doctors, internists, gynecologists—are not fully aware of all the different treatments used for the multitude of childhood cancers, and their late effects.

It is imperative that survivors be informed advocates for their own healthcare. They need to be educated, in a supportive and responsible way, of the risk for future physical adversities, so that if a problem does arise, it will be recognized early and receive prompt attention. Young adults who have survived childhood cancer need to be fully cognizant of their unique medical history and able to share this information with all future doctors who will care for them.

A few months before the end of treatment, ask the oncologist to fill out the booklet at the back of this book. This health history will become an indispensable part of your child's medical records for the rest of his life. It should be kept in a safe place and a copy should be given to each medical caregiver. When your child leaves home to begin her adult life, this booklet should go with her.

If you do not have a copy of the health history booklet, write down the following important information in your child's health history:

- Name of disease
- Date of diagnosis and relapse, if any
- Place of treatment
- Dates of treatment
- Names of attending oncologist and primary nurse
- Names and total dosages of chemotherapeutic agents used
- Type, areas treated, and amount of radiation used
- Name of radiation center
- Date(s) radiation received
- Number of rads and to what location, e.g., whole body, cranial, etc.
- Dates and types of any surgeries
- Date and type of bone marrow or stem cell transplant, if any
- Any major treatment complications
- Any persistent side effects of treatment
- Recommended medical follow-up
- Contact numbers for treating institutions

If your child will not be periodically examined at a long-term follow-up clinic, write down this information, and make sure that your child has a copy to give to any future doctor who will be treating her.

Employment

The population of adults who have survived childhood cancer is growing at a rapid rate. It is estimated that by the year 2000, 1 in every 900 young adults will be a cancer survivor. Thousands of survivors are staying well, growing up, graduating from high school or college, and successfully entering the workforce. Survivors of childhood cancer are educators, sports figures, radio announcers, doctors, social workers, dancers, lawyers, and professionals of all types.

Diane Komp, MD, in *A Child Shall Lead Them*, writes:

> I lecture about long-term survivors to each new group of medical students that comes through pediatrics at Yale. I can see from their faces that most of them prefer memorizing the odds that someone will make it than tasting the sweetness of individual victories. "That's very nice, but how representative is that case?"
>
> Not all of them feel that way, though. I watch their faces and can now pick out from their ranks a special type of young person who is being seen in increasing numbers in medical classrooms. Although their classmates cannot tell who they are, I can spot a long-term survivor of childhood cancer five minutes into that lecture.

Despite their numbers, some survivors still face job discrimination due to fears about cancer and its treatment. Under US federal law, and many state laws, an employer cannot treat a survivor differently from other employees because of a history of cancer except in certain circumstances involving health, life, and disability insurance. The Americans with Disabilities Act (ADA) prohibits many types of job discrimination by employers, employment agencies, state and local governments, and labor unions. In addition, most states have laws that prohibit discrimination based on disabilities, although what these laws cover varies widely.

The Americans with Disabilities Act of 1990 (ADA) prohibits discrimination based on actual disability, perceived disability, or history of a disability. Any employer with fifteen or more workers is covered by the ADA.

The ADA requires that:

- Employers may not make medical inquiries of an applicant, unless the applicant has a visible disability, e.g., amputation, or the applicant has voluntarily disclosed his cancer history. Such questions must be limited to asking the applicant to describe or demonstrate how she would perform essential job functions. Medical inquiries are allowed after a job offer has been made or during a pre-employment medical exam.

- Employers must provide reasonable accommodations unless it causes undue hardship.

- Employers may not discriminate because of family illness.
- Employers are not required to provide health insurance.

The Equal Employment Opportunity Commission (EEOC) enforces Title 1 (employment) of the ADA. Call (800) 669-4000 for enforcement information and (800) 669-3362 for enforcement publications. Other sections are enforced, or have their enforcement coordinated by, the US Department of Justice (Civil Rights Division, Public Access Section). The Justice Department's ADA web site is at *http://www.usdoj.gov/crt/ada.html*.

The Job Accommodation Network (JAN) is an international consulting service that provides free information about how employers can accommodate people with disabilities. The service also provides information about the Americans with Disabilities Act (ADA). They can be reached by calling (800) 526-7234 (USA), or (800) 526-2262 (Canada).

In the United States, JAN is a service of the President's Committee on Employment of People with Disabilities. In Canada, (JANCANA) it is a service of Human Resources Development Canada and the Canadian Council on Rehabilitation and Work.

In Canada, the Canadian Human Rights Act provides essentially the same rights as the ADA. The act is administered by the Canadian Human Rights Commission. You can get further information by calling the national office at (613) 995-1151.

If you feel that you have been discriminated against due to your disability or a relative's disability, contact the EEOC or the Canadian Human Rights Commission promptly. In the US, a charge of discrimination generally must be filed within 180 days of the notice of the discriminatory act.

If a survivor of cancer or a member of the family feels that he has been denied a job, fired, forced from a job, denied reasonable accommodation, or discriminated against for promotions or medical leave because of cancer history, contact the Childhood Cancer Ombudsman Program (listed in Appendix C, *Resource Organizations*) for help. They can provide the following free services:

- Outside review by experts
- Citations to medical and legal literature
- Mediation

- Analysis of employment contracts
- Instructions in appeal procedures
- Assistance with filing complaints
- Explanations of how to respond to questions on job applications and at interviews

The military

Some survivors of childhood cancer wish to enlist in the military, or qualify for ROTC, the reserves, or the service academies. The Childhood Cancer Ombudsman Program can research federal regulations and research previous cases to help the survivor get accepted into the military.

Insurance

Job discrimination can spell economic catastrophe for cancer survivors because most health insurance is obtained from employment. As survivors mature, seek employment, and move away from home, many encounter barriers to obtaining health insurance, such as rejection of application based on cancer history, policy reductions, policy cancellation, pre-existing condition exclusions, increased premiums, or extended waiting periods. As current discussions about national healthcare reform are extremely contentious, it seems unlikely that major reforms of the American health insurance system will occur in the near future.

> I realize that I must do whatever is necessary to stay covered on my parent's insurance as long as possible. I don't particularly like that, but it is important. As long as I remain a full-time student, it will be okay.

Twenty-five states offer high-risk individuals, like survivors, access to comprehensive health insurance plans (CHIPS). CHIPS, also called "high-risk pools," are a means for individuals to obtain insurance regardless of their physical condition or medical history. For more information on CHIPS, call your state Office of the Insurance Commissioner. The NCI publication *Facing Forward* lists contacts by state for insurance coverage for the hard to insure. See Appendix D, *Books and Online Sites*, for ordering information.

Although neither the US federal nor the state governments mandate a legal right to insurance, there are some legal remedies to insurance discrimination:

- COBRA. The Comprehensive Omnibus Budget Reconciliation Act (COBRA) is a federal law which requires public and private companies employing more than twenty workers to provide continuation of group coverage to employees if they quit, are fired, or work reduced hours. Coverage must extend to surviving, divorced, or separated spouses, and to dependent children. You must pay for your continued coverage, but it must not exceed by more than 2 percent the rate set for your former co-workers. By allowing you to purchase continued coverage, you have time to seek other long-term coverage.

- ERISA. The Employee Retirement and Income Security Act (ERISA) is a federal law which protects workers from being fired because of the cancer history of the employee or beneficiaries (spouse and children). ERISA also prohibits employers from encouraging a person with a cancer history to retire as a "disabled" employee. ERISA does not apply to job discrimination (denial of new job due to cancer history), discrimination which does not affect benefits, and employees whose compensation does not include benefits.

- Health Insurance Portability and Accountability Act of 1996. This law allows individuals to change to a new job without losing coverage if they have been insured for at least twelve months. It prevents group health plans from denying coverage based on medical history, genetic information, or claims history, although insurers can still exclude those with specific diseases or conditions. It also increases portability if you change from a group to an individual plan.

ERISA, COBRA, and parts of the Health Insurance Portability and Accountability Act of 1996 are enforced by the Pension and Welfare Benefits Administration in Washington, DC, (202) 219-8776.

For detailed information on the ADA, COBRA, ERISA, and the Health Insurance Portability and Accountability Act of 1996, read *A Cancer Survivor's Almanac: Charting Your Journey*, edited by Barbara Hoffman, JD.

Appendix C contains an extensive list of resource organizations which can help if you or your child faces job discrimination or problems with insurance due to treatment for cancer.

CHAPTER 26

Relapse

Hold fast to dreams
For if dreams die
Life is a broken winged bird
That cannot fly.

—Langston Hughes

PARENTS FREQUENTLY DESCRIBE the return of their child's cancer as more devastating than the original diagnosis. Parents feel betrayed. They think that they put their child through hell for nothing. They are scared, for they know that any recurrence is serious. The anger is back—since they did everything the doctors said, why did the cancer return? They are afraid that if the first battery of treatments didn't work, what will? And the unspoken but most crushing feeling of all: "If my child dies, how will I survive?"

If your child has relapsed, one point is well worth remembering: you are not the same person that you were at diagnosis. You've been through this before so you know how to get medical and emotional support. You have a relationship with the medical team, and you can speak the language now. You have developed friendships with other families of children with cancer. You know that something that seems insurmountable can be overcome, one day at a time.

This chapter explains how doctors determine if a relapse has occurred, emotional responses of the parents, and how to decide on a treatment plan.

Signs and symptoms

Relapse can happen at any time during treatment or after therapy ends. The signs and symptoms of relapse can include many or all of the indicators that were present at diagnosis:

- Discomfort
- Shortness of breath

- Pain

- Bruises

- Pale skin

- Back, leg, or joint pain

- Loss of appetite

- Fatigue

- A lump or mass

- Enlarged abdomen caused by a large spleen or liver

- Changes in behavior, such as excessive irritability

- Dizziness

- Headaches

- Limping

Remember that many of these symptoms are also seen with normal childhood illnesses. However, persistent loss of appetite or fatigue or unusually severe symptoms require a call to your oncologist.

> Zack (age six) was in remission after thirteen rounds of chemo for stage IV neuroblastoma. He had scans every three months and everything was looking good. Nine months later, Zack started to complain that his hair hurt. "Hair pain" seemed weird to me, so we went to the doctor. Blood test results came back abnormal, and the worry intensified. We admitted Zack to the hospital feeling fine, with the exception of his sore hair! The doctor ordered a bunch of tests and scans which came back fine, but when the bone marrow aspiration was done, the news was not good. His cancer had come back.

In some cases, parents have no warning. After they bring their child in for a routine examination, they receive a totally unexpected telephone call from the doctor with the news.

> I am a long-term survivor (30 years old), who first was diagnosed with cancer at age 8 and subsequently relapsed three times, at ages 13, 15, and 16. The first relapse was by far the worst to deal with emotionally. It had been five years since my diagnosis, so I went in for my last bone marrow aspiration. I had been off treatment with good counts for two years. My mother and I didn't even wait for the test results; we went out to lunch and went shopping. Later that day, I called the clinic, and my

doctor told me the bone marrow was fine, but she needed to talk to my
mother. I heard my mother say, "No, no, oh no," and she started to cry. I
just stood there feeling numb, knowing the news was bad. The cancer had
returned. We held each other and cried.

The site of relapse depends on the type of solid tumor. The disease can recur in the area of the original tumor, or it may develop elsewhere.

Jody was complaining about pain and a feeling of pressure in his leg
bones. I kept bringing him back to the oncologist, saying that something
was wrong, that he was in great pain, but the doctor kept insisting that it
was just growing pains. He didn't even examine his legs for a month.
When he did, he could feel parts of the bone radiating heat. The bone
scan showed the cancer in the exact spots that Jody had pointed out.

Some children develop an entirely different type of cancer than they had in the beginning. These second cancers can be caused by some types of chemotherapy or radiation. Evidence also shows that some children may have a genetic predisposition to cancer.

Emotional responses

Parents who have children with cancer in remission think or speak of relapse with an almost palpable dread. Just the thought can cause the emotions which surged in them at diagnosis to erupt. The depth of the emotions generated by relapse is very hard for parents and survivors to relive and describe. As one survivor said in a shaky voice when being interviewed, "It's been eleven years since I finished treatment, but talking about it shows that you scratch the surface and those overwhelming feelings are still right there."

Parents feel a wide array of emotions at relapse: numbness, guilt, dread, anger, fear, confusion, denial, and grief. Physical symptoms such as dizziness, nausea, fainting, and shortness of breath are common. Parents wonder how they can ask their child to endure it again. They wonder how they will survive it themselves. They oscillate between optimism and panic.

I found that relapse was far worse than the original diagnosis. At
diagnosis, after a certain period of adjustment, you think that treatment
has a beginning, a middle, and an end. But relapse creates a bigger bur-
den to accept. You begin to feel that maybe the disease is more powerful
than the medicine. I found that for a while I just stopped functioning and

thinking rationally. I felt that all the hell of treatment had been just a waste of time. I felt guilt and a tremendous sense of loss of control. I felt like I was on a runaway freight train, hurtling towards an end that didn't look so good anymore. This is the point at which people are willing to use any type of unconventional therapies because they are desperate. I know one mom in our support group who was even willing to try coffee enemas. She looks back on it now and says, "I just went crazy."

· · · · ·

My first relapse was the worst emotionally. Neither my parents or I ever thought that after five years it would be back. I also had been so young when I was first treated that I didn't really think of cancer as cancer and didn't understand that I could die from it. But at thirteen, I remembered clearly what I had been through and all I could think was that it hadn't worked. I told my parents that I wouldn't do it again. My father sat me down and gave me a reality check. He explained that I would die if I didn't get treatment. He said, "If you don't do it for yourself, please do it for me and your mom." The next morning I went into the clinic and started all over again.

Deciding on a treatment plan

A rapid response is necessary when faced with a recurrence of childhood cancer. Treatment plans for a first relapse may be specified in your child's protocol, or your physician may suggest a different approach. Suggestions for treatment may include radiation, more intensive chemotherapy, surgery, immunotherapy, or bone marrow or stem cell transplantation.

Physicians make recommendations based on knowledge, experience, and consultations with other experts in the field. Do not hesitate to ask your physician why she has suggested a certain approach to your child's relapse. Ask your doctor about treatment goals, methods, and possible side effects. Ask your doctor if she has consulted with others in the decision-making process, and if so, whom. Older children and teens need to be involved in decisions regarding their care and treatment choices.

Health Canada's publication, *This Battle Which I Must Fight: Cancer in Canada's Children and Teenagers*, states:

> *This (relapse) is a time of crisis and ambivalence. The decision to be made is whether to continue to try to achieve a remission or to replace*

this hope with the hope for comfort for the child and a special time together. Each parent, and the child who is old enough to understand, requires differing amounts of time to reach a decision about how to proceed. Careful and frequent discussions with the medical team, as well as with trusted friends and relatives, may help clarify issues and bring some peace-of-mind.

Just like at diagnosis, time is a pressing concern. Parents know that treatment should begin as soon as possible. But beware rushing into a new treatment plan if you feel uncomfortable. Your child needs to know that you are 100 percent in favor of proceeding, and children have radar for parents' feelings. There is always time for answers to all of your questions and time to get a second opinion.

Refer to Chapter 4, *Forming a Partnership with the Medical Team*, for ways to obtain a second opinion. One excellent resource is the Childhood Cancer Ombudsman Program (see Appendix C, *Resource Organizations*, for contact information). Panels of volunteer pediatric oncologists volunteer to give second medical opinions or medical record reviews at the request of families or the treating oncologist. The program is particularly valuable in helping families make well-informed treatment choices, as well as becoming comfortable with the therapeutic approach chosen.

The Physician's Data Query (800) 4-CANCER or *http://cancernet.nci.nih.gov/pdq.htm* lists protocols for recurrent disease currently being used as well as ongoing clinical trials. The information gleaned from second opinions and/or research may reinforce what your doctor recommended, or it might provide you with some additional treatment options. Either way, it may increase your comfort level during the treatment planning process.

The following are questions that you might want to ask your doctor when discussing the treatment plan:

- What is the goal of this treatment? Is it likely to cure my child, or is it meant to keep him comfortable?

    After my son relapsed, we set immediately back to work trying to determine what the best treatment option for him should be. His oncologist was very committed to making him well again. As it turned out, the best option was a phase II study drug that wasn't yet available in our area. The hospital social worker helped us with travel arrangements and accommodations, and within a day we were on a plane headed for another hospital. Meanwhile, the oncologist completed all the necessary paperwork so that by the time the next course of chemotherapy was due, it was able to be administered at our own hospital. It was obvious to us from the very beginning of relapse that we had a wonderful medical team that was dedicated to helping our son get well again.

Unfortunately, after two courses of chemotherapy, it was clear that the drug wasn't getting rid of the cancer. Once again, we all rolled up our sleeves and tried to find another protocol that might help him. Some of the options we tried were protocols that I had found. I would gather the information and then his oncologist and I would sit and review all the data. As long as the therapy was reasonable and had the potential to help without further diminishing his quality of life, it was worth considering. One of the most comforting things that my son's oncologist ever said to me was, "I will always be in your corner."

- Why do you think that this treatment is the best option? What are the other choices, and why did you choose this one?

- Have you consulted with other physicians? If so, whom? Did you all agree on this treatment, or was there a range of choices suggested?

- Is there a standard treatment for this type of relapse? What is it?

- What clinical trials are ongoing for this type of relapse?

- Explain the potential benefits and possible side effects of the suggested treatment.

- What are the known or potential risks of the treatment?

- How often will my child need to be hospitalized?

- How long will my child need this treatment?

- If the treatment is investigational, is there scientific evidence that it works for her type of cancer?

- Does insurance cover this type of investigational treatment?

When Greg relapsed, they threw his protocol in the trash can, and our oncologist started making phone calls to other doctors in the Children's Cancer Group network to decide on a plan. Greg was put successively on three different relapse protocols in an attempt to keep him in remission.

· · · · ·

*After another relapse, they wanted to try a chemotherapy with lim-
ited possible results, and we really didn't want our eleven-year-old Caitlin to go through any more. But she talked it over with the doctor and
concluded, "Of course I have to do it, I'm a fighting Irish."*

When older children and parents disagree on the details of how to proceed,
use the hospital social worker or psychologist to help you negotiate and
make compromises. These discussions will help clarify each family member's thoughts and feelings, and will allow the child's emotional and physical
well-being to be part of the equation.

In the Spring 1995 issue of the Candlelighters newsletter, Arthur Ablin, MD
(Director Emeritus of Pediatric Clinical Oncology at the University of California, San Francisco) wrote of the importance of goal setting in the decision-making process after relapse:

*Before determining which treatment is to be chosen, a decision must
be made to determine the goal of treatment—in other words, what is it
that we are trying to achieve. This crucial first step is the basis upon
which any decision concerning treatment must be made. But it is too often
omitted from consideration and/or discussion, even by the most experienced. The frustrations accompanying the previous failure of treatment,
the fear of the loss of the hope for cure, the pressure of urgency to find
solutions, the new awareness of the possibility or probability of death,
lead us all to want to consider treatments first rather than these more difficult considerations involved in establishing goals. These also force us to
deal with reality earlier, which could mean the almost intolerable confrontation with the death of a very-much-loved child, a tragedy to be avoided
at all cost.*

After you have set goals, received answers to all of your questions, obtained
a second opinion if desired, and decided on a treatment plan, it is time to
proceed. Your knowledge and experience may prove to be a double-edged
sword. You have no illusions about the difficulties ahead because you've
done it before, but you also will be strengthened by your ties with the cancer community, your comfort with your physicians and hospital routines,
and your ability to work with the system to get what your child needs. Many
parents shared how their child took the lead about relapse treatment. While
the parents agonized, their child said simply, "Let's just do it." And they did.

I encourage people to try to keep things in perspective. Attitude is a big part of survival. As difficult as it is, try to maintain a good attitude and keep focused on the future. I always thought, "I have cancer, this is a bad thing, but I am going to beat it." My analogy was a boxing match. When I relapsed, I was knocked down. But I always got up and kept fighting.

I had a total of three relapses, two of which were on treatment. Every time we relapse, statistics say our chances of survival are less likely. But I survived those three relapses, and now I live a life as normal as if cancer never touched it. After cancer, I finished high school and went to college. I gave birth to a beautiful, healthy baby girl. My daughter (still beautiful) is now seven years old, and with her I'll have a chance to relive some of the childhood I missed. For me, life does go on after cancer.

CHAPTER 27

Death and Bereavement

*In this book I have tried to capture a few
remembered strains of the brief, glad music of
my son's life. These are all I have of him now,
and they comfort me even as they
break my heart.*

—Gordon Livingstone, MD
Only Spring

THE DEATH OF A CHILD causes almost unendurable pain and anguish for loved ones left behind. Death from cancer comes after months or years of debilitating treatment, emotional swings, and financial crises. The family begins the years of grief already exhausted from the years of fighting cancer. It is truly every parent's worst nightmare.

In this chapter, many parents share their innermost thoughts and feelings about their decisions to end treatment, death at home or in the hospital, and grief. It didn't matter whether the parents had recently lost their child or it had happened decades ago—tears flowed when talking about it. Because family members and friends can be strong sources of support, or casualties of the grieving process, parents describe things that really helped them, and they make suggestions on what to avoid. Grief has as many facets as there are grieving parents, so what follows are the experiences of a few.

Making the decision to end treatment

For children or teenagers who have had a series of relapses, medical caregivers and parents need to decide when to end active treatment and begin to work toward making the child comfortable for his remaining days. This is an intensely personal decision. Some families want to try every available treatment and exhaust all possible remedies. Others reach a point where they feel they have done all they can and they simply do not want their child to suffer any more. They hope for time to share memories, express love, and prepare for death.

> *When Cienna was found to have tumors metastasized to her brain, I knew that I was not so desperate for her to live that I would sacrifice the last bit of quality life she had left, dragging her from doctor to doctor, putting her through treatment after treatment, so that I could hope to have one more day with her. Doing that would not have been for her, but for me. If Cienna had been older and was able to choose for herself it would have been one thing, but she could not. I struggle with the "quantity versus quality" issue and usually keep it to myself. A lot of people, including some doctors, think quantity is more important. I believe it's not how much time you have, but what you do with it that matters most. I loved her so much that I wanted the remainder of her life to be happy and not filled with more suffering than she was already enduring from her cancer.*

Although no child is a statistic, at relapse it is important to look at probabilities of cure, tumor control, and impact of the disease and treatment options on the child's emotional and physical well-being. Older children and teenagers need to be an integral part in these discussions. Their thoughts and feelings are crucial during the decision-making process. Age, coping mechanisms, culture, and communication styles within families all affect discussions. Honest, thorough communication between the ill child or teen, family members, and involved professionals helps everyone work toward the same endpoint.

Dr. Arthur Ablin, Director Emeritus of Pediatric Clinical Oncology at the University of California, San Francisco, wrote in the Spring 1995 Candlelighters newsletter about the difficulties of deciding to end active treatment:

> *All too often, the decision to abandon the goal for cure and, reluctantly, accept the reality of inevitable death of a child is too painful and, therefore, never made. This paralyzing pain occurs with equal frequency, perhaps, for the family and the doctor. We of the medical profession have no equal in our ability to prolong dying. We have a powerful array of mechanical, electronic, pharmaceutical, and biotechnical interventions at our command. We can keep people dying for months and even years. Applying or withholding this armamentarium is an awesome responsibility, and it requires infinite wisdom to know how to manage wisely and correctly. We can do great good by applying these tools correctly, but can also do incalculable harm through over-utilization. Physicians and families alike must work together to avoid the possible pitfalls. When cure is beyond all of us, then the challenge is to make the rest of life as worth-*

while and rich as possible. There is much to do for the terminally and critically ill child and his or her family. They have that right, we have the privilege, to be of service.

Many children know when it is time to stop. In the Spring 1995 issue of the Candlelighters newsletter, Grace Powers Monaco describes how her four-year-old daughter told her that it was time to stop treatment:

> *I don't think I can come home, Mommy! All my machinery is worn out, and I don't think they have any more parts.*

Another parent relates how her son felt it was time to stop:

> *When my six-year-old son Greg was in the hospital in intensive relapse treatment, he would repeat over and over again, "I want to go home." When he was finally well enough to come home for awhile, he kept saying, "I want to go home." In frustration, I said, "Greg, you are home, why do you keep saying that?" He looked up and quietly said, "I want to go to my heavenly home. I want to go to God." I said, "Honey, please don't say that," and, knowing how much we loved him, he replied, "Okay, Mom, I'll fight, I won't go." And he did fight hard for several more months. But he was way ahead of us in acceptance, he was at peace, and he knew it was time to let go.*

When it is clear that death is inevitable, parents struggle with the thought of how to "tell" the ill child and siblings. All too often in our culture, children are perceived as having to be protected from death, as if this somehow makes their last days better. On the contrary, any pediatric nurse, oncologist, or social worker can tell you that children, often as young as four, know that they are dying. If the parents are trying to spare the child, an unhealthy situation develops. The child pretends everything is okay to please the parents, and the parents try to mask their deep grief with false smiles. Everyone loses.

This scenario is replayed on a daily basis at hospitals all over the country: scared, lonely children die without being able to tell the people they love the most how they are feeling. This type of denial keeps children and parents alike from finishing up business—distributing belongings, telling each other how much they love one another, and saying good-bye. It also strips parents of their ability to prepare their child for the journey from life to death. Children need to know what to expect. They need to know that they will be surrounded by those they love, that their parents will be holding them, and they need to know the family's beliefs about what happens after death.

Jennifer contracted a respiratory fungal infection that resulted in her being hospitalized on a ventilator. She was given lots of morphine so that she wouldn't feel air hungry. She was alert off and on for a few days. We read to her and played tapes. After one week on the respirator, she took a turn for the worse. She didn't respond to me after that. Her kidneys were ceasing to function, and she started to get puffy. Her liver was deteriorating, and her painful pancreatitis had come back. After ten days on the respirator, I couldn't bear it any longer. I lay down in her bed, took her in my arms, and kissed her at least 200 times. I talked to her for a long time, and told her that we would take care of her cats, and that I was sorry that she had to suffer so much, and how beautiful Heaven is. I told her to go be with Jesus, her Grandpa, and her dog. I also told her how much we all loved her and how proud we were of her. I got off the bed to change positions, and the nurse rushed in. Her heart had suddenly stopped the second I got up. I believe she heard me and just needed to know it was okay to go. She didn't want to leave until she knew her mommy was ready.

Because of her Christian upbringing, Jennifer knew all about Heaven. She had told me that she wasn't afraid to die, and this has been a great source of comfort to us. I believe that she was preparing for her death, even as we hoped for her remission. Before she went to the hospital, she spent all her money, gave away some of her possessions to her sisters, and said a final good-bye to her home, cats, teachers, and friends.

Supportive care

In the US and Canada, there are very active and effective hospice systems. Hospices ease the transition from hospital to home and provide support for the entire family. Hospice personnel ensure adequate pain control, allow the patient to control the last days or weeks of his life, and provide active bereavement support after death.

Usually, if the family wishes the child to die at home, a smooth transition occurs from the oncology ward to hospice care. Unfortunately, sometimes pediatric patients are not referred to hospice, and the parents are left to deal with their child's last days at home with no experienced help and no clear idea of what is to come. Before you leave the hospital, it is wise to find out the name of a contact person at the agency that will be taking over the home care of your child.

When Jody came home, he was assigned both a pediatric visiting nurse and a hospice nurse. On their first visits, I was handed a great deal of literature to read, including a whole notebook from hospice. I lacked both the desire and energy to read the literature and learn a whole new medical system—let alone two. I just wanted one phone number to call for help, with two or three consistent people to answer.

In actuality, the care we received was wonderful. The primary nurse would call, offer to visit if we wanted it, assess Jody's condition over the phone, handle any questions we had, and would ask if we wanted a call the next day. She would tell us who would be calling if she was not working at the appointed time. Interestingly, the service that I found most beneficial at that time was the nurse running interference for us with the doctor. The pain medications needed to be adjusted and changed at times; advice was needed about his intake, his mouth sores, and his hand and foot inflammation. As I, along with Jody, became quieter and more removed from outside activities, even the thought of calling the clinic and being made directly aware of the bustle and demands of that world was very unappealing.

If you have questions about hospice or what support is available, you can contact Children's Hospice International at (800) 2-4-CHILD.

Dying in the hospital

Some children die in the hospital suddenly, while others slowly decline for weeks or months. If your child is slowly dying, you may have choices about where she will spend her last days. There are no right or wrong choices. Much depends on the number of people available to provide care at home, and how comfortable they are doing so. Many parents ask their child where he prefers to be. Some children and teens like to be with the nurses in a hospital environment, while others want to stay at home with brothers, sisters, friends, and pets. Parents, children, and staff need to talk honestly to decide on the appropriate place for the child, and then obtain the support (hospice, private nurses in the hospital, family members) needed to make the choice a comfortable reality. Remain flexible so that as the situation changes, options remain open.

Although we had been advised that it didn't look good for Greg, we were trying one last time to get him to transplant. He was sleeping qui-

*etly in his hospital bed. He had been complaining of severe head pain, and
was on a low morphine drip. The afternoon nurse woke him to take vitals,
and he chatted with her. He told me, "Mom, I'm going to go back to sleep,
I love you." Two hours later the night nurse tried to wake him up to give
him some medicine, and she couldn't wake him. They called the doctor in
from his home, and he ordered a CAT scan. When the film came up to the
floor, the doctor took me out in the hall and said, "He's not going to live
through the night." He held up the film showing a massive cerebral infarc-
tion; Greg was bleeding into the brain. He quietly died less than an hour
later. Family and staff were in total shock. Nobody expected it. But, looking back, Greg had decided that he had had enough, he was ready to go. I
am grateful that he didn't die on a transplant floor in a strange city. We
were able to call in friends and family, and we were surrounded and supported by the wonderful nurses whom we knew so intimately. I couldn't
leave him until three nurses promised to stay with him and escort him to
the morgue. They are still dear friends.*

• • • • •

*I felt bad for my daughter, because like any good child, she wanted
permission, even to die. My husband had promised her that he would
never give up. He kept on saying, "Fight. Fight. Don't give up, don't leave
me. We'll do another transplant, we'll try different medicine. It's too early
to give up." I looked at him and said, "She's not going anywhere until you
tell her that it's okay." Then he told her, and she took her last breath. He
still feels guilty to this day because of his promises. He just doesn't understand that it was time; that she needed to know that it was okay with us.*

Parents of children who died in the hospital stressed the importance of clear
communication. Parents need to be strong advocates for adequate pain control, and they need to clearly tell the staff how they would like things to be.
For instance, in most hospitals, patients are routinely resuscitated using CPR
and electric shocks to the heart (this is called a "code"). Parents need to discuss their wishes with the oncologist and ensure that an order of "NO
CODE" is put in the chart and on the child's door. Parents also should discuss whether they want nurses or doctors present when their child dies.
Many families feel very close to the hospital staff and feel supported by their
presence, while others prefer to have only family and close friends at the
bedside. Advance planning helps to ensure that as death approaches, the
family's wishes are understood and respected.

Dying at home

A child's death at home can be a peaceful or a frightening experience, depending on the extent of preparation and the quality of support provided to the family.

We decided to bring Jody home to die for several reasons. First of all, the medical profession was offering no more realistic hope. Secondly, Jody was young enough and small enough to be easily held, carried, cared for by us. Thirdly, nothing violent or terrifying happened to make us seriously debate whether to go back in the hospital with him.

I saw many life values in a new way from the experience of Jody dying at home. What comes to my mind is a sunny, breezy afternoon, September 13. Only Jody and I were home. I held him outside under the plum tree for perhaps an hour and a half or longer. I couldn't support him well and read to him at the same time, so we didn't do anything. I spoke to him some, but mostly just held him quietly. I was aware as I looked up into the sky that my normal reaction on such a day would be to want to be hiking, biking, "doing" something. A surprise recognition burst and spread gently through my consciousness: I was exactly where I wanted to be and no doing of anything could mean as much as being there with Jody.

Jody's last day, September 16, was peaceful. A spiritual healer, whom Jody had known for two years, came and spent time with him. A massage therapist/healer/friend, who had visited him several times during the five weeks he was home, gave him a long, gentle massage. My husband Tom stayed home from teaching that day (by chance?). Jody lay in his arms or on my lap most of the day. The visiting home nurse came by briefly, offered to stay, but we preferred to be alone. I was holding Jody; Tom was next to me holding his feet. His breathing became labored and irregular. His eyes were unblinking long before he took his last breath, then a heartbeat, then another, then silence.

· · · · ·

Martin (three years old) died very peacefully at home in our bed. He was so weak, but he still managed to drink by himself. We were all in the bed together, my husband and me, our little three-month-old daughter, and Martin. His dad was reading him Winnie-the-Pooh, and Martin just stopped breathing. The most difficult time for us was when they came to take his body away. I feared that moment and it was so very horrible.

Siblings

Whether your child is dying at home or in the hospital, any siblings should be included in the family response. Being part of things and having jobs to do helps brothers and sisters remain involved, contributing members of the family. Young children can answer the doorbell, go on errands, or make tapes to play for the sibling. Older children can help with meals, stay with the ill child to give parents a break, answer the phones, or help make funeral arrangements. These jobs should not be "make-work"—children should truly be helping. This allows them not only to clarify their role in the family, but helps them to prepare for the death as well as have an opportunity to say good-bye. These jobs help siblings feel themselves to be a useful part of the family rather than a forgotten and perhaps less loved brother or sister.

The Compassionate Friends, an organization for both parents and siblings, is listed in Appendix C, *Resource Organizationss*.

The funeral

Funerals and related rituals (memorial services, wakes, burial, shiva) are important not only as a times to say good-bye and to begin to accept the reality of death, but they also provide an opportunity to recognize the relationships and impact that the child or teen has had on others. Funerals allow friends and family to gather together to share memories and to show support for the remaining family members. A funeral is a tangible demonstration of love.

> *When Michael died, we wanted to plan a perfect memorial service for him. We were disappointed, however, that there wasn't much available in the way of children's materials. Most of it pertained to adults. So, we did things our own way. I had been thinking about how things would be done long before Michael died. Nick and I had some ideas, but we also asked Michael what he would like at his memorial service. One point he made quite clear was that he wanted balloons instead of flowers since "flowers are for girls." He also told me exactly what he wanted to wear— his 101 Dalmatians shirt with his favorite black sweat pants and Batman socks—which we granted. He even helped with an idea for his gravestone. He was familiar with them since we had visited his Grampa's grave a lot. In fact, they're buried beside each other. Michael wanted a little lamb and a cross on his stone. A lamb because Jesus was the shepherd and*

we were the sheep, and a cross because that was what Jesus died on for our sins. He was very mature in the way he handled his impending death, even though he was only four years old. Never did he fear it, nor dwell on it, nor become angry about it. The way Michael put it was, "Well, Mom. Some people die and some people don't."

Children of all ages should be allowed to attend the funeral if they wish, but only after they have been prepared about what to expect. They need an explanation of where they will be going (funeral, shiva, wake, memorial service, burial) and what it means. They need to know what type of room they are going to, if the casket will be there, if it will be open, if there will be flowers, who will be there, how the mourners will be acting, who will stay with the them, what they will be expected to say, and how long they will be there. All questions should be answered honestly and children's feelings respected.

Many siblings also benefit from giving one last gift to the departed, such as writing a private note and dropping it in the casket, or bringing some of their sister's favorite flowers to put in her hands. If you have any questions or concerns about what to tell the remaining children or whether they should attend the services or burial, read *How Do We Tell the Children? A Parent's Guide to Helping Children Understand and Cope when Someone Dies* by Dan Schaefer and Christine Lyons, which is listed in Appendix D, *Books and Online Sites*.

One of our pastors was a very close personal friend who stayed with us for the last three days in the hospital at Jesse's bedside. When she died, we were physically and emotionally weary; we just couldn't think. He and the other pastors planned the whole service and walked us through it.

There were hundreds of people there—Jesse had touched so many lives. The pastors had known Jesse her whole life and they loved her, truly loved her. They told personal stories, reminisced about the last hugs they had shared with her. They told the story of her faith and of her death, which comforted many of those who attended. Each family member walked up during the service and brought some of her favorite flowers.

We had given our children free rein to pick out the clothes that Jesse would be buried in. They made very thoughtful choices: her favorite, very comfortable pajamas with little tea cups on them, and her teddy bear. The service was very special—a celebration, a testament to her faith and ours.

Ministers, priests, and rabbis have a unique opportunity to provide support, love, and comfort to the grieving family and friends. They usually know the family well, and can evoke poignant memories of the deceased child or teen during the service. Members of the clergy often have excellent counseling skills, and can visit the family after the funeral to provide ongoing help during mourning.

The role of family and friends

Family members and friends can be a wellspring of deep comfort and solace during grieving. Some people seem to know just when a hug is necessary or when silence is most welcome. Unfortunately, in our society there are few guidelines for handling the social aspects of grief. Many well-meaning people voice opinions concerning the time it is taking to "get over it" or question the parents' decision to not give away their child's clothing. Others do not know what to say, so they are silent, pretending that life's greatest catastrophe has not occurred. Many friends never again mention the deceased child's name, not knowing that this silence, as if the cherished child never existed, only adds to parents' pain. Holidays can become uncomfortable, as they bring sadness as well as joy.

In an attempt to alleviate these difficulties, bereaved parents helped compile the following lists of what helps, and what does not, in the hope that it may guide those family members and friends who deeply care, but just don't know how to help. These suggestions are offered with the understanding that what works for one person may not work for another. Try to use your knowledge of the bereaved family to choose options that you think will make them comfortable. If in doubt, ask them. As Mother Theresa said, "Kind words can be short and easy to say, but their echoes are truly endless."

Things that help

The long lists of things that help from Chapter 3, *Family and Friends*, (e.g., keeping the household running, feeding the family, and helping with bills) are still appropriate here. The following lists are specific suggestions for grief:

Helpful things to say:

- I am so sorry.

- I cannot imagine the pain you are feeling, but I am thinking about you.

- I really care about you.

- You and your family are in my thoughts and prayers.

- We would like to hold a memorial service at the school for your son if you think that it would be appropriate.

- I will never forget John's sunny smile.

- I will never forget Jane's gentle way with children and animals.

Parents also offer a list of helpful things to do:

- Go to the funeral or memorial service.

   We were overwhelmed and touched by all of the people who came to the funeral. Even people that I had not seen in years—like some of my college professors—attended. Her oncologist and nurse drove 100 miles to be there.

- Show genuine concern and caring by listening.

   What has helped me the most is for people to just listen. Finding time to remember and reminisce is sometimes very difficult and painful, yet other times I feel much pride and happiness. Friends whose children also have cancer have been the greatest help to me during my daughter's illness and after her death.

- Help the siblings.

   We had friends just call and say, "We will pick up Nick on Saturday and take him to Water World, then to our house for dinner. We were hoping he could spend the night. Will that be all right?" They did this many times, and it not only was fun for him, but gave us a chance to be alone with each other and our grief.

- Write the parents a note instead of sending just a preprinted sympathy card with your signature. Include special things you remember about their child or your feelings about their child. Letters, poems, or drawings from classmates and friends allow children to share their feelings with the family of the deceased, as well as provide poignant testimonials that the family will cherish.

- Talk about the child who has died. Parents forever carry cherished memories of their child and enjoy hearing others' favorite recollections.

Months after the funeral, we gathered family members and some close friends to share memories on tape. We did a lot of laughing as well as shed a few tears. But I will always cherish those tapes.

. . . . .

I think most of all parents want their child to be remembered. It really comforts me to go to Greg's grave and find flowers, notes, or toys left by others.

- When parents express guilt over what they did or did not do, reassure them that they did everything they could. Remind them that they provided their child with the best medicine had to offer.

- Remember anniversaries. Call or send a card or flowers on the anniversary of the child's death.

- Respect the family's method of grieving.

- Give donations in the child's name to a favorite charity of the child or parents, for instance, the child's school library, Candlelighters, the local children's camp, The American Cancer Society, or US Children's Hospice International.

Every year we still get a card saying that Caitlin's occupational therapist donated money to Camp Goodtimes. It makes me feel good that she is remembered so fondly and that the money will help other kids with cancer and their brothers and sisters.

- Commemorate the child's life in some tangible way. Examples of this are: planting trees, shrubs, or flowers, erecting a memorial or plaque, or displaying a picture of the child.

The spring after Matthew's death, his school contacted me and said they wanted to do something special in his honor. They planted a little leaf linden tree in front of the building and built a wonderful seat around its base. They picked this particular tree because of its wonderful fragrance, and because the leaves were shaped like little hearts. A plaque beside the tree proclaims that this is Matthew's Friendship Tree. In addition to his name and the date of his birth and death, it reads: "When you remember me, please have a smile and cherish the good times we shared. And in these memories I will live with you forever."

- Be patient. Acute grief from the loss of a child lasts a long, long time. Expectations of a rapid recovery are unrealistic and hurtful to parents.

- Encourage follow-up from medical personnel.

Caitlin had a very kind, very gentle radiation oncologist. I went back to see her after Caitlin died; she said, "We were so happy when we saw the progress that Caitlin made, from a stretcher to sitting to talking and walking again; and then our hearts broke when she relapsed. I wept." It was so human and so wonderful for her to let me know that she cared.

Things that do not help

Please do not say the following to the parents:

- I know exactly how you feel.
- It's a blessing her suffering has ended.
- Thank goodness you are young enough to have another child.
- At least you have your other children.
- Be brave.
- Time will heal.
- God doesn't give anyone more than they can bear.
- It was God's will.
- He's in a better place now.

Every time someone approached me at the funeral home with the words, "He's gone to a better place," I felt as if I would scream. Matthew's place was with me, his mother. Seven-year-old boys need their mother. It also really angered me when people repeatedly said, "Oh, with all he suffered, you wouldn't wish him back if you could." Well, yes, I would wish my child back! I would wish him back healthy and well. To this very day I would wish my child back, even if I could hold him for just a moment or hear the sound of his laughter one more time.

- God must have needed another angel.
- It's lucky this happened to someone as strong as you.
- Don't worry, in time you'll get over it.
- Why did you decide to cremate him?
- How is your marriage holding up?
- You need to be strong for your other children.

Please do not say to the siblings:

- You need to be strong for your mom and dad.

- Don't cry, it upsets your parents.

- You're the man of the house now.

- How does it feel to be the big sister?

Even if a bereaved parent has deep religious faith, it is often tested by their child's death. Parents are not comforted by well-meaning friends who assume faith is making the grief bearable; indeed, many parents find it to be infuriating. It's better to just say "I'm sorry."

In the months and years following the child's death, any of the following might not be appreciated:

- Don't you think it's time to get over it?

- It's been six months; it's time to put the past behind you.

- Life goes on.

- You need to get on with your life.

- You shouldn't be feeling that way.

- Don't you think you should give away all of his clothes?

- Don't cry.

- Don't be sad.

- Don't worry.

- Doesn't it bother you to have her pictures around?

- Please don't talk about Johnnie, it just stirs up all those memories.

- It's not good to just sit around, you need to get out and have some fun.

Don't let your own sense of helplessness keep you from reaching out. Pretending that nothing is wrong or being afraid to talk about the child who has died hurts grieving parents.

The following are suggestions from parents on what not to do:

- Don't remove anything which belonged to the child who died, unless specifically asked to by the parents.

    *One family member took my son's toothbrush out of the bathroom
    and threw it away. I missed it immediately. She probably felt that she was*

doing me a favor, but it made me so angry. I needed to keep things. I have his hair from the second time it fell out, because he wanted to save it, and I've kept his teeth which had to be pulled during treatment. I just need to have those things, and I resent people who insist you must clear out a child's things. Parents should be able to keep things or get rid of them—whichever is comfortable—regardless of others' opinions.

- Don't offer advice.

    Christie's room is still her room. We still refer to it as Christie's room. People just don't have the right to say you shouldn't leave that room empty: it's not empty, it's full of her life. I know that they are not trying to hurt us. It just bothers them to see that room. Sometimes it is just a reminder of death; yet, there are times when being in there and surrounded by all her things brings us closer to her and her time with us.

- Don't say anything which in any way suggests that the child's medical care was inadequate. Parents already feel intense guilt over what should have been or could have been.

    I can't tell you how many people said things like "If only you had gone to a different treatment facility," or "If only you had used this or that treatment." What people need most is support for what they are doing or did do.

- Don't look on the bright side or find silver linings.

    I became unexpectedly pregnant the month after my daughter died. I can't tell you how many people said things like "The circle of life is complete," or "God is taking one and giving you another," or "God is replacing her." She can never be replaced. It was horrible to hear those things, and I felt it was unfair to both the unborn baby and to my daughter who died.

- Don't come and pray over the child who is dying unless you have been asked.

    The mother of one of my son's friends called and asked to pray. I said okay, but was surprised when she showed up in person with a friend, and in a very loud voice, began exhorting the devil to leave. My son was only seven, and very sick, and it was scary for him.

· · · · ·

The sister of my son's bus driver, whom I had never met, came by the hospital with a bit of holy cloth to put under my son's pillow. It required us to say a special prayer over and over again. We declined, but it was awkward. People need to respect the parents' beliefs, not push their own.

- Don't drop bereaved parents from the support group. Talk about your options; grief-stricken parents have enough silence in their lives.

When my daughter was terminal, in really bad shape, I went to the support group. We had all bonded and were very close. I felt guilty because I really wanted to cry and was trying to hold it back because I didn't want to upset everybody else. All of the sudden, I felt like I was the alien, like you feel when your child is diagnosed. Here I was in a room full of people I loved, where I had felt safe. Now I was alone again, this time with no hopes of Christie's recovery. It was truly the end. I never felt more scared or alone.

- Don't make comments about the parents' strength.

People would say things to me like "You're so strong," or "I just couldn't live through what you have." It makes me want to scream. Do they mean I loved my child less than they love theirs because I have physically survived?

Sibling grief

Siblings are sometimes called the "forgotten grievers" because attention is typically focused on the parents. Children and teens hesitate to express their own strong feelings in an attempt to prevent causing their parents additional distress. Indeed, adult family members and friends may advise the brothers and sisters to "be strong" for their parents or to "help your parents by being good." These requests place a terribly unfair burden on children who have already endured months or years of stress and family disruption. Siblings need continual reinforcement that each of them is an irreplaceable member of the family and that the entire family has suffered a loss. They have a right to mourn openly, in their own way, and in their own time (which may be delayed or intermittent).

The family requires such reorganization after a child's death, and there is nowhere to look for an example. Each person in the family constellation has different feelings and different ways of grieving; there is just no way to reconcile all of this when the supposed leaders of the group are totally out of it. Not to mention the fact that both my husband and I wanted more understanding and compassion from each other than we were possibly able to give.

Children express grief in many ways, including physically (changes in eating habits, toileting, sleeping, stomachaches); emotionally (regression to earlier behaviors, risk taking); fear (of the dark, being away from parents); guilt (once said "I wish you would die," to the sibling, and the sibling died); and emotional changes (tantrums, crying, sadness, anxiety, withdrawal, depression). Older children and teens may appear nonchalant, angry, withdrawn, or take risks involving alcohol and drugs.

In families with siblings of different ages, parents need to engage them at their developmental level. Sometimes private times together or individual outings with the parent can be very helpful for siblings.

Many families pull apart because it is too painful to share their deep, but different feelings of grief. Some parents worry that if they start talking, they will "break down" in front of the children. But children who are excluded from the family's mourning may begin to feel alienated from the family. Here are suggestions from families about how to help pull together while mourning:

- Let the siblings go to the funeral. They have suffered a loss; they need to say good-bye; they need support for their grief just as much as adults.

- Children and teens experience the same feelings as adults. By sharing your own feelings, you can encourage them to identify their own. (For example, "I'm really feeling sad today. How do you feel?")

- Some families establish a regular meeting time to talk about their feelings. Both tears and laughter erupt when family members talk about funny or touching memories of the departed child. One family even had theme nights, such as trying to remember every practical joke he ever pulled, or things that he did that were not so nice (no need to remember the child as a saint).

- Jointly discuss how holidays and anniversaries should be observed. Some families hang a Christmas stocking every year for the departed child, while others merely mention her name during the blessing. Each family devises different ways to handle the child's birthday and the anniversary of her death.

Last year we marked our first Christmas since Matthew's death. It was so incredibly hard for me to open the boxes of decorations knowing that inside I would find treasures he had made for me over the years with his own two little hands. I cried when I found his stocking, because I didn't know what to do with it. Somehow it didn't seem right to not hang it as usual.

I decided that I would continue to place Matthew's stocking beside David's and Kristina's. Instead of Santa filling it with treats, I asked my family to fill it for me. A few weeks before Christmas, I ask members of my family to write a memory of Matthew on a piece of paper. The only stipulation is that it must be a happy memory. On Christmas morning I look forward most of all to the gifts my children have made for me in school, and the memories that fill Matthew's stocking. Matthew will always be included in our Christmas. That's because he will always be an important member of our family.

- Encourage all family members to join a group such as a Candlelighters bereavement group or Compassionate Friends, listed in Appendix C.

Parental grief

There are as many ways to grieve as there are bereaved parents. There is no timetable, no appropriate progression from one stage to the next, no time when parents should "be over it." Losing a child is one of life's most horrific and painful events. Therese A. Rando, in her book, *Grieving: How to Go On Living When Someone You Love Dies*, writes:

Parental grief is particularly intense. It is unusually complicated and has extraordinary up-and-down periods. It appears to be the most long lasting grief of all.

The death of a child shatters the very order of the universe—children are not supposed to die before their parents. It seems unnatural, incomprehensible. Losing a child entails mourning not only the child herself, but all of our hopes, dreams, wishes, fantasies, and needs relating to her. When you lose a child, you lose part of yourself, part of your future.

This book will not go through psychological descriptions of the grieving process. There are excellent reference books available, several of which are listed in Appendix D. Here, the parents themselves will tell you about grief.

I truly think that it is the worst thing in the entire world. Nothing worse can happen than losing your child. There is no reprieve. None.

. . . . .

I was having a very hard time grieving when a wonderful therapist that I was seeing said to me, "You are beating yourself up about grieving. Think about it. When you enter marriage, what are you called? A wife. When your spouse dies, what are you called? A widow. When you don't have a home and you are living on the street, what is the name for that? A homeless person. When you lose a child, what's it called, what's the name?" I said, "I don't know." She said, "Exactly. There is not even a word in our vocabulary. That's how terrible it is. It doesn't even have a name."

. . . . .

Every day when I walk out of my house I tell myself to grab the mask. I feel like I walk different than everybody and talk different than everybody and look different than everybody. It's the worst part of bereavement, the isolation caused by people who just don't know how to talk to you, when really all they need to do is listen and remember with you.

. . . . .

I found myself getting busier and busier, thinking that I could outrun the pain. I realized that I couldn't avoid the hurt; I just had to grit my teeth, cry, and live through it.

. . . . .

I felt like our sick daughter was the center of our universe for so long, that now I need to start feeling some responsibility for my other kids whom I've been away from for so long, both physically and emotionally. I told my husband the other night that I didn't even know if I loved the three kids anymore. I cannot feel a thing. Pinch me, I don't feel it. Hug me, I don't feel it. I'm numb.

. . . . .

It's hard to admit, but there was an element of relief when my daughter died. Not relief for myself, but for her. I was almost glad that she wouldn't face a life full of disabilities, that she wouldn't face the numerous orthopedic surgeries that would have been required to repair the damage from treatment, that she wouldn't face the pain of not having children of her own. I just felt relief that she would no longer feel any pain.

. . . . .

At first we didn't feel like a family anymore. Now it's better, but it's still not the family that I was used to, that I want. I still feel like the mother of four children, not three. I find it very hard to answer when someone asks me how many children I have. I also can't sign cards like I used to, with all of our names, so now I just write "from the gang." I guess that's not fair to the boys, but I just can't bear to leave her name off.

• • • • •

Birthdays are hard for us. Greg's birthday was June 10, and his brother's is June 9. So it's pretty hard to ignore. On Greg's birthday and the anniversary of his death, we blow up balloons, one for every year he would have been alive, write messages on them with markers, and release them at his grave.

• • • • •

It seems like just about every holiday has some difficult memory attached to it now. He was diagnosed on Easter, and then relapsed the next year on Valentine's Day. I hate them both now. Christmas is always hard. And Halloween is tough because he so loved to dress up. I see all those little ones in their costumes and I'm just flooded with pain.

• • • • •

This evening my heart was so saddened. I paced up and down in front of the mantel pausing to look at each picture of my daughter. Something that I cannot describe catches in my chest, and I can't breathe right. I look at her face and try to will it to life for a kiss and a touch, for softly spoken endearments at night. How we love all of our children, yet one missing leaves such a stabbing pain.

• • • • •

It's hard when people I have just met ask, "How many children do you have?" In the beginning I always felt that I had to explain that I had two but one died. Now, I just say one. I don't want their sympathy, I don't want their pity, but most of all I just don't want to have to explain. After two years or so, I started to feel uncomfortable giving out my life history and then having to deal with other people's discomfort. So now I just say one, and yet it still feels like I'm betraying him every time I do it.

• • • • •

On the anniversary of Ryan's death we all went to the cemetery, and his girlfriend's parents planted a cherry tree at the foot of his grave. That *was on a Sunday. I woke up on Monday feeling just as bad as I did the day before. All I could think was, "Oh hell, I have to go through that whole cycle again." The first year did not bring me any peace.*

Bereaved parents are frequently reassured that "time will ease the pain." Most find that this is not the case. Time helps them understand the pain; the passage of time reassures them that they can adjust and they will survive. The acute pain becomes more quiescent, but still erupts when parents go to what would have been their child's graduation, hear their child's favorite song, or just go to the grocery store. Grief is a long, difficult journey, with many ups and downs. But, with time, parents report that laughter and joy do return. They acknowledge that life will never be the same, but it can be good again.

Judith Barrington wrote in her book *Grief Postponed*:

> *Certain smells, certain moments when I feel unloved, certain aspects of the Christmas rituals, and hundreds of other ordinary details of life, will reopen the wound. But at least now I can let it bleed for a while and go on. At least now I can be open, not only to those painful moments, but also to the many joys of my life.*

Looking back after many years

Parents whose children died years ago share their thoughts on grief and how they changed.

> *Life does go on after the death of someone you love, even if it's your child. It isn't always easy or fun or purposeful, but it's like anything else, life is what YOU make of it.*

> *My son Cory died on Mother's Day 1985 after five and a half years of battling cancer. When he left this existence, a big part of my heart died with him. At first, the sky wasn't as blue as it once was, the mountains weren't as majestic, the ocean wasn't as magnificent, and yeah, it was hard to get out of bed and put one foot in front of the other. But I had to do it. I had to go on, not only for my daughter, but for myself, too.*

> *One day the fog lifted, and I knew in what remained of my heart that my little boy wanted me to continue on loving life and all it has to offer. Before he died, Cory told me, "Don't weep for me, Mama. Just remember me and all the love I brought with me. I chose this life to be with you, but I was never meant to grow up."*

I wrote a poem based on the things he said to bolster my courage and to help me cope with his leaving. I hope anyone who reads it can derive some comfort from it as well.

The Freedom of Flight

Don't weep for me when I have gone away...
Death is not like the end of the play.
It's like the freedom of the butterfly's first flight.
I won't really be gone—only from sight.
All the love that I brought with me from birth,
Will always be with you, while you are on earth.
I will be back in God's loving embrace...
So please wipe those tears of sadness off of your face.

Be happy I'm free from pain and despair,
Free like the birds that soar through the air.
I will always be with you, in everything you see...
Wherever you look it will remind you of me...
A flower in bloom, a new bud on a tree...
Or even a dandelion growing in the lawn,
But please don't think of me as gone.
A kid's game of soccer, a familiar song you will hear...
Comic books, cartoons, and "Danger," my favorite bear.
Don't think of death as the end of me.
It's just the beginning of my flight to be free.
Don't mourn my passing, because I will be
As one with God, all knowingness and light.
I will dance on the stars that shine in the night,
Or glide like a leaf caught in a gentle breeze...
Or soar on the wind with a bird's grace and ease...
Maybe hitch a ride on the tail of a kite,
All with the magic and freedom of a butterfly's first flight.

I will never stop missing him. Thankfully he gave me the strength to move forward. Cory loved life so much and fought so courageously during the short time he was here, it would be an insult to his memory if I didn't cling to and enjoy life as tenaciously as he taught me to. The memories of the fun we had, the love we shared, and the vision of him dancing on the stars sustain me.

· · · · ·

The old adage that "time heals" is a myth. You need to choose to heal and then find out how to help yourself. As I look back on our journey, our first instinct was to huddle as a family, to bask in what was left. We were hurting together; we loved him; we missed him; we needed to celebrate who he was. We intuitively knew that we were going to make it, we just didn't know how.

When Donnie died thirteen years ago, we didn't know much about grief. There wasn't as much written about it then as there is now. But we were committed to healing individually and as a family. One of the important things that we did for one another was to give each other lots of space. My husband and I knew the distancing was necessary but temporary. We were on a teeter-totter. We each had a different schedule, a different way of handling pain. He allowed me my "craziness," and I respected his silence. I found that it helped me to wallow in it, to feel it all, to cry. I've grieved clean.

If you have children, learn about how kids grieve. They revisit their grief at each developmental stage. Keep the door open so that they can talk about it.

After Donny's death, I found that I just had to be with kids. I volunteered at the school, and followed all of his friends until they graduated from high school. A friend carried his cap and gown, and they made a speech about how a very important person was missing from the ceremony. I cried, but it was good.

I think it is very important for people to choose to feel. If you attend a grief support group or Compassionate Friends, or read about the grief process, you will quickly realize that your feelings are normal and that each person goes through grief differently. Another good reason to go to a group is that other people can give voice to your feelings when you just don't have any words. In the beginning you are just a ball of pain. You learn that every person feels that way; that it is normal, human. Many people come to group and never speak, but they are comforted. I found it was far better for me to be in the same room with real people who had walked down the same road, rather than just to read about it in books. Feel the pain and you will heal.

I just wish that I had armfuls of time.

—Four-year-old with cancer
Armfuls of Time

Photographs of Our Children

Children during and after treatment

YOUR CHILD WILL PROBABLY be changed in appearance or attitude by the drugs that he takes for treatment. However, when treatment ends, your child's appearance, energy, and personality will recover. The parents of the children below make these photos public so that you can more fully believe that you will "get your child back" after chemotherapy is over.

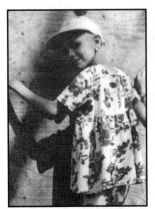
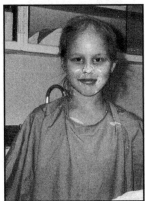

ELIZABETH

MATTHEW

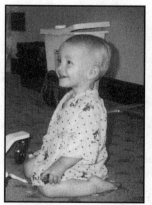 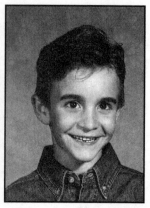

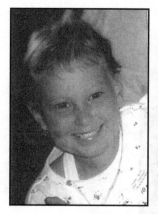 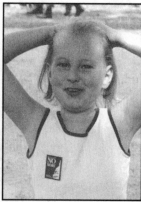

DESTINY

SCOTT

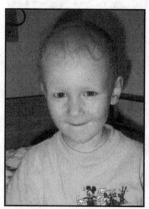 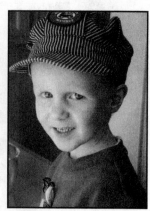

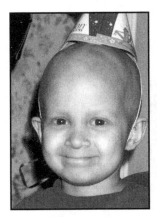 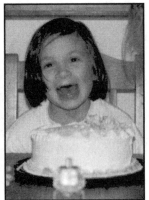 PAIGE

ERIC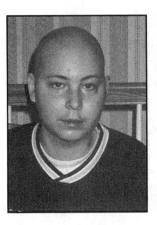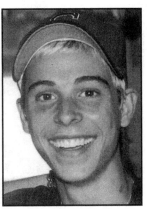

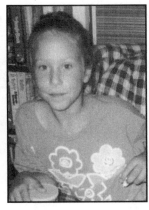 ELIZABETH

EVAN

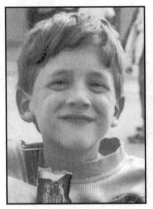 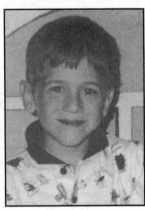

COURTNEY

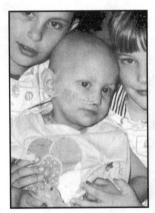 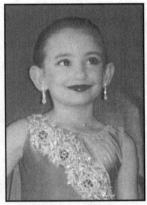

LEEANN

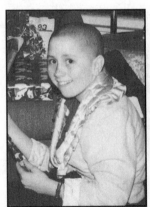 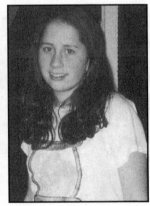

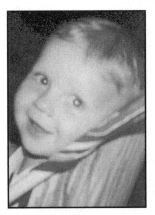 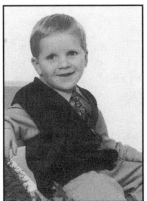

JOHN ALLEN

JOSEPH

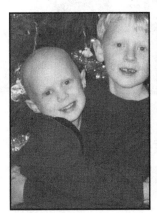 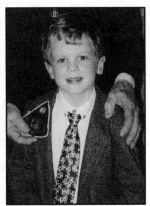

HAILEE

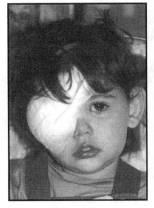 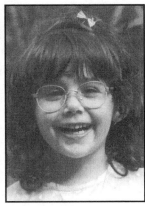

In memoriam

Despite major advances in treatment, some children still die from childhood cancer. Some of the grieving parents who helped create this book wished to share a photograph of their beloved child. In loving memory, we dedicate these pages to them—departed but not forgotten.

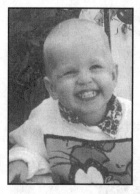
CIENNA EVANS

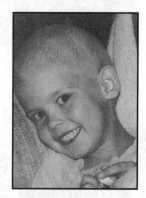
MIKEY HARRISON

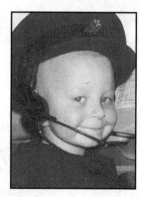
MATTHEW HODDER

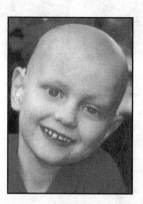
ZACKARY JORDAN

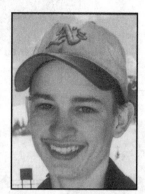
GREGGORY KAISER

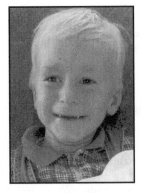

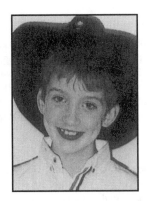

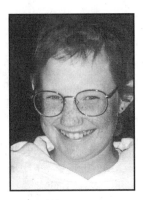

MARTIN LEHRMAN   LEVI LINDEKUGEL   MICHELLE RIEF

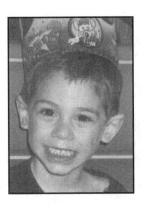

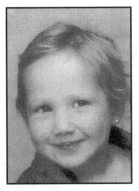

MICHAEL
KARANICOLA

MOLLY THOMPSON

APPENDIX B

Blood Counts and What They Mean

KEEPING TRACK OF THEIR CHILD'S BLOOD COUNTS becomes a way of life for parents of children with cancer. Unfortunately, misunderstandings about the implications of certain changes in blood values can cause unnecessary worry and fear. To help prevent these concerns, and to better enable parents to help spot trends in the blood values of their child, this appendix explains the blood counts of healthy children, the blood counts of children being treated for cancer, and what each blood value means.

Values for healthy children

Each laboratory and lab handbook has slightly different reference values for each blood cell, so your lab sheets may differ slightly from those that appear later in this appendix (see figure B-1). There is also variation in values for children of different ages. For instance, in newborn to four-year-old children, granulocytes are lower and lymphocytes higher than the numbers listed below. Geographic location affects reference ranges as well. The following table lists blood count values for healthy children:

Blood count type	Values for healthy children
Hemoglobin (Hgb.)	11.5–13.5 g/100ml.
Hematocrit	34–40%
Red blood count	3.9–5.3 m/cm or 3.9-5.3 x 10^{12}/L
Platelets	160,000–500,000 mm^3
White blood count	5,000–10,000 mm^3 or 5–10 K/ul
WBC differential:	
Segmented neutrophils	50–70%
Band neutrophils	1–3%
Basophils	0.5–1%
Eosinophils	1–4%
Lymphocytes	12–46%
Monocytes	2–10%
Bilirubin (total)	0.3–1.3 mg./dl
Direct (conjugated)	0.1–0.4 mg./dl
Indirect (unconjugated)	0.2–0.18 mg./dl
AST (SGOT)	0–36 IU./l.

Blood count type	Values for healthy children
ALT (SGPT)	0–48 IU./l.
BUN	10–20 mg/dl
Creatinine	0.3–1.1 mg/dl

Values for children on chemotherapy

Blood counts of children being treated for cancer fluctuate wildly. White blood cell counts can go down to zero, or be above normal. Red cell counts decrease periodically during treatment, necessitating transfusions of packed red cells. Platelet levels also decrease, requiring platelet transfusions. Absolute neutrophil counts (ANC) are closely watched as they give the physician an idea of the child's ability to fight infection. ANCs vary from zero to in the thousands.

Oncologists consider all of the blood values to get the total picture of the child's reaction to illness, chemotherapy, radiation, or infection. Trends are more important than any single value. For instance, if the values of three tests were 5.0, 4.7, 4.9, then the second result was insignificant. If, on the other hand, the values were 5.0, 4.7, 4.2, then there is a decrease in the cell line.

The explanations below will describe each blood value. If you have any questions about your child's blood counts, ask your child's doctor for a clear explanation. Especially in the beginning, many parents agonize over whether the rapid changes in blood counts (often requiring transfusions, changes in chemo dosages, and changes in whether the child can have visitors) are normal or expected. The only way to address your worries, and prevent them from escalating, is to ask what the changes mean.

What do these blood values mean?

The following sections explain each line of the table of blood values shown earlier. See Figure B-1 to get an idea of the different ways these values might be displayed on the actual lab reports prepared for your child.

Hemoglobin (Hgb)

Red cells contain hemoglobin, the molecules that carry oxygen and carbon dioxide in the blood. Measuring hemoglobin gives an exact picture of the ability of the blood to carry oxygen. Children may have low hemoglobin levels at diagnosis and during the intensive parts of treatment. This is because both cancer and chemotherapy decrease the bone marrow's ability to produce new red cells. Signs and symptoms of anemia—pallor, shortness of breath, fatigue—may start to show if the hemoglobin gets very low.

Hematocrit (HCT)
also called packed cell volume (PCV)

The purpose of this test is to determine the ratio of plasma (clear liquid part of blood) to red cells in the blood. Blood is drawn from a vein, finger prick, or from a Hickman or Port-a-cath and is spun in a centrifuge to separate the red cells from the plasma. The hematocrit is the percentage of cells in the blood; for instance, if the

```
NAME:                                          LOCATION: 6000
DOB:                          SEX: F           REQUEST#: 342491
COLLECTED: 08/25/1992   08:34                  ACCOUNT#:
REPORTED: 08/25/1992 @ 11:02                   DR:
PATIENT PHONE#:                                COPY TO:
TESTS: **CBC**
ORDERED:
```

TEST	RESULTS		UNITS	REFERENCE RANGE			
Collection Cmt.	–						
*CBC**							
White Blood Count	1.7	L	x10-3	3.8	–	12.5	JK
Red Blood Cnt	3.02	L	x10-6	3.90	–	5.30	JK
Hemoglobin	8.9	L	g/dl	11.5	–	13.5	JK
Hematocrit	26.1	L	%	34.0	–	40.0	JK
MCV	86.0		um3	75.0	–	87.0	JK
MCH	29.4		uug	24.0	–	30.0	JK
MCHC	34.1		%	32.0	–	36.0	JK
Segs	33		%	30	–	70	JK
Bands	1		%	0	–	5	JK
Lymphocytes	19	L	%	20	–	70	JK
Monocytes	42	H	%	0	–	6	JK
Eosinophiles	5	H	%	0	–	3	JK
Morphology Cmt 1 Anisocytosis	2+						
Platelets	34	L	x10-3	250	–	550	JK

```
Speciman ID:                        August 20 1992 11:36
Patient:                            Operator ID      SVT
Sex:          DOB:                  Sequence #       7358
DR:                                 Open Sampler
Param Set 1    Limit Set 4

  WBC:  0.7 K/uL
  NEU:  0.4   68.6 %N              S                    D
  LYM:  0.1   17.8 %L              I                    E
 MONO:  0.1   10.9 %M              Z                    P
  EDS:  0.0    2.2 %E              E                    O
 BASO:  0.0    0.5 %B                                   L

  RBC:  3.03 M/uL                    COMPLEXITY        ORTHOGONAL
  HGB:  9.2 g/dL
  HCT: 26.9 %
  MCV: 88.7 fL
  MCH: 30.4 pg
 MCHC: 34.2 g/dL
  RDW: 13.6 %


  PLT: 147. K/UL                      RBC               PLT
```

```
          INTERPRETATION           MANUAL DIFFERENTIAL   RBC MORPHOLOGY
--------WBC--------RBC--------PLT--------
```

NEU	META	NORMAL	MICRO
BAND	MYELD	PLYCHROM	MACRO
LYMPH	PRO	HYPCHROM	ANISO
MONO	BLAST	POIK	BASOSTIP
EOSIN	VAR LYM	TARGET	
BASO	TOXGRAN	SPHERO	NRBC

```
SUSPECTED ABNORMAL POPULATIONS:
  Variant Lymphocytes

USER-DEFINED ABNORMALITIES:
  Leukopenia       Anemia
  Neutropenia      Macrocytic RBC
  Lymphopenia

            PATIENT LIMITS SET 4

WBC:  5.0-13.0          RBC:  4.20-5.20  PLT: 142.-424.
NEU:  1.0-6.6  35.0-75.0 %N  HGB: 12.5-15.0  MPV: 0.0-99.9
LYM:  2.5-9.0  16.0-56.0 %L  HCT: 33.0-45.0
MONO: 0.0-1.2   0.0- 8.0 %M  MCV: 76.0-87.0
EDS:  0.0-0.8   0.0- 5.0 %E  MCH: 24.0-33.0
BASO: 0.0-0.4   0.0- 3.0 %B  MCHC: 31.4-35.8
                             RDW:  8.0-14.0
```

```
COMMENT:

DIFF BY
```

Figure B-1. Sample lab data sheets

child has a hematocrit of 30 percent, it means that 30 percent of the amount of blood drawn was cells and the rest was plasma. When the child is on chemotherapy, the bone marrow does not make many red cells, and the hematocrit will go down. The child may be given a transfusion of packed red cells when the hematocrit goes below 18 to 19 percent. This results in less oxygen being carried in the blood, and your child may have less energy.

Red blood cell count (RBC)

Red blood cells are produced by the bone marrow continuously in healthy children and adults. These cells contain hemoglobin which carries oxygen and carbon dioxide throughout the body. To determine the RBC, an automated electronic device is used to count the number of red cells in a liter of blood.

Red cell indices (MCV, MCH, MCHC) are mathematical relationships of hematocrit to red cell count, hemoglobin to red cell count, and hemoglobin to hematocrit. They give a mathematical expression of the degree of change in shape found in red cells and the concentration of hemoglobin within each cell. The higher the number (low teens are fine), the more distorted the red cell population is.

White blood cell count (WBC)

The total white blood cell count determines the body's ability to fight infection. Treatment for cancer kills healthy white cells as well as diseased ones. Parents need to expect prolonged periods of low white counts during treatment. To determine the WBC, an automated electronic device counts the number of white cells in a liter of blood. If your lab sheet uses K/ul instead of mm³, multiply by 1000 to get the value in mm³. For example, on the lab sheet in Figure B-1, the total WBC is 0.7 K/ul. Therefore, $0.7 \times 1000 = 700$ mm³.

White blood cell differential

When a child has blood drawn for a complete blood count (CBC), one section of the lab report will state the total white blood cell (WBC) count and a "differential," in which each type of white blood cell is listed as a percentage of the total. For example, if the total WBC count is 1500 mm³, the differential might appear as in the following table:

White blood cell type	Percentage of total WBCs
Segmented neutrophils (also called polys or segs)	49%
Band neutrophils (also called bands)	1%
Basophils (also called basos)	1%
Eosinophils (also called eos)	1%
Lymphocytes (also called lymphs)	38%
Monocytes (also called monos)	10%

You might also see cells called metamyelocytes, myelocytes, promyelocytes, and myeloblasts listed. These are immature white cells usually only found in the bone marrow. They may be seen in the blood during recovery from low counts.

Absolute neutrophil count (ANC)

The absolute neutrophil count (also called the absolute granulocyte count or AGC) is a measure of the body's ability to withstand infection. Generally, an ANC above 1,000 means that the child's infection fighting ability is near normal.

To calculate the ANC, add the percentages of neutrophils (both segmented and band) and multiply by the total WBC. Using the example above, the ANC is 49% + 1% = 50%. 50% of 1,500 (.50×1,500) = 750. The ANC is 750.

Platelet count

Platelets are necessary to repair the body, and stop bleeding through the formation of clots. Because platelets are produced by the bone marrow, platelet counts decrease when a child is on chemotherapy. Signs of lowering platelet counts are small vessel bleeding such as bruises, gum bleeding, or nosebleeding. Platelet transfusions may be given when the count is very low or when there is bleeding. Platelets are counted by passing a blood sample through an electronic device.

Approximately one third of all platelets spend a great deal of time in the spleen. Any splenic dysfunction such as enlargement may cause the counts to drop precipitously. If the spleen is removed, platelet counts may skyrocket. This transient thrombocytosis (elevated platelet count) will abate within a month.

ALT (alanine aminotransferase)
also called SGPT (serum glutamic pyruvic transaminase)

When doctors talk about "liver functions," they are usually referring to tests on blood samples that measure liver damage. If the chemotherapy is proving to be toxic to your child's liver, the damaged liver cells release an enzyme called ALT into the blood serum. ALT levels can go up in the hundreds or even thousands in some children on chemotherapy. Each institution and protocol has different points at which they decrease dosages or stop chemotherapy to allow the child's liver to recover. If you notice a change in your child's ALT, ask for an explanation and plan of action (for example, "John's ALT is now 450—what are your thoughts about reducing or stopping the chemotherapy to allow his liver to recover?").

AST (aspartate aminotransferase)
also called SGOT (serum glutamic oxaloacetic transaminase)

SGOT is an enzyme present in high concentrations in tissues with high metabolic activity, including the liver. Severely damaged or killed cells release SGOT into the blood. The amount of SGOT in the blood is directly related to the amount of tissue damage. Therefore, if your child's liver is being damaged by the chemotherapy, the SGOT can rise into the thousands. In addition, there are other causes for an elevated SGOT, such as viral infections, reaction to an anesthetic, and many others. If your child's level jumps unexpectedly, ask the physician for an explanation and a plan of action.

Bilirubin

The body converts hemoglobin released from damaged red cells into bilirubin. The liver removes the bilirubin from the blood, and excretes it into the bile, which is released into the small intestine to aid digestion.

Normally there is only a small amount of bilirubin in the bloodstream. Bilirubin rises if there is excessive red blood cell destruction or if the liver is unable to excrete the normal amount of bilirubin produced.

There are two types of bilirubin: indirect (also called unconjugated) and direct (also called conjugated) bilirubin. An increase in indirect (unconjugated) is seen when destruction of red cells has occurred, while an increase of direct (conjugated) is seen when there is a dysfunction or blockage of the liver.

If excessive amounts of bilirubin are present in the body, the bilirubin seeps into the tissues producing a yellow color called jaundice.

If your child's total bilirubin rises above normal levels, ask the physician for an explanation and plan of action.

AFP (alpha fetoprotein)

Alfa-fetoprotein (AFP) is a type of protein that is normally produced by the liver and the yolk sac of the fetus. It is found in the blood of pregnant women, and in those with some liver disorders, including cancer. For children with hepatoblastoma and hepatocellular carcinoma, AFP levels are usually increased. Measuring the AFP in the blood can be a a useful tool for the oncologist to assess the child's response to treatment.

LDH (lactate dehydrogenase)

Lactate dehydrogenase (LDH) is an enzyme that is present in many body tissues, such as the heart, liver, kidney, skeletal muscle, brain, blood cells, and lungs. Several types of childhood solid tumors—neuroblastoma, hepatoblastoma, hepatocellular carcinoma, osteosarcoma, and Ewing's sarcoma—can cause elevated levels of LDH found in the blood. Measuring LDH can be used to assess the child's response to treatment.

ALP (alkaline phosphatase)

Alkaline phosphatase is an enzyme that is found in all body tissues with high concentrations normally found in the liver, bile ducts, and bone cells. There are several different types of ALP, called isoenzymes. For example, liver ALP and bone ALP are structurally different from each other.

Diseased tissue releases ALP into the bloodstream. Based on its structural appearance, the doctor is able to locate the area of damaged or diseased tissue.

Catecholamines

Catecholamines are hormones produced by the adrenal medulla. The main catecholamines are dopamine, norepinephrine, and epinephrine. Catecholamines, which can be measured in the blood or urine, are tested to diagnose and monitor therapy of neuroblastoma. Since the catecholamine metabolic end products vanillylmandelic acid

Blood Counts								
Date:								
WBC *ref. range* _____								
Neutrophils *(polys or segs)*								
Neutrophils *(bands)*								
ANC *(polys + bands, multiplied by WBC)*								
Hematocrit *ref. range* _____								
Platelets *ref. range* _____								
Chemistries								
Chemotherapy								
Side Effects								

Figure B-2. Example of a record-keeping sheet

(VMA) and homovanillic acid (HVA) are measured in the urine, urine catecholamines are measured more frequently than serum (in the blood) catecholamines. Approximately 95 percent of neuroblastomas create abnormal levels of catecholamines. This makes the test particularly useful in detection and monitoring of the disease.

Blood urea nitrogen (BUN)

Blood urea nitrogen (BUN) is a blood test used to assess kidney function. It is also used to detect liver disease, dehydration, congestive heart failure, gastrointestinal bleeding, starvation, shock, or urinary tract obstruction by a tumor. The test measures the amount of an end product of protein metabolism, called urea nitrogen, in the blood. For children with kidney or liver disease, BUN is often found in abnormal levels.

Creatinine

Creatinine is the breakdown product of protein metabolism found in the urine and the blood. Creatinine is measured to assess kidney function and to determine the presence and severity of suspected kidney disease. An elevated blood creatinine level is often seen in children with kidney insufficiency and renal failure. Doctors use a creatinine clearance test to assess kidney function, particularly to see how efficiently the kidney filters and excretes creatinine.

Your child's pattern

Each child develops a unique pattern of blood counts during treatment, and observant parents can help track these changes. This appendix contains a record-keeping sheet that you can use to record your child's blood values (see Figure B-2 on the previous page). If there is a change in the pattern, show it to your child's doctor and ask for an explanation. Doctors consider all of the laboratory results to decide how to proceed, but they should be willing to explain their plan of action to you so that you better understand what is happening and worry less.

If your child is participating in a clinical trial and you have obtained the entire clinical trial protocol (discussed in Chapter 5, *Clinical Trials*), it will contain a section that clearly outlines the actions that should be taken by the oncologist if certain changes in blood counts occur.

Resource Organizations

Service organizations

American Cancer Society
1599 Clifton Road NE
Atlanta, GA 30329-4251
(800) ACS-2345
http://www.cancer.org/

Its programs include patient-to-patient visitation, transportation to appointments, housing near treatment centers, equipment and supplies, support groups, educational literature, and summer camps for children with cancer.

Canadian Cancer Society
565 W. 10th Avenue
Vancouver, BC Canada V5Z 4J4
(604) 872-4400
http://www.bc.cancer.ca/

Provides same services as the US Cancer Society.

Candlelighters Childhood Cancer Foundation
7910 Woodmont Avenue, Suite 460
Bethesda, MD 20814
(800) 366-CCCF
Fax: (301) 718-2686
http://www.candlelighters.org
email: *info@candlelighters.org*

Founded in 1970, Candlelighters has more than 40,000 members worldwide. Free of charge, it provides yearly bibliography and resource guides, quarterly newsletters, youth newsletters, and various handbooks to help families of children with cancer.

Candlelighters Childhood Cancer Foundation Canada
National Office
55 Eglinton Avenue E., Suite 401
Toronto, ON Canada M4P 1G8
(800) 363-1062 (Canada only)
(416) 489-6440
Fax: (416) 489-9812
http://www.candlelighters.ca
email: *staff@candlelighters.ca*

Provides the same services as US Candlelighters.

Ronald McDonald House Coordinator
c/o Golin Communications Inc.
111 E. Wacker Drive
Chicago, IL 60601
(312) 729-4000

Organizations that provide information

The Academy for Guided Imagery
P.O. Box 2070
Mill Valley, CA 94942
(800) 726-2070

This organization can assist in locating a professional in your area to help your child learn visualization.

The American Society of Clinical Hypnosis
33 West Grand Avenue, Suite 402
Chicago, IL 60610
(847) 297-3317

A membership organization for doctors, psychologists, and dentists who use hypnosis in their practices. For referral to a local member, send a request with a self-addressed stamped envelope.

Childhood Cancer Ombudsman Program
P.O. Box 595
Burgess, VA 22432
Fax: (804) 580-2502
email: *gpmonaco@rivnet.net*

This free service helps children with cancer and their families who are experiencing difficulties gain access to appropriate education, medical care, healthcare cost coverage, and meaningful employment. Services include medical library searches, a second opinion program, and help resolving insurance or discrimination problems.

The Disability Rights Education and Defense Fund
2212 Sixth Street
Berkeley, CA 94710
(800) 466-4232

Answers questions about the Americans with Disabilities Act, explains how to file a complaint, and provides dispute resolution.

The Institute for Families of Blind Children
Attention: Nancy
P. O. Box 54700 MS# 111
Los Angeles, CA 90054-0700
(213) 669-4649

Supports and provides information to families affected by retinoblastoma and visual impairment.

Job Accommodation Network
West Virginia University
918 Chestnut Ridge Road, Suite 1
P.O. Box 6080
Morgantown, WV 26516
(800) 526-7234 or (800) ADA-WORK

Provides information about on-the-job accommodations for persons with disabilities.

National Cancer Institute (NCI)
Cancer Information Service
Building 31, Room 10A16
9000 Rockville Pike
Bethesda, MD 20892
(800) 4-CANCER
Fax: (301) 231-6941
CANCERFAX: (301) 402-5874

Provides a nationwide telephone service for people with cancer, their families, friends, and the professionals who treat them. It provides answers and sends out informational booklets on a variety of cancer-related topics.

CANCERFAX provides treatment guidelines, with current data on prognosis, staging, and histologic classifications. To use CANCERFAX, you need a fax machine with a telephone set to touch tone dialing. A recording will give you instructions.

National Childhood Cancer Foundation
440 E. Huntington Drive
P.O. Box 60012
Arcadia, CA 91066-6012
(626) 447-1674
Fax: (626) 447-6359
http://www.nccf.org/

Supports pediatric cancer treatment and research in more than 115 hospitals in North America and Australia. Their newsletter, *Childhood Cancerline*, provides information on new treatments and psychosocial support.

National Coalition for Cancer Survivorship
1010 Wayne Avenue
Silver Spring, MD 20910
(301) 650-8868
Fax: (301) 565-9670

Organization that addresses the needs of long-term cancer survivors and advocates for changes in healthcare to maximize survivors' access to optimal treatment and support. The coalition has an extensive publications list.

National Information Center for Children and Youth with Disabilities (NICHY)
P.O. Box 1492
Washington, DC 20013
(800) 695-0285

A clearinghouse that provides free pamphlets and information on disabilities and the rights of disabled children and their parents.

Neuroblastoma Children's Cancer Society
P.O. Box 957672
Hoffman Estates, IL 60195
(800) 532-5162
Fax: (847) 490-0705
http://www.granitewebworks.com/nccs.htm

Supports neuroblastoma research and provides information to families about the disease.

PDQ (Physician Data Query)
(800) 4-CANCER
http://cancernet.nci.nih.gov/

PDQ is the National Cancer Institute's computerized listing of accurate and up-to-date information for patients and health professionals about cancer treatments, research studies, clinical trials, organizations, and doctors.

The Retinoblastoma Society
c/o St. Bartholomew's Hospital
West Smithfield
London, England EC1A 7BE
0171 600 3309
Fax: 0171 600 8579

Supports and provides information to those with retinoblastoma.

Starbright Foundation
1990 South Bundy Drive, Suite 100
Los Angeles, CA 90025
(310) 442-1560
Fax: (310) 442-1568
http://www.starbright.org

Co-chaired by Steven Spielberg and Gen. Norman Schwarzkopf, Starbright Foundation is best known for its online network of interactive, virtual-reality playgrounds where seriously ill, hospitalized children across the country meet, talk, and play to help cope with the pain, stress, and anxiety of treatment. For teens who are ill, "Videos with Attitude" offer guidance from peers who have "been there." The videos are free to families and come with a parent guide.

Organizations that provide emotional support

Association of the Care of Children's Health (ACCH)
7910 Woodmont Avenue, Suite 300
Bethesda, MD 20814
(609) 224-1742

A nonprofit, multidisciplinary organization of health professionals and parents that promotes psychosocial health of children and their parents. It sponsors conferences, provides advocacy resources, and publishes journals, newsletters, and booklets.

Cancer Care, Inc.
1180 Avenue of the Americas
New York, NY 10036
(800) 813-4673
(212) 302-2400
Fax: (212) 719-0263
http://www.cancercare.org

A national, nonprofit organization that provides referrals, one-on-one counseling, specialized support groups, and educational programs.

Cancer Cured Kids
P.O. Box 189
Old Westbury, NY 11568
(800) CCK-7525
(516) 484-8160
Fax: (516) 484-8160 (call first)

An organization dedicated to the quality of life of kids who have survived cancer, it supplies information about educational and psychosocial needs.

Center for Attitudinal Healing
33 Buchanan Drive
Sausalito, CA 94965
(415) 331-6161

A nonprofit, nonsectarian group that sponsors local and national workshops for children with catastrophic or life-threatening diseases and their siblings. It promotes the use of the arts in a loving, supportive program to help children ages six to sixteen share their feelings about their situation. It has published several excellent books.

Chai Lifeline/Camp Simcha
National Office
48 West 25th Street, 6th Floor
New York, NY 10010
(212) 255-1160 or (800) 343-2527
Fax: (212) 255-1495

A national, nonprofit Jewish organization that provides support service programs to children and their families in crisis, including medical referrals, support groups, visits to hospitalized and housebound children, financial aid, transportation, a kosher camp for kids with cancer, and more.

ChemoCare
231 North Avenue West
Westfield, NJ 07090
(800) 55-CHEMO (outside New Jersey)
(908) 233-1103 (within New Jersey)
Fax: (908) 233-0228

Provides one-to-one emotional support to cancer patients and their families under-going chemotherapy, radiation, and/or surgery, from trained and certified volunteers who have undergone the treatments themselves.

Child Life Council
11820 Parklawn Drive, Suite 202
Rockville, MD 20852
(301) 881-7090
Fax: (301) 881-7092

Promotes the well-being of children and families in healthcare settings by support-ing the development and practice of the child life profession with training confer-ences, publications, and information.

Children's Hopes and Dreams Foundation
280 Route 46
Dover, NJ 07801
(973) 361-7348

This organization operates a free, worldwide pen-pal program for children ages five to seventeen with disabilities, chronic illnesses, or life-threatening illnesses.

Coping Magazine
P.O. Box 682268
Franklin, TN 37068
(615) 790-2400
Fax: (615) 794-0179

A bimonthly publication devoted to people whose lives have been touched by cancer.

Famous Phone Friends
9109 Sawyer Street
Los Angeles, CA 90035
(310) 204-5683

Links children who are confined to the hospital or home due to injury or illness with entertainers and athletes by telephone. Obtain a referral from a physician, nurse, hospital volunteer, or treatment center social worker.

Friends Network
P.O. Box 4545
Santa Barbara, CA 93140
Attention: Kenon Neal

A national, nonprofit organization that distributes *The Funletter,* a full-color activities newsletter, to children with cancer.

Love Letters, Inc.
P.O. Box 416875
Chicago, IL 60641
(630) 620-1970

This free service, started by a mother whose son died of cancer, is run by a group of volunteers who send letters, cards, and gifts to catastrophically ill children. This is not a pen-pal organization. Confidentiality is guaranteed.

National Children's Cancer Society
(800) 532-6459
http://www.children-cancer.com/

Advocates for children affected by childhood cancer and their families by providing financial assistance, education, and emotional support.

Parents Caring and Sharing
c/o Chumie Bodek
109 Rutledge Street
Brooklyn, NY 11211
(718) 596-1542 or 596-9002 (call during business hours, Eastern time)

Provides outreach, a support network, and newsletter for Jewish Orthodox families with children with cancer. Holds monthly meetings and links families of children with similar diseases.

Songs of Love Foundation
P.O. Box 750809
Forest Hills, NY 11375
http://www.songsoflove.org

A nonprofit organization that has a volunteer group of more than 200 artists who produce personalized musical portraits for children and teens with chronic or life-threatening diseases.

Bone marrow and stem cell transplantation

Additional resources for bone marrow or stem cell transplant families are listed at *http://www.bmtnews.org/*.

The Barbara DeBoer Foundation
2069 S. Busse Road
Mount Prospect, IL 60056
(800) 895-8478 or (847) 981-0130

Helps to identify and utilize resources in your community to raise necessary funds for transplants.

BMT Family Support Network
P.O. Box 845
Avon, CT 06001
(800) 826-9376

Provides information, resources, and telephone links to families involved in bone marrow transplants. Also serves grieving families.

Children's Organ Transplant Association
2501 Cota Drive
Bloomington, IN 47403
(800) 366-2682
http://www.cota.org

Provides fundraising help.

National Bone Marrow Transplant Link
29209 Northwestern Highway #624
Southfield, MI 48034
(800) LINK-BMT or (810) 932-8483

Operates a hot-line, and provides peer support, a library, clearinghouse, and suggestions for financial assistance.

National Marrow Donor Program (NMDP)
3433 Broadway Street, NE, Suite 500
Minneapolis, MN 55413
Donor Information: (800) MARROW-2
Patient Search Information: (800) 526-7809
Corporate Recruitment Programs: (800) 526-7809
Fax: (612) 627-8195
http://www.marrow.org

The NMDP has developed the world's largest computerized listing of potential marrow donors.

The National Transplant Assistance Fund
6 Bryn Mawr Avenue
P.O. Box 258
Bryn Mawr, PA 19010
(800) 642-8399 or (610) 527-5056
http://www.transplantfund.org

Provides fundraising assistance and donor awareness material to transplant patients nationwide.

Financial Help

Cancer Fund of America
2901 Breezewood Lane
Knoxville, TN 37921
(800) 578-5284
Fax: (615) 938-2968

Helps defray cancer-related expenses not covered by insurance.

The Sparrow Foundation
1155 N. 130th, Suite 310
Seattle WA 98104
(206) 745-5403

Provides help with fundraising for any medical needs.

Free air services

Air Care Alliance
(800) 296-1217
http://www.angelflightfla.org/aircareall.org/acahome.html
ACA is a nationwide association of humanitarian flying organizations.

Corporate Angel Network, Inc. (CAN)
Westchester County Airport, Building 1
White Plains, NY 10604
(914) 328-1313
Fax: (800) 328-4226

A nationwide, nonprofit program designed to give patients with cancer the use of available seats on corporate aircraft to get to and from recognized cancer treatment centers. Patients must be able to walk and travel without life-support systems or medical attention. A child may be accompanied by up to two adults. This service will also fly donors. There is no cost or financial need requirements.

DreamLine, Inc.
Contact: Bob Iverson
1701 N. Clybourn
Chicago, IL 60614
(312) 202-9000
Fax: (312) 202-0188
http://www.bobiverson.com/dreamline.htm

Provides free airline travel for children with serious illnesses needing transportation for emergency medical treatment or vacation.

Mission Air Transportation Network
Proctor & Gamble Building
4711 Young Street
North York, ON Canada M2N 6K8
(416) 222-6335
Fax: (416) 222-6930

An organization that provides free air transport to Canadians in financial need who must travel from their own communities to recognized facilities for medical care.

National Patient Air Transport Hotline
24-hour hotline: (800) 296-1217

Specialists refer callers to the most appropriate, cost-effective charitable or commercial services, including volunteer pilot organizations and airline transport programs.

Wish fulfillment organizations

In addition to the large organizations listed below, there are many smaller and local organizations that grant wishes to seriously ill children. A comprehensive list of wish fulfillment organizations can be found on the Web at *http://www.patientcenters.com/ childcancer/*.

Children's Wish Foundation International
7840 Roswell Road, Suite 301
Atlanta, GA 30350
(770) 393-WISH
(800) 323-WISH
FAX: (404) 393-0683

Fulfills wishes of terminally ill children in the US and Europe.

The Children's Wish Foundation of Canada
95 Bayly Street, Suite 404
Ajax, Ontario
Canada L1S 7K8
(905) 426-5656
Fax: (905) 426-4111

Its goal is to provide a once-in-a-lifetime experience for children ages three to eighteen with high risk, life-threatening diseases. There are chapters throughout Canada. Parents can call for the location of the chapter nearest to them.

The Dream Factory, Inc.
P.O. Box 3942
Louisville, KY 40202
(800) 456-7556
Fax: (502) 584-0023

Grants wishes of children ages three to thirteen who are seriously or chronically ill. There are chapters in 30 states.

Make A Wish Foundation of America
100 W. Clarendon, Suite 2200
Phoenix, AZ 85013
(602) 279-WISH or (800) 722-WISH
Fax: (602) 279-0855

Grants wishes to children under the age of eighteen with life-threatening illnesses. US and international chapters and affiliates exist.

The Starlight Foundation
International Headquarters
12424 Wilshire Boulevard, Suite 1050
Los Angeles, CA 90025
(310) 207-5558

Fulfills wishes for seriously ill children ages four to eighteen. There are chapters in the United States, Canada, Australia, and the United Kingdom.

Sunshine Foundation
P.O. Box 255
5400 County Road 547 N
Loughman, FL 33858
(813) 424-4188 or (800) 457-1976

Grants wishes to chronically or terminally ill children ages three to twenty-one. It has no geographic boundaries.

Bereavement

The Centering Corporation
1531 N. Saddle Creek Road
Omaha, NE 68104
(402) 553-1200

Publishes a free catalog which contains an extensive listing of books, cards, and audio and videotapes on death and grieving.

Children's Hospice International
2202 Mt. Vernon Avenue, Suite 3C
Alexandria, VA 22301
(703) 684-0330
(800) 24-CHILD

The Compassionate Friends National Office
P.O. Box 3696
Oak Brook, IL 60522-3696
(630) 990-0010
Fax: (630) 990-0246
http://www.compassionatefriends.org

A self-help organization that offers understanding and friendship to bereaved families through support meetings at local chapters and telephone support (they match persons with similar losses). It publishes a newsletter for parents and one for siblings, and offers a Resource Catalog with a comprehensive list of books, audio, and video materials on adult and sibling grief.

Books and Online Sites

A wealth of information is available through libraries and computers. This appendix briefly describes how to get the most from these resources and lists specific books and online sites that you might find helpful when researching your child's medical condition or treatment.

How to get information from your library or computer

Most libraries now have a computerized database of all materials available in their various branches. Some libraries may still use a manual card catalog system. Ask a librarian if you need help learning to use these systems. A librarian can also tell you how to request a book from another branch and how to put a book on hold if it is currently checked out.

If a book is not in your library's collection, ask the librarian if she can obtain it from another library by requesting an inter-library loan. This is a common practice, and you might be able to get medical texts from university or medical school libraries.

In addition to books, you can find relevant magazine and medical journal articles at the library. The librarian can show you how to use the database to search for relevant articles and where to find the periodicals. Public libraries usually subscribe to only the most popular medical journals such as the *New England Journal of Medicine*. If you are able to visit a university or medical school library, you will find many more medical journals available. To find the nearest medical library open to the public, call the National Network of Libraries of Medicine at (800) 338-7657. If you do not live close to one of these libraries, ask your local librarian if she can help you obtain copies of the articles you want.

There is an astonishing amount of information available through the Internet. Libraries from all over the world can be accessed, and you can download information in minutes from huge databases like MedLine or Cancerlit. Obtaining information from large medical databases, established journals, or large libraries is exceedingly helpful for parents at home with sick children. However, the huge numbers of people using the Internet has spawned chat rooms, bulletin boards, and thousands of FAQs (frequently asked questions), which may or may not contain accurate information. You may want to adopt the motto "Let the buyer beware."

If you do not have a home computer, many libraries provide Internet access. Ask the librarian to help you connect to MedLine, Physician's Data Query (PDQ), or other databases you wish to search. Don't hesitate to ask for assistance in finding web sites or whatever else you need on the Internet.

General

Candlelighters Childhood Cancer Foundation. *Bibliography and Resource Guide.* 1998. (800) 366-CCCF, or for CCCF-Canada, (800) 363-1062. Extensive listing of books and articles on childhood cancer, coping skills, death and bereavement, effects on family, long-term side effects, medical support, and terminal home care. Excellent resource.

Centering Corporation. *Creative Care Package.* (402) 553-1200. Lists more than 300 books and videos on coping with serious illness, loss, and grief.

Compassionate Friends. *Resource Guide.* (630) 990-0010. Contains hundreds of books, pamphlets, videos, and audiotapes on all aspects of grief.

Cousins, Norman. *Head First: The Biology of Hope and the Healing Power of the Human Spirit.* New York: E.P. Dutton, 1989. Cousins presents mounting volumes of evidence that positive attitudes help combat disease. Also contains excellent information on enhancing the doctor/patient relationship.

Johnson, Joy, and S. M. Johnson. *Why Mine?: A Book for Parents Whose Child Is Seriously Ill.* Omaha, NE: Centering Corporation, 1981. To order, call (402) 553-1200. Quotes from parents about fears, feelings, marriages, siblings, and the ill child.

Kushner, Harold. *When Bad Things Happen to Good People.* Boston: G.K. Hall, rev. ed. 1997. A rabbi wrote this comforting book on how people of faith deal with catastrophic events.

Lerner, Michael. *Choices in Healing: Integrating the Best of Conventional and Complementary Approaches to Medicine.* Cambridge, MA: The MIT Press, 1996. A comprehensive overview of both conventional and complementary approaches to cancer treatment. Available online at *http://www.commonweal.org/choicescontents.html.*

National Institute of Health. *Young People With Cancer: A Handbook for Parents.* This booklet describes the different types of childhood cancer, medical procedures, coping skills, and family issues, and gives sources of information. (800) 4-CANCER.

CANSearch
http://www.cansearch.org/canserch/canserch.htm

This guide to cancer resources is produced by the National Coalition for Cancer Survivorship.

GrannyBarb and Art's Leukemia Links
http://www.acor.org/diseases/hematology/Leukemia/leukmain.html

Covers mostly leukemia information, but also has links to useful resources such as CancerNet, PDQ, abstracts, cancer lit, Internet support groups, bone marrow transplant sites, cord blood transplant sites.

Yahoo
http://dir.yahoo.com/Health/Diseases_and_Conditions/Cancer/

Steve Dunn's CancerGuide
http://www.cancerguide.org

A great place to start when looking for information. Steve Dunn, a cancer survivor, clearly explains cancer types and staging, chemotherapy, pathology reports, and the advantages and disadvantages of researching your own cancer. He also recommends books, includes inspirational patient stories, and has links to many of the best cancer sites on the Web.

Reading for children/teens/siblings

Children

Chernus-Mansfield, Nancy, MA, and Marilyn Horn, LCSW. *My Fake Eye: The Story of My Prosthesis,* and *My New Glasses: A Book for Parents and Children.* Published by the Institute for Families of Blind Children, Los Angeles, 1991 and 1993. For free copies, call (213) 669-4649.

Crary, Elizabeth. *Dealing with Feelings.* I'm Frustrated; I'm Mad; I'm Sad Series. Seattle: Parenting Press, 1992. Fun, game-like books to teach preschool and early elementary children how to handle feelings and solve problems.

Foss, Karen. *The Problem with Hair: A Story for Children Learning about Cancer.* Centering Corporation, 1996. A poem about a group of friends and what happens when one of them loses her hair from chemotherapy.

Hairballs on my Pillow. CARTI. Little Rock, AR, (800) 482-8561. Video interviews of children with cancer and their friends, about friendship and returning to school. $35 includes video plus newsletters, exercises and activities for students, a teacher's notebook about cancer, its treatment, and dealing with returning students.

Hautzig, Deborah. *A Visit to the Sesame Street Hospital.* New York: Random House, 1985. Grover, his mother, Ernie, and Bert visit the Sesame Street Hospital in preparation for Grover's upcoming operation.

Krishner, Trudy. *Kathy's Hats.* Concept Books, 1992. Written by a mother of a nine year old with Ewing's sarcoma, this attractively illustrated book explains how Kathy used different hats to cope with her treatments.

Leukemia Society of America. *I'm Having a Bone Marrow Transplant.* For a free copy, call (800) 955-4LSA. Coloring book for young children that helps to explain what to expect during the BMT.

Nessim, Susan, and Barbara Wyman. *Draw Me a Picture.* A coloring book for children with cancer (ages three to six). Marty Bunny talks about how it was when he was in the hospital for cancer and invites readers to draw about their experiences. Send $7.45 to Cancervive, 6500 Wilshire Blvd., #500, Los Angeles, CA 90048.

Richmond, Christina. *Chemo Girl: Saving the World One Treatment at a Time.* Jones and Bartlett Publishers, 1996. Written by a twelve-year-old with rhabdomyosarcoma, this book describes a superhero who shares hope and encouragement.

Rogers, Fred. *Going to the Hospital.* New York: G. P. Putnam's Sons, 1997. With pictures and words, TV's beloved Mr. Rogers helps children ages three to eight learn about hospitals.

Rogers, Fred. *Some Things Change and Some Things Stay the Same.* American Cancer Society. Order by calling (800) ACS-2345. Very comforting book for preschool-age children with cancer and their siblings.

Mr. Rogers Talks About Childhood Cancer. 1990. Videotapes (2), guidebook, storybook. 45 mins. VHS. Available from American Cancer Society. (800) ACS-2345. Mr. Rogers talks to children and uses characters from the land of make believe to stress the importance of talking about feelings.

Teens

Child Life Council. *For Teenagers: Visiting the Hospital*. 1996. Helps acquaint adolescents with hospital routines, policies, staff, and common medical terms. $2.00. Can be ordered at *www.childlife.org/*.

Gravelle, Karen and Bertram A. John. *Teenagers Face to Face with Cancer*. New York: Julian Messner, 1986. Seventeen teenagers talk openly about their cancer.

Lazar, Linda and Bonnie Crawford. *My Journal: Reflections on Life*. Centering Corporation. (402) 553-1200. Journal for teens coping with life threatening or terminal illness.

Richter, Elizabeth. *The Teenage Hospital Experience: You Can Handle It*. New York: Coward, McCann, and Geohegan, 1982.

Siblings

American Cancer Society. *When Your Brother or Sister Has Cancer*. For a free copy, call (800) ACS-2345. Sixteen-page booklet which describes the emotions felt by siblings of a child with cancer.

O'Toole, Donna. *Aarvy Aardvark Finds Hope: A Read Aloud Story for People of All Ages About Loving and Losing, Friendship and Hope*. Compassion Books, 1988. Aarvy Aardvark and his friend Ralphie Rabbit show how a family member or friend can help another in distress.

Peterkin, Allan. *What About Me? When Brothers and Sisters Get Sick*. Magination Press, 1992. Describes the conflicted feelings of siblings when their brother or sister is hospitalized.

Medical Treatment

Diseases

Kingston, Judith, MD. *Understanding Retinoblastoma: An Information Booklet for Parents and Those Looking After Children with Eye Cancer*. Produced by The Retinoblastoma Society, London, England. To receive a copy of this or their quarterly newsletter, *ORbS,* call 0171-600-3309, fax: 0171-600-8579, or email: *rbnews@ rbsociety.org.uk.*

Neuroblastoma Hope. An informative newsletter produced quarterly by The Neuroblastoma Children's Cancer Society to educate, support, and increase awareness. Call (800) 532-5162 or fax: (847) 490-0705.

Pizzo, Phillip A., MD, and David G. Poplack, MD, eds. *Principles and Practice of Pediatric Oncology*. Philadelphia: Lippencott-Raven, 1996. Chapter 29, "Neuroblastoma." Chapter 28, "Wilms Tumor." Chapter 30, "Rhabdomyosarcoma and the Undifferentiated Sarcomas." Chapter 31, "Ewing's Sarcoma Family of Tumors." Chapter 32, "Other Soft Tissue Sarcomas of Childhood." Chapter 33, "Osteosarcoma." Chapter 27, "Hepatic Tumors." Chapter 26, "Retinoblastoma." Extremely technical.

Retinoblastoma Support News. A quarterly newsletter distributed by The Institute for Families of Blind Children. Call (213) 669-4649.

Wagner, D., S. Kreissman, and L. Wiriek. *Neuroblastoma: A Handbook for Families*. Association of Pediatric Oncology Nurses, 1997. $5. Call (847) 375-4724 or email: *info@apon.org.*

Coping with procedures

Benson, Herbert, MD. *The Relaxation Response*. New York: Avon Books, 1990. This is an excellent resource for the relaxation method of pain relief.

Kuttner, Leora, PhD. *A Child In Pain: How to Help, What to Do*. Point Roberts, Washington: Hartley & Marks, 1996. Thoroughly explains how to understand, assess, and alleviate pain. Excellent resource.

Kuttner, Leora, PhD. *No Fears, No Tears*. Videotape. Available through the Canadian Cancer Society, (604) 872-4400 or *http://www.bc.cancer.ca/ccs/*. Documentary of eight young children and their parents as they learn how to manage the pain of cancer treatment. 27 minutes.

Kuttner, Leora, PhD. *No Fears, No Tears—13 Years Later*. Videotape. To order, fax request to: (604) 294-9986, or email: *leora_kuttner@sfu.ca*. Thirteen years after learning how to manage their painful cancer treatments, seven survivors of childhood cancer make sense of their early traumatic experiences, and demonstrate the power of mind-body pain relief. 46 minutes.

Partnership with medical team

Center for Attitudinal Healing. *Advice to Doctors and Other Big People from Kids*. Berkeley, CA: Celestial Arts, 1991. Written by children with catastrophic illnesses; offers suggestions and expresses feelings about healthcare workers. Wise and poignant.

Keene, Nancy. *Working with Your Doctor: Getting the Healthcare You Deserve*. Sebastopol, CA: O'Reilly & Associates, Inc., 1998. Practical guidance to help patients take an active role in maintaining health, and steps to help improve the doctor/patient relationship.

Hospitalization

Keene, Nancy. *Your Child in the Hospital: A Practical Guide for Parents*. Sebastopol, CA: O'Reilly & Associates, rev. ed. 1999. A pocket guide full of parent stories to help others prepare their children physically and emotionally for hospitalizations.

Kellerman, Johnathan. *Helping the Fearful Child*. New York: W.W. Norton, 1981. Although this book was written as a guide for everyday and problem anxieties, it is full of excellent advice for parents of children undergoing traumatic procedures. This book is out of print, but may be available in your local library.

Clinical trials

Finn, Robert. *Cancer Clinical Trials: Experimental Treatments and How They Can Help You*. Sebastopol, CA: O'Reilly & Associates, 1999. Excellent guide that explains the structure, ethics, and types of clinical trials. Also covers how to evaluate a trial and deal with financial issues.

McAllister, Robert M., MD, and Sylvia Horowitz, PhD. *Cancer*. New York: Basic Books, 1993. Includes an excellent and detailed chapter on all aspects of clinical trials and a good basic description of how cancer cells operate.

National Cancer Institute. *What Are Clinical Trials All About?* For a free copy call (800) 4-CANCER. 22-page booklet covers basic information about clinical trials.

The Centerwatch Clinical Trials Listing Service at *http://www.centerwatch.com* contains a searchable database of 7,500 current clinical trials in all areas of medicine, including cancer.

Chemotherapy

Dodd, Marylin J., RN, PhD. *Managing the Side Effects of Chemotherapy & Radiation Therapy: A Guide for Patients and Their Families.* UCSF Nursing, 1996. This book contains thorough explanations of possible side effects of chemotherapy and radiation and suggestions for managing them.

National Institutes of Health. *Chemotherapy & You: A Guide to Self-Help During Treatment.* For a free copy, call (800) 4-CANCER. 56-page booklet includes answers to commonly asked questions about chemotherapy, its side effects, emotions while on chemotherapy, and nutrition.

Physicians Desk Reference. Oradell, New Jersey: Medical Economics Data, 1996. Issued yearly, lists authoritative information on all FDA approved drugs. Technical language. Available at reference desk in most libraries.

Pizzo, Phillip A., MD, and David G. Poplack, MD, eds. *Principles and Practice of Pediatric Oncology.* Philadelphia: Lippencott-Raven, 1997. Chapter 9, "General Principles of Chemotherapy." Chapter 44, "Management of Nausea and Vomiting." Extremely technical.

USP DI, Volume II, *Advice for the Patient: Drug Information in Lay Language.* United States Pharmacopeial Convention, Inc., 1995. Contains detailed drug information in non-medical language. Available in most libraries.

Radiation

McKay, Judith and Nancee Hirano. *The Chemotherapy and Radiation Survival Guide.* Oakland, CA: New Harbinger, 1998. Basic, understandable guide to chemotherapy and radiation and their side effects.

National Cancer Institute. *Radiation Therapy and You: A Guide to Self-help During Treatment.* For a free copy, call (800) 4-CANCER. 52-page booklet clearly defines radiation, explains what to expect, describes possible side effects, and discusses follow-up care.

O'Connell, Avice, MD, and Norma Leone. *Your Child and X-Rays: A Parents' Guide to Radiation, X-Rays and Other Imaging Procedures.* Rochester, NY: Lion Press, 1988. 89-page book explains x-ray treatments in easy-to-understand language.

Pizzo, Phillip A., MD, and David G. Poplack, MD, eds. *Principles and Practice of Pediatric Oncology.* Philadelphia: Lippencott-Raven, 1997. Chapter 11, "General Principles of Radiation Therapy." Extremely technical.

Surgery

O'Neill, James A., ed. *Pediatric Surgery.* St. Louis: Mosby-Year Book, 1998. Extremely technical.

Pizzo, Phillip A., MD, and David G. Poplack, MD, eds. *Principles and Practice of Pediatric Oncology.* Philadelphia: Lippencott-Raven, 1997. Chapter 10, "General Principles of Surgery." Extremely technical.

Bone marrow and stem cell transplantation

Johnson, F. Leonard, MD, and 31 others. *The Candlelighters Guide to Bone Marrow Transplants in Children.* Bethesda, MD: Candlelighters, 1994. (800) 366-CCCF. Straightforward, informative guide designed to educate parents about what a BMT is, types of BMTs, long-term medical effects, financial issues, psychosocial effects, impact on schooling and family life, what happens if the transplant fails, and seven family stories on their experiences.

National Cancer Institute. *Bone Marrow Transplantation and Peripheral Blood Stem Cell Transplantation.* 1994. To obtain free copy, call (800) 4-CANCER and ask for NIH Pub. No. 95-1178. Excellent 50-page booklet covers the purpose of BMTs, the types of BMTs, complications, long-term effects, financial considerations, psychosocial considerations, the future of BMTs, clinical trials and PDQ, and resources.

Pizzo, Phillip A., MD, and David G. Poplack, MD, eds. *Principles and Practice of Pediatric Oncology.* Philadelphia: Lippencott-Raven, 1997. Chapter 14, "Bone Marrow Transplantation in Pediatric Oncology." Extremely technical.

Stewart, Susan. *Bone Marrow Transplants: A Book of Basics for Patients.* Published by BMT Newsletter, (888) 597-7674 or (847) 433-3313. Explains all medical aspects of bone marrow transplantation. Technically accurate, yet easy to read. Find the *BMI Newsletter* on the Internet at *http://www.bmtnews.org/.*

Terminal illness

Callanan, Maggie, and Patricia Kelley. *Final Gifts: Understanding the Special Awareness, Needs, and Communications of the Dying.* New York: Poseidon Press, 1992. Written by two hospice nurses with decades of experience, this book helps families understand and communicate with terminally ill patients. Highly recommended.

Modlow, D. Gay, and Ida M. Martinson. *Home Care for the Seriously Ill Child: A Manual for Parents.* 1991. $7.95 from Children's Hospice International, (703) 684-0330. Helps parents explore the possibility of home care for the dying child.

Pizzo, Philip A., MD, and David G. Poplack , MD, eds. *Principles and Practice of Pediatric Oncology.* Philadelphia: Lippincott-Raven Publishers, 1997. Chapter 52, "Care of the Dying Child."

Online medical resources

CancerNet
(800) 4-CANCER
http://pdqsearch@icicc.nci.nih.gov/
email: *CancerNet@icicc.nci.nih.gov*

To subscribe, send a message. Leave the subject line blank, or use a dash if required. In the message body, type: help (if you use a signature, delete it). You will receive a list of available publications and instructions on how to get the information you want.

By far the most comprehensive and up-to-date source of information about cancer. It is maintained by the U.S. National Cancer Institute. Many of the resources listed in this book are available from the database.

TeleSCAN-Telmatics Services in Cancer
http://telescan.nki.nl/

The first European Internet service for cancer research, treatment, and education, providing a hypermedia interface to primarily European information resources and services related to cancer.

Oncolink
http://cancer.med.upenn.edu/

A text and multimedia service available through the Internet. This service was started by E. Loren Buhle, Jr., PhD, the parent of a child with leukemia. Oncolink offers a wide variety of cancer-related information, including articles, handbooks, case studies, writings by patients and their families, and visual images, including a children's art gallery.

Medicine Online
http://www.meds.com/

Provides patients and professionals with in-depth educational information on specific diseases. Also includes information on reimbursement and a treatment guide.

American Cancer Society
http://www.cancer.org/

Provides useful information about cancer treatments, news, and research.

Canadian Cancer Society
http://www.cancer.ca/

Provides useful information about cancer and includes a link to its research partner, the National Cancer Institute of Canada.

Pediatric Oncology Resource Center
http://www.acor.org/ped-onc/

Site provides useful information on diseases, treatments, signs of childhood cancer, family issues, and activism. Also includes information on bereavement. Numerous links to helpful medical resources.

Med help International
http://medhlp.netusa.net/
telnet: *medhlp.netusa.net*
ftp: *medhlp.netusa.net*
or dial up modem to 516-423-0472 (N81-ANSI)

A nonprofit organization that provides medical information written in nontechnical language. The all-volunteer staff is comprised of physicians and other healthcare professionals.

MedWeb: Oncology
http://www.medweb.emory.edu/MedWeb/

Hypermedia Clinical Practice Guidelines for Cancer Pain
http://www.statsci.com/talaria/talaria.html

The Multimedia Medical Reference Library
http://www.med-library.com/medlibrary/

PharmInfoNet

http://pharminfo.com/

Devoted to delivering useful, up-to-date, and accurate pharmaceutical information to healthcare providers, pharmacists, and patients.

Preventing Central Venous Catheter Infections

http://www.med.umkc.edu/cvcsite/

Patient Support.com

http://www.patientsupport.com/

Rx List—The Internet Drug Index

http://www.rxlist.com/

Alternative Medicine Homepage

http://www.pitt.edu/~cbw/altm.html

The Anthony Nolen Bone Marrow Trust

http://www.anthonynolan.org.uk/index.html

A leading research center and the United Kingdom register for potential donors. This site references other international BMT sites.

The BMT Newsletter

http://www.bmtnews.org/

All issues of the *BMT Newsletter* are online, as well as the book *Bone Marrow Transplants: A Book of Basics for Patients.*

Bone Marrow Donors Worldwide

http://bmdw.leidenuniv.nl

The National Marrow Donor Program

http://www.marrow.org/

CancerWEB Online Medical Dictionary

http://www.graylab.ac.uk/omd/index.html

One of the most complete medical dictionaries available on the Internet.

Emotional Support

Family Portrait: Coping with Childhood Cancer. Videotape. 25 minutes. VHS. Purchase from Films for the Humanities and Sciences, (800) 257-5126. Five family portraits cover issues such as guilt, sibling rivalry, divorce, the adopted child, and involvement of other family members.

Mr. Rogers Talks with Parents About Childhood Cancer. 1990. Videotapes (2), guidebook, and pamphlet. 47 minutes. VHS. Available from American Cancer Society, (800) ACS-2345. Interviews with parents. The first tape illustrates ways to deal with emotions during diagnosis and treatment The second tape sensitively deals with bereavement.

Sourkes, Barbara M., PhD. *Armfuls of Time: The Psychological Experience of the Child with a Life-Threatening Illness*. University of Pittsburg Press, 1995. Features the voices and artwork of children with cancer. Highly recommended.

Support groups

American Psychological Association. *Finding Help: How to Choose a Psychologist*. To obtain free brochure, send self-addressed stamped envelope to *Finding Help*, APA Public Affairs Office, 750 First St. NE, Washington, DC 20002-4242. Covers psychotherapy, the types of problems people discuss, and how to choose a therapist.

Bogue, Erna-Lynne, ACSW, and Barbara K. Chesney, MPH. *Making Contact: A Parent-to-parent Visitation Manual*. Bethesda, MD: The Candlelighters Childhood Cancer Foundation, 1987. (800) 366-CCCF. For parents of children with cancer. Includes guidelines for selection of parent visitors, training to improve parent-visitor contact, developing referral systems, and support resources.

Chesler, Mark A., PhD, and Barbara Chesney. *Cancer and Self-Help: Bridging the Troubled Waters of Childhood Illness*. Madison, WI: The University of Wisconsin Press, 1995. Explains how self-help groups are formed, how they function and recruit, and why they are effective.

National Cancer Institute. *Taking Time: Support for People with Cancer and the People Who Care About Them*. NIH Publication No. 88-2059. (800) 4-CANCER. 61-page booklet includes sections on sharing feelings, coping within the family, and when you need assistance.

Pizzo, Philip A., MD, and David G. Poplack, MD. *Principles and Practice of Pediatric Oncology*. Philadelphia: Lippincott-Raven, 1997. Chapter 47, "Psychiatric and Psychosocial Support for the Child and Family." Chapter 48, "The Other of Side of the Bed: What Caregivers Can Learn from Listening to Patients and Their Families."

Speigel, David, MD. *Living Beyond Limits*. New York: Random House, 1993. This book is an excellent guide for coping with cancer, strengthening family relationships, controlling pain, dealing with doctors, and evaluating alternative medicine claims. Out of print, but may be available at your local library.

ACOR, The Association of Cancer Online Resources, Inc.
http://www.acor.org/

ACOR has information and electronic support groups for patients, caregivers, or anyone affected by cancer. To join a discussion group, send a message addressed to *listserv@listserv.acor.org*. Leave the subject line blank (or add a dash if necessary). In the message body, type: subscribe <list name> <your first and last name> (if you have an automatic signature, turn it off). For example, to subscribe to PED-ONC, type: subscribe PED-ONC John Smith.

Sickkids Mailing List
email: *listserv@maelstrom.stjohns.edu*

Moderated (with adult supervision) email support group for children under eighteen who have serious illnesses. The children share information, establish friendships, ask questions, and exchange humor. There is a team of children who serve as discussion managers. To subscribe, leave the subject line blank. In the message body, type: subscribe SICKKIDS <your first and last name> (if you have an automatic signature, turn it off). Although adults may not participate in the group, they can email questions or concerns to an adult advisor at: *Sickkids-request@maelstrom.stjohns.edu.*

Touchstone Support Network
http://www-med.stanford.edu/touchstone/

A nonprofit, nonsectarian, volunteer organization that provides emotional and practical support services for families and their children with chronic and life-threatening illnesses.

SpeciaLove
http://www.speciallove.org/

A resource devoted to parents and children with cancer to facilitate networking. This resource is oriented to the family aspects of childhood cancer. SpeciaLove, Inc. was started in 1983 by Tom and Sheila Baker, who lost their thirteen-year-old daughter to leukemia.

Patient Advocacy Numbers
http://infonet.welch.jhu.edu/advocacy.html

Siblings

Faber, Adele, and Elaine Mazlish. *Siblings Without Rivalry: How to Help Your Children Live Together So You Can Live Too.* New York: Avon Books, 1998. Required reading for parents with fighting siblings. Offers dozens of simple yet effective methods to reduce conflict and foster a cooperative spirit.

Leukemia Society of America. *Emotional Aspects of Childhood Leukemia.* (800) 955-8484. 32-page booklet deals with the gamut of emotions experienced by all members of the family, including siblings.

Murray, Gloria, and Gerald Jamplosky, eds. *Straight from the Siblings: Another Look at the Rainbow.* Millbrae, CA: Celestial Arts, 1982. Written by sixteen children who have brothers and sisters with a life-threatening illness who met at the Center for Attitudinal Healing. A must-read for both parents and siblings.

Feelings, communication, and behavior

Faber, Adele, and Elaine Mazlish. *How to Talk So Kids Will Listen...and Listen So Kids Will Talk.* New York: Rawson, Wade Publishers, 1995. The classic book on developing new, more effective ways to communicate with your children, based on respect and understanding. Highly recommended.

Kurcinka, Mary Sheedy. *Raising Your Spirited Child: A Guide for Parents Whose Child Is More Intense, Sensitive, Perceptive and Energetic.* New York: Harper Collins, 1992. Many of the strategies in this reassuring guide are very effective for children stressed by cancer treatment.

Nelsen, Jane. *Positive Discipline.* rev. ed. New York: Ballantine Books, 1996. Written by a psychologist, educator, and mother of seven, this book teaches parents how to promote self-discipline and personal responsibility.

Practical support

Finances

Leeland, Jeff. *One Small Sparrow: The Remarkable Real-Life Drama of One Community's Compassionate Response to a Little Boy's Life*. Sisters, OR: Multnomah Books, 1995. Contains numerous ideas for methods to raise funds. Christian perspective.

Peterson, Sheila. *A Special Way to Care*. 1988. Available from Friends of Karen, Box 217, Croton Falls, NY 10519. Free guide for those who wish to provide financial/emotional support for families of ill children. Discusses how to differentiate between interference and advocacy. Explains how to organize, manage, and perpetuate a support fund. Excellent resource.

Pizzo, Philip A., MD, and David G. Poplack, MD, eds. *Principles and Practice of Pediatric Oncology*. Philadelphia: Lippincott-Raven Publishers, 1997. Chapter 53, "Financial Issues in Pediatric Cancer."

Nutrition

Bohannon, Richard, and others. *Food for Thought: The Cancer Prevention Cookbook*. Contemporary Books: 1889. Written by an oncologist, a chef, and a writer, this book follows American Cancer Society guidelines. Contains many tasty recipes.

National Cancer Institute. *Managing Your Child's Eating Problems During Cancer Treatment*, and *Eating Hints for Cancer Patients*. (800) 4-CANCER. These booklets cover how cancer treatments affect eating, how to cope with side effects, special diets, family resources, and recipes.

Pizzo, Philip A., MD, and David G. Poplack, MD, eds. *Principles and Practice of Pediatric Oncology*. Philadelphia: Lippincott-Raven Publishers, 1997. Chapter 42, "Nutritional Supportive Care."

Wilson, J. Randy. *Non-Chew Cookbook*. Glenwood Springs, CO: Wilson Publishing, Inc., 1986. P.O. Box 2190, 81602. (303) 945-5600. Contains recipes for patients unable to chew due to the side effects of chemotherapy and/or radiation.

School

American Cancer Society. *Back to School: A Handbook for Parents of Children with Cancer*. (800) ACS-1234. 16-page introductory booklet covers school re-entry, classroom presentations, the importance of advocates, legal issues, IEPs, and special needs.

Anderson, Winifred, Stephen Chitwood, and Deidre Hayden. *Negotiating the Special Education Maze: A Guide for Parents and Teachers*. Bethesda, MD: Woodbine House, 3rd ed. 1997. Step-by-step guide to obtaining help for your child. If you only read one book on this subject, this should be the one.

Candlelighters Childhood Cancer Foundation Canada. *School Reentry Resource Manual*. 1992. (416) 489-6440. For parents, educators, and healthcare professionals, addresses siblings, adolescence, survivor's quality of life, programs, bereavement, and grief.

Chai Lifeline. *Back to School: A Handbook for Educators of Children with Life-threatening Diseases in the Yeshiva/Day School System*. 1995. (212) 465-1300. Covers diagnosis, planning for school re-entry, infection control, needs of junior and senior high school students, children with special educational needs, and saying good-bye when a child dies.

The Compassionate Friends. *Suggestions for Teachers and School Counselors.* P.O. Box 3696, Oak Brook, IL 60522. (630) 990-0010.

Deasy-Spinetta, Patricia, and Elisabeth Irvin. *Educating the Child With Cancer.* Candlelighters Childhood Cancer Foundation. (800) 366-CCCF. 137-page book discusses all aspects of educating the child with cancer.

Gliko-Braden, Majel. *Grief Comes to Class: A Teacher's Guide.* Centering Corporation, 1531 N. Saddle Creek Rd., Omaha, NE 68104. (402) 553-1200. Comprehensive guide to grief in the classroom.

Peterson's Guides. *Peterson's Guides to Colleges with Programs for Learning Disabled Students or Attention Deficit Disorders.* 5th ed. Princeton, NJ: Peterson's Guides, 1997. Excellent reference, available at most large libraries.

Pizzo, Philip A., MD, and David G. Poplack, MD, eds. *Principles and Practice of Pediatric Oncology.* Philadelphia: Lippincott-Raven Publishers, 1997. Chapter 51, "Educational Issues for Children with Cancer."

After Treatment ends

Harpham, Wendy Schlessel. *After Cancer: A Guide to Your New Life.* Harperperennial, 1995. Written in a question and answer format, doctor/cancer survivor Harpham addresses the medical, psychological, and practical issues of recovery.

Hoffman, Barbara, J.D., ed. *A Cancer Survivor's Almanac: Charting Your Journey.* National Coalition for Cancer Survivorship, 1998. Comprehensive guide to the issues of cancer survivorship.

Keene, Nancy, Wendy Hobbie and Kathy Ruccione. *Childhood Cancer Survivors: A Guide to the Future.* Sebastopol, CA: O'Reilly & Associates, 2000. A user-friendly, comprehensive guide on late effects of treatment for childhood cancer.

Pizzo, Philip A., MD, and David G. Poplack, MD, eds. *Principles and Practice of Pediatric Oncology.* Philadelphia: Lippincott-Raven Publishers, 1997. Chapter 50, "Late Effects of Childhood Cancer and Its Treatment." Chapter 54, "Pediatric Cancer: Advocacy, Legal, Insurance, and Employment Issues." Chapter 57, "Preventing Cancer in Adulthood: Advice for the Pediatrician."

Bereavement

Parental grief

Bereavement: A Magazine of Hope and Healing. Provides support for the grieving, allows for feedback from professionals, and teaches nonbereaved how to help. (719) 282-1948. Other grief-related publications are also available.

Kubler-Ross, Elisabeth, MD. *On Children and Death.* New York: Macmillan, 1983. This comforting book offers practical help in living through the terminal period of a child's life with love and understanding.

Morse, Melvin, MD. *Closer to the Light: Learning from Near Death Experiences of Children.* New York: Villard Books, 1990. About startlingly similar spiritual experiences of children who almost die.

Rando, Therese, PhD, ed. *Parental Loss of a Child.* Champaign, IL: Research Press, 1986. Addresses death from a serious illness; guilt and grief; advice to physicians, clergy and funeral directors; professional help and support organizations.

Wild, Laynee. *I Remember You: A Grief Journal.* San Francisco: HarperCollins, 1994. A journal for written and photographic memories during the first year of mourning. Beautiful book filled with quotes and comfort.

Sibling grief (adult reading)

Doka, Kenneth, ed. *Children Mourning, Mourning Children.* Hemisphere Publications, 1995. Topics include children's understanding of death, answering grieving children's questions, and the role of the schools. Write to Taylor and Francis, 1900 Frost Road, Suite 101, Bristol, PA, 19007. Include $14.95 plus $2.50 for shipping and handling.

Grollman, Earl. *Talking About Death: A Dialogue Between Parent and Child.* Boston, MA: Beacon Press, 1990. This very comforting book teaches parents how to explain death, understand how children react to specific types of death, and when to seek professional help. Highly recommended.

Schaefer, Dan, and Christine Lyons. *How Do We Tell the Children?: A Step-by-Step Guide for Helping Children Two to Teen Cope When Someone Dies.* updated ed. New York: Newmarket Press, 1993. If your terminally-ill child has siblings, read this book.

Sibling grief (young child reading)

Buscaglia, Leo. *The Fall of Freddy the Leaf: A Story of Life for All Ages.* New York: Holt, Rinehart and Winston, 1982. This wise yet simple story about a leaf named Freddy explains death as a necessary part of the cycle of life. This book is out of print, but may be available in your local library.

Hickman, Martha. *Last Week My Brother Anthony Died.* Abingdon, TN: 1984. Touching story of a preschooler's feelings when her infant brother dies.

Mellonie, Bryan, and Robert Ingpen. *Lifetimes: The Beautiful Way to Explain Death to Children.* New York: Bantam Books, 1983. Paintings and simple text explain that dying is as much a part of life as being born.

Sibling grief (school-aged children)

Houston, Gloria. *My Brother Joey Died.* New York: J. Messner, 1982. Simple, caring book describes one child's journey through grief after the death of her sibling.

Temes, Roberta, PhD. *The Empty Place: A Child's Guide Through Grief.* Far Hills, NJ: New Horizon Press, 1992. (402) 553-1200. Explains and describes feelings after the death of a sibling, such as the empty place in the house, at the table, in a brother's heart.

White, E.B. *Charlotte's Web.* New York: Harper, 1952. Classic tale of friendship and death as a part of life. (The videotape is widely available to rent.)

Sibling grief (teenagers)

Gravelle, Karen, and Charles Haskins. *Teenagers Face to Face with Bereavement.* Englewood Cliffs, NJ: J. Messner, 1989. The perspectives and experiences of seventeen teenagers coping with grief.

Grollman, Earl. *Straight Talk About Death for Teenagers: How to Cope with Losing Someone You Love.* Boston, MA: Beacon Press, 1993. Wonderful book that talks to teens, not at them. Discusses denial, pain, anger, sadness, physical symptoms, and depression.

Audio/video

Drying Their Tears. Produced by CARTI, Communication Division, Markham University, P.O. Box 55050, Little Rock, AR 72215. (800) 482-8561. Video and manual to help counselors, teachers, and other professionals help children deal with the grief, fear, confusion, and anger that occur after the death of a loved one.

The Healing Path. The Compassionate Friends sibling video addresses concerns of surviving siblings, such as sadness, pain, anger, and fear. Call (630) 990-0010 or fax: (630) 990-0246.

Glossary

Abdomen
The area of the body that lies between the chest and the pelvis.

Absolute neutrophil count (ANC) (also known as absolute granulocyte or AGC)
Total count of the neutrophils in the blood, which provides an indication of a person's ability to fight infection. To calculate the ANC, add the percentages of seg neutrophils and band neutrophils, divide by 100, and multiply by the total white blood count.

Acute
Occurring over a short period of time.

Adjuvant chemotherapy
Chemotherapy given with surgery or radiation.

Adrenalectomy
Surgical removal of one or both adrenal glands.

Alkylating agents
A family of anticancer drugs that work by interfering with the DNA of a cell to prevent normal division.

Allogenic transplant
Type of bone marrow transplant in which the marrow is donated by another person.

Alopecia
Hair loss; a common side effect of chemotherapy.

Alfa-fetoprotein
A protein that is elevated in the blood of children with liver cancer.

Ambulatory
Able to walk.

Amputation
Surgically removing a part of the body.

Anaphalaxis
An acute allergic reaction which can be life-threatening.

Analgesic
A drug used to relieve pain.

Anaplastic
A tumor that has no resemblance to the normal tissue of the involved organ when viewed under a microscope.

Anemia
Condition in which there is a reduction in the number of circulating red blood cells.

Anesthesia
    Partial or total loss of sensation, with or without loss of consciousness, induced by the administration of a drug.

Anesthesiologist
    A doctor who specializes in the study and administration of anesthesia.

Anorexia
    Loss of appetite.

Antibiotic
    A drug used to treat bacterial infections.

Antibody
    A protein that works to defend the body against bacterial and viral infections.

Antiemetic
    A drug given to prevent or reduce nausea and vomiting.

Antigen
    A foreign substance that stimulates the lymphocytes to produce antibodies.

Antihistamine
    A drug used to treat allergic reactions.

Antimetabolites
    A family of anticancer drugs that replace normal vitamins to starve cancer cells.

Apheresis
    The collection of blood components from a patient or donor in which desired elements are removed and the remainder returned to the body.

Artery
    A blood vessel that carries oxygen-rich blood from the heart to other tissues.

Ascites
    An abnormal collection of fluid in the abdomen.

Asepsis (Aseptic)
    Free of infection.

Ataxia
    Loss of balance.

Attending physician
    Doctor on the staff of a hospital who has completed medical school, residency, and fellowship.

Asymptomatic
    Without symptoms.

Atypical
    Not usual or ordinary.

Autologous
    From the same person. An autologous bone marrow transplant is a procedure in which bone marrow that has been removed from a patient is given back to that patient.

Axilla
    The armpit.

Bacteria

A group of one-celled organisms that can be viewed only through a microscope. Most do no harm; however, if the immune system is lowered, some can cause disease.

Benign

Noncancerous.

Bilateral

Occurring on both sides of the body.

Bilirubin

A pigment that is produced by the liver as it processes waste products. When elevated, bilirubin causes yellowing of the skin.

Biopsy

Removal of a small sample of tissue for examination under a microscope.

Blood-brain barrier

A network of blood vessels located around the central nervous system with very closely spaced cells that make it difficult for potentially toxic substances—including anticancer drugs—to enter the brain and spinal cord.

Blood type

Identification of the proteins in a person's blood cells so that transfusions can be given with compatible blood products. Possible blood types are A+, A–, B+, B–, AB+, AB–, O+, and O–.

Bone marrow

Soft, inner part of large bones that makes blood cells.

Bone marrow aspiration

Process in which a sample of fluid and cells is withdrawn from the bone marrow using a hollow needle.

Bone marrow biopsy

The removal of a sample of solid tissue from the bone marrow.

Bone marrow transplant

A procedure in which doctors replace bone marrow that has been destroyed by high doses of chemotherapy and/or radiation.

Brachytherapy

Radioactive seeds implanted directly at a tumor site allowing high dose radiation to be delivered to the tumor while sparing surrounding tissue from exposure.

Bypass

A surgical procedure used to maneuver around an organ or area that may be blocked by a tumor.

CBC (Complete blood count)

Measurement of the numbers of white cells, red cells, and platelets in a cubic millimeter of blood.

Cachexia

The wasting away of the body; extreme weight loss, usually caused by disease or malnutrition.

Cancer

A term for diseases in which abnormal cells divide without control.

Carcinogen
A substance or agent that produces cancer.

Cardiac
Pertaining to the heart.

Catheter
A tube that can be placed into the body to deliver fluids or medications, or to drain fluid.

Centigray
Measurement of radiation-absorbed dose; same as a rad.

Central nervous system (CNS)
Brain, spinal cord, and nerves.

Cerebrospinal fluid (CSF)
Fluid which surrounds and bathes the brain and spinal cord and provides a cushion from shocks.

Chemotherapy
Treatment of disease with drugs. The term usually refers to cytotoxic drugs given to treat cancer.

Chromosome
A structure in the nucleus of a cell that contains genetic material. Normally, 46 chromosomes are inside each human cell.

Chronic
Lasting over a long period of time.

Clinical trial
A carefully designed and executed investigation of a drug, drug dosage, combination of drugs, or other method of treating disease. Each trial is designed to answer one or more scientific questions and to find better ways to prevent or treat disease.

Colony-stimulating factors
A substance that is used to stimulate the production of some types of bone marrow cells.

Coma
A deep, prolonged state of unconsciousness.

Combination chemotherapy
Using two or more chemotherapy drugs at the same time.

Combined modality therapy
Treatment that consists of two or more types of therapy, such as chemotherapy with surgery, radiotherapy, or immunotherapy.

Conditioning
The treatment given before a bone marrow or stem cell transplant. Conditioning can include high-dose chemotherapy with or without total body irradiation. Also called preparative regimen.

Congenital
Any condition that is present at birth.

Contralateral
Referring to the opposite side of the body.

Cryosurgery
A cold probe that is used as a surgical tool to kill cancer tissues.

Culture
To grow in a test tube; cultures can be taken from blood, urine, and throat secretions when an infection is suspected.

Cytokine
Proteins secreted by immune system cells which enable them to communicate with each other.

Cytomegalovirus (CMV)
One of a group of herpes viruses that can cause fatal infections in immunosuppressed patients.

Cytotoxic
Causing the death of cells.

Debulking
A surgical procedure to remove as much of a tumor as possible without removing it entirely.

Differentiation
The process by which cells mature and become specialized.

Distal
Further away from any point of reference, as opposed to proximal.

Diuretics
Drugs used to help rid the body of excess water and salt through the urine.

Dysphagia
Difficulty in swallowing.

Dysplasia
Abnormal changes in a cell which sometimes indicate that cancer may occur.

Dyspnea
Shortness of breath.

Dysuria
Painful or difficult urination.

Edema
The abnormal collection of fluid within tissues.

Embolization
A treatment that is delivered to a localized area by blocking the flow of blood to the area, such as the blood supply to a tumor.

Emesis
Vomiting.

Engraftment
During bone marrow or stem cell transplant, the point at which the infused marrow is accepted by the patient and begins to produce blood cells.

Enteral feeding
Delivering nutrients through a tube inserted into the stomach or intestine.

Enucleation
The surgical removal of an eye.

Epideral
    The space immediately outside the spinal cord.

Erythrocytes
    Red blood cells.

EUA
    Examination under anesthesia. EUAs are often used to evaluate children that
    have been diagnosed with retinoblastoma.

Excision
    Surgery to remove tissue.

External catheter
    Indwelling catheter in which one end of the tubing is in the heart and the other
    end of the tubing sticks out through the skin, for example, a Hickman catheter.

Extraosseous
    Occurring outside of the bone.

Febrile
    A fever.

Fellow
    A physician who has completed four years of medical school, several years of
    residency, and is pursuing additional training in a specialized field.

Fine needle aspiration (FNA)
    Removing small samples of tissue, usually while under a local anesthetic,
    through a fine needle.

Finger poke
    When a laboratory technician pricks the finger tip to obtain a small sample of
    blood.

Gastritis
    An inflammation of the stomach.

Gastrointestinal
    Pertaining to the stomach and intestines.

Gene
    A unit of DNA that transmits a single trait from a parent to a child.

Graft
    Tissue taken from one person (donor) and transferred to another person (recipi-
    ent or host).

Graft-versus-host disease
    A condition that may develop after allogenic bone marrow transplantation in
    which the transplanted marrow (graft) attacks the patient's (host's) organs.

Granulocytes
    A type of white cell which destroys foreign substances in the body such as
    viruses, bacteria, and fungi.

Hematocrit
    The measurement of the proportion of cells to plasma in a sample of blood.
    Sometimes called packed cell volume (PCV).

Hematologist
Physician who specializes in the diagnosis and treatment of disorders of blood and blood-forming tissues.

Hematoma
A localized collection of blood.

Hematuria
Blood in the urine.

Hemoglobin
The protein found in red blood cells that carries oxygen.

Hemorrhagic cystitis
Bleeding from the bladder, which can be a side effect of the drug cytoxan.

Hepatectomy
Surgical removal of all or part of the liver.

Hepatic
Pertaining to the liver.

Hepatitis
Inflammation of the liver by virus or toxic substance. Fever and jaundice are usually present, and sometimes the liver is enlarged.

Hickman catheter
An indwelling catheter that has one end of the tubing in the heart and the other end outside the body.

Histology
Appearance of tissue when viewed under a microscope.

HIV (Human immunodeficiency virus)
The virus that causes AIDS.

Host
In bone marrow transplantation, the person who receives the marrow.

Human leukocyte antigens (HLAs)
Proteins on the surface of cells that are important in transplantation and transfusion. For BMTs, the HLAs on white cells of the patient and potential donor are compared. A perfect HLA match occurs only between identical twins.

Hyperalimentation
Artificial feeding which delivers nutrients through the use of a special catheter or intravenously.

Hypercalcemia
Abnormally high levels of calcium in the blood.

Infusion Pump
A small, computerized device that allows drugs to be given at home through an IV or indwelling catheter.

Intraocular
Occurring within the eye.

Immune System
Complex system by which the body protects itself from foreign invaders.

Immunosuppression
　　Suppression of the immune system, which leaves the body susceptible to infection.

Immunotherapy
　　A type of cancer therapy that uses the body's own immune system to attack cancerous cells.

Induction
　　The first part of the chemotherapy protocol for treating some types of cancer in which several powerful chemotherapy drugs are given to kill as many cancer cells as possible.

Infusion
　　Giving fluids or medications through a vein over a period of time.

In situ
　　An early stage of cancer in which the tumor is localized to one area.

Institutional review board (IRB)
　　Group made up of scientists, clergy, doctors, and citizens from the community, which approves and reviews all research taking place at an institution.

Intern
　　Recent medical school graduate who is receiving her first year of supervised practical training in medical and surgical care of patients in hospitals.

Intramuscular (IM)
　　Injection of drugs into the muscle.

Intrathecal
　　Injection of drugs into the cerebrospinal fluid during a spinal tap.

Intravenous-access line (IV)
　　A hollow metal or plastic tube which is inserted into a vein and attached to tubing, allowing various solutions or medicines to be directly infused into the blood.

Ipsilateral
　　On the same side of the body.

Jaundice
　　A yellowing of the skin and the whites of the eyes caused by too much bilirubin in the blood. Jaundice is indicative of liver problems.

Laparotomy
　　Surgical procedure in which the abdominal cavity is opened.

Lesion
　　A tissue abnormality.

Leukocytes
　　White blood cells.

Leukokoria
　　A white dot seen in the center of the eye of very young children which may be indicative of retinoblastoma. Leukokoria is sometimes called a "cat's eye reflex."

Leukopenia
　　A below-normal number of white cells.

Localized
Cancer that has not spread to other areas within the body.

Lumbar puncture (Spinal tap)
Procedure in which a needle is inserted between the vertebrae of the back to obtain a sample of cerebrospinal fluid and/or inject medication.

Lymph
A clear, colorless fluid found in lymph vessels throughout the body that carries cells to fight infection.

Lymph nodes
Rounded bodies of lymphatic tissues found in lymph vessels.

Lymph system
A system of vessels and nodes throughout the body that help filter out bacteria and perform numerous other functions.

Lymphocytes
Type of white cell formed in the lymphoid tissues that prevents infection and helps provide immunity to disease.

Lytic
A bone lesion. Lytic lesions may appear as a "hole" on an x-ray.

Malaise
Tiredness.

Malignant
Cancerous.

Mediastinum
The area of the middle of the chest.

Medical student
Student who has completed four years of college and is enrolled in medical school.

Metastasis
The spread of cancer from one area of the body to another through the lymph system or the blood.

Mitosis
The process of cell division or reproduction.

Modality
A method of treatment.

Monocytes
Type of white blood cell.

Mucositis
Inflammation of the mucous membranes.

Multifocal
Arising from more than one location.

Myelosuppression
Low blood counts caused by chemotherapy or radiation.

Nadir
The lowest point that blood counts will fall after chemotherapy.

Necrosis
> The death of tissues caused by chemotherapy, radiation, or a lack of blood supply.

Neoplasm
> A new abnormal growth that may be benign or malignant.

Nephrectomy
> The surgical removal of a kidney.

Neuropathy
> A condition sometimes caused by chemotherapy. Neuropathy is the malfunctioning of a nerve, which can cause numbness or weakness.

Neurotoxic
> Substance which is poisonous to the brain, spinal cord, and/or nerve cells.

Neutropenia
> Condition when the body does not have enough neutrophils (a type of infection-fighting white cell).

Neutrophils
> The most numerous of the granulocytic white cells, they migrate through the bloodstream to the site of infection, where they ingest and destroy bacteria.

Nutritionist
> A professional who analyzes nutritional requirements and gives advice on how to eat an appropriate diet for any condition.

Oncogenes
> Any gene that contributes to the transformation of a normal cell into a cancerous cell.

Oncologist
> Doctor who specializes in the treatment of cancer.

Oncology
> Study of cancer.

Ototoxicity
> Damage to the ears which can result in a ringing in the ears or permanent hearing loss.

Palliative
> Treatment given with a primary goal of adequate pain control.

Palpation
> Examining an area of the body, such as the abdomen, by feeling with the fingers to detect abnormalities.

Pancreatitis
> Inflammation of the pancreas which can cause extreme pain, vomiting, hiccoughing, constipation, and collapse.

Pathologist
> Doctor who specializes in examining tissue and diagnosing disease.

Pediatrician
> Doctor who specializes in the care and development of children and the treatment of their diseases.

Petechiae
> Small, reddish spots under the skin caused by hemorrhage.

Phlebitis
Inflammation of a vein.

Plasma
The liquid part of the lymph and the blood.

Platelet
Disc-shaped blood cell which aids in blood clotting.

Poorly differentiated
Cancerous cells that have little resemblance to the normal tissue from the same organ when viewed under a microscope.

Port-a-cath
Indwelling catheter which has a small portal under the skin of the chest attached to tubing which goes into the heart.

Preparative regimen
See conditioning.

Primary tumor
The original site where cancer first begins to grow.

Prognosis
Expected or probable outcome.

Progression
A worsening of disease by the continued growth of cancer.

Prophylaxis
An attempt to prevent disease.

Proptosis
A forward projection of the eyeball.

Prosthesis
An artificial replacement for a part of the body that has been surgically removed, such as a limb or an eye.

Protocol
Document which outlines the drugs that will be taken, when they will be taken, and in what dosages. Also includes the dates for procedures.

Proximal
Closest to any point of reference, as opposed to distal.

Pulmonary
Pertaining to the lungs.

Purging
A process to remove certain components found in bone marrow or stem cell harvests. In an autologous harvest, purging may be used to remove any remaining cancerous cells. In an allogeneic harvest, purging may be used to remove components of the donor collection that can cause graft-versus-host disease.

Rad
Radiation absorbed dose. A unit of measurement of the absorbed dose of radiation. Same as a centigray (cGy)

Radiation
High-energy rays which are used to kill or damage cancer cells.

Radiologist
> Doctor who specializes in using radiation and radioactive isotopes to diagnose and treat disease.

Radiosensitive
> A type of cancer that usually responds well to radiation.

Randomized
> Chosen at random. In a randomized research project, a computer chooses which patients receive the experimental treatment(s), and which patients receive the standard treatment.

Recurrence
> See Relapse.

Regression
> The shrinking or disappearance of cancer cells, usually as a result of therapy.

Relapse
> A return of cancer after its apparent complete disappearance.

Remission
> Disappearance of detectable disease.

Renal
> Pertaining to the kidney.

Resection
> The surgical removal of tissue.

Resident
> Physician who has completed four years of medical school and one year of internship, and who is continuing his or her clinical training.

Residual disease
> The cancerous cells that are left behind after a tumor has been surgically removed.

Right atrial catheter
> Indwelling catheter with tubing that extends into the heart that provides access for drawing blood and injecting medication.

Second-look surgery
> An operation performed after an initial surgery to allow the surgeon to view the area of the original procedure.

Seizure
> Uncontrollable shaking of the body, often with loss of consciousness. Also called convulsion.

Sepsis
> Bacterial growth found within the bloodstream.

Side effect
> Unintentional or undesirable secondary effect of treatment.

Somnolence syndrome
> Syndrome which can occur from three to twelve weeks after cranial radiation. It is characterized by drowsiness, prolonged periods of sleep (up to twenty hours a day), low-grade fever, headaches, nausea, vomiting, irritability, difficulty swallowing, and difficulty speaking.

Spinal tap
> Procedure in which a needle is inserted between the vertebrae of the back to obtain a sample of cerebrospinal fluid and/or inject medication. Also called lumbar puncture (LP).

Staging
> A process involving many procedures to determine the extent of disease. Staging is important in deciding the most appropriate treatment and prognosis.

Staphylococcus epidermidis
> Bacteria normally present on the skin which can infect the blood through an indwelling catheter.

Stem cells
> Cells from which all blood cells develop.

Stomatitis
> Soreness and inflammation of the mouth that can sometimes be caused by chemotherapy or radiation.

Strabismus
> A visual disorder in which one eye cannot focus with the other.

Stroke
> Injury or death of brain tissue caused by bleeding into the brain or clotting that blocks blood flow to a portion of the brain.

Subcutaneous port
> Type of indwelling catheter comprised of a portal under the skin of the chest attached to tubing leading into the heart.

Systemic
> Affecting the body as a whole.

TBI
> Total body irradiation. TBI is sometimes used as part of the conditioning regimen before bone marrow or stem cell transplantation.

Thoracotomy
> A surgical procedure in which the chest wall is opened.

Thrombocytes
> Platelets.

Thymus
> Small gland located behind the breast bone and between the lungs that plays a major role in the immune system.

Tissue
> A collection of cells that are of the same type.

Tumor
> A benign or cancerous lump, mass, or swelling.

Tumor board
> A meeting held at hospitals, attended by oncologists, pathologists, radiologists, fellows, and residents, in which complicated cases are discussed to develop a treatment plan.

Tumor burden
> The number of cancerous cells found in an organ or tissue; the size of a tumor.

Unilateral
Affecting one side of the body.

Venipuncture
Obtaining blood samples, starting an intravenous infusion, or giving a medication by inserting a needle into a vein.

Vital signs
Term which describes a patient's pulse, rate of breathing, and blood pressure.

White blood cells
Cells that help the body fight infection and disease.

Xerostomia
Dry mouth caused by salivary gland dysfunction.

X-ray
High-energy electromagnetic radiation used in low doses to diagnose disease or injury, and in high doses to treat cancer.

X-ray technician
Certified technician who positions patients for x-rays, monitors equipment, and takes x-rays of the body.

Index

H

hair loss, 245–247, 278
health insurance. *See* insurance
Health Insurance Portability and
    Accountability Act of
    1996, 417
helplessness, 6–7
    See also emotional responses
hemangiopericytoma, 137, 148–151
hematocrit (packed cell volume (PCV)),
    459
hemihypertrophy, 128
hemoglobin (Hgb), 459
hepatic arterial chemoembolization, 179
hepatitis, 23, 33, 172, 412
hepatoblastoma. *See* liver cancers
hepatocellular carcinoma. *See* liver
    cancers
hereditary Wilms tumor, 129
herpes zoster, 252–254
Hexadrol, 234
Hickman catheters, 91
    See also catheters
high-dose chemotherapy, 179, 291
    See also chemotherapy
HIV/AIDS, 23–24, 32–33, 412
hope, importance of, 10
hormones, 211
Horner syndrome, 116
hospitals and hospitalization
    choice of hospital, 3, 68
    coping with, 106–112
    financial assistance, sources of, 52–
        53, 317–320, 473
    food, 108
    parking arrangements, 108–109
    play areas, 111–112
    role of parents, 109–111
    rooms, 106–108
    siblings' concerns about, 365–366
    social workers, 194–196
    staff of, 3, 109
    See also doctors; insurance; nurses
Hycamtin, 229–230
hydromorphone, 238–239
hydroxyurea, 225
hypnosis, 17

I

I-MIBG (radiotherapy), 124
Idamycin, 225–226
idarubicin, 225–226
Ifex, 226
IFF (ifosfamide), 226
ifosfamide, 226
imagery, 17–18
immobilization devices, 271–272
    See also radiation
immune system
    reactions to radiation, 278
    reactions to transfusions, 23–24,
        32–33
    reactions to transplantation, 300–
        301
    See also blood counts; infections;
        side effects; *under specific*
        names of chemotherapeutic
        drugs
immunizations, 251, 253, 411
immunotherapy, 150
implanted catheters, 91
    See also catheters
Individual Education Plans (IEPs), 355–
    357
Individuals with Disabilities Education
    Act (IDEA), 352
indwelling catheters. *See* catheters
infections
    from catheters, 93–94, 99, 102
    chicken pox, 252–254, 347–348
    cytomegalovirus, 24, 33, 300
    detection of, 249–252
    following transplantation, 300–301
    hepatitis, 23, 33, 412
    HIV/AIDS, 23–24, 32–33, 412
    immunizations, 251, 253, 411
    from pets, 254–255
    pneumonia, 252
    prevention of, 249–252, 300–301,
        347–348, 411–412
    sexually transmitted, 411–412
    shingles (herpes zoster), 252–254
insurance, 314–317
    Americans with Disabilities Act
        (ADA), 414–415
    challenging claims, 316–317

osteosarcoma (*continued*)

    signs and symptoms, 154–155

    staging, 156

    treatments, 157–162

        chemotherapy, 161–162

        new and experimental, 162

        surgery, 157–161

oxycodone, 240–241

oxycotin, 240–241

P

pain

    distraction from, 18

    drugs for, 19–21, 236–241

    hypnosis, 17

    imagery, 17–18

    management and relief of during procedures

        pharmacological method, 19–21

        psychological method, 16–18

palliation, 283

paraplatin, 216–217

parent-to-parent visitation, 200–201

parenting stressed children, checklist for, 400–401

parents. *See* family and friends

Percoset, 240–241

peripheral primitive neuroectodermal tumor (PPNET). *See* Ewing's sarcoma family of tumors (ESFT)

pets, possible infections from, 254–255

pharmaceuticals. *See* drugs

Phenergan, 236

photocoagulation, 191

physicians. *See* doctors

Physician's Data Query (PDQ), 477

PICC lines, 91

    See also catheters

pill-taking, 36–38

platelet count, 462

platelet transfusions, 32–33

Platinol, 217–218

pneumonia, 252

Port-a-cath, 91

    See also catheters

ports. *See* catheters

prayer, 241

    See also religious support

procedures

    adjunctive therapies during, 18

    pain relief during, 16–21

    planning for, 13–15

    presence of parents at, 15

    questions before, 21–22

    specific types of

        audiogram, 22

        blood draws, 22–23

        blood transfusions, 23–24

        bone marrow aspiration, 24–25

        bone scan, 25–26

        computed tomography, 26–27

        conventional x-rays, 27

        echocardiagram, 27–28

        finger pokes, 28

        gallium scan, 29

        gastronomy, 29

        intravenous lines (IV), starting, 35–36

        intravenous pyelogram (IVP), 29

        magnetic resonance imaging (MRI), 30

        MIBG scan, 30–31

        MUGA scan, 31–32

        needle aspiration biopsy, 32

        pill-taking, 36–38

        platelet transfusions, 32–33

        pulmonary function test, 33

        spinal tap (lumbar puncture/LP), 34

        subcutaneous injections, 36

        surgical, 280–283

        temperature-taking, 38–39

        ultrasound imaging, 39–40

        urine specimens, 40

        x-rays, conventional, 27

prochlorperazine, 236

Procrit, 232–233

promethazine, 236

propofol, 20

psychological counseling. *See* emotional responses; support and self help

puberty, effect of treatment on, 303
pulmonary function test, 33

R

radiation
    description and types of, 266–268,
        274–277
    immobilization during, 271–272
    liver cancers, not generally used to
        treat, 178
    oncologists, therapists, 270–271
    questions to ask about, 269–270
    sedation during, 272–274
    side-effects
        coping with, 245–265
        long-term, 279, 302–304
        short-term, 278–279
    simulation, 274–275
    total body irradiation (TBI), 277,
        302–304
    treatment centers, choice of, 270
    treatments for
        bone sarcomas, 167
        Ewing's sarcoma family of
            tumors (ESFT), 167
        hepatoblastoma, not generally
            used to treat, 178
        hepatocellular carcinoma, not
            generally used to treat,
            178
        neuroblastoma, 122–123
        non-rhabdomyosarcoma soft
            tissue sarcomas, 149
        osteosarcoma not very
            responsive to, 157
        retinoblastoma, 191–192
        rhabdomyosarcoma, 147–148
        soft tissue sarcomas, 147–148,
            149
        Wilms tumor, 135
radiation oncologists, 270
radiation simulation, 274–275
radiation therapists, 270–271
radioactive iodine meta-
                iodobenzylguanidine
                (I-131 MIBG), 268
radioactive plaque therapy, 192

radioimmunotherapy, 268
    See also radiation
radiotherapy. *See* radiation
Rando, Therese A.
    on intensity of parental grief, 443
record keeping
    blood counts, chart for, 464
    financial records, 309–314
    medical records, 305–309
    special education records, 358
recurrence after transplant, 302
    See also relapse
red blood cells (RBCs), 23–24, 461
    See also blood counts
relapse
    emotional responses, 420–421
    recurrence after transplant, 302
    signs and symptoms, 418–420
    treatment plans, 421–425
relaxation therapy, 18
religious support, 54, 201–202
renal cell carcinoma, 136
researching medical condition or
        treatment, 467–469, 477
resection, 282–283
resource organizations, list of, 466–476
resources, 466–491
retinoblastoma, 181–193
    description, 181–185
    diagnosis, 186–187
    environmental risk factors, 185
    genetic risk factors, 183–185
    prognosis, 187
    signs and symptoms, 185–186
    staging, 186–187
    treatments, 187–193
        chemotherapy, 192–193
        new and experimental, 193
        radiation, 191–192
        surgery/local eye methods,
            188–191
rhabdoid tumor (of kidney), 135–136
rhabdomyosarcoma, 137–148, 151
    description, 137–140
    diagnosis, 142
    environmental risk factors, 140
    genetic risk factors, 139–140
    prognosis, 143–144

About the Authors

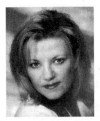

Honna Janes-Hodder's youngest son Matthew was diagnosed with neuroblastoma on his third birthday, and passed away at age seven on September 3, 1997. She loved, cared for, and advocated for Matthew throughout his long struggle with cancer. Currently, she lives with her husband, fourteen-year-old son, and eleven-year-old daughter, in beautiful Paradise, Newfoundland and Labrador, Canada. Honna is founder of ChildCan, The Childhood Cancer Research Association of Newfoundland and Labrador, Inc., and president of the International Pediatric Cancer Alliance, Inc.

Honna also manages most of the pediatric discussion groups for ACOR, the Association of Cancer Online Resources, Inc. ACOR, based in New York, provides accurate and timely medical support and information for all those affected by cancer, in both the pediatric and adult communities. She is the administrator for five online discussion groups, providing support and reliable information to families dealing with childhood cancers globally. In addition, Honna sits on the Public Issues Committee for the Newfoundland and Labrador division of the Canadian Cancer Society, and writes a regular health section for a national newspaper in Canada.

Honna spends a great deal of time advocating on behalf of children diagnosed with cancer. She does not view this as a job, but as an important part of her identity. Honna attends Memorial University of Newfoundland as a part-time student when time permits, working toward a PhD in biochemistry.

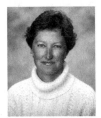

Nancy Keene is one of the original developers of the Patient-Centered Guides series. Nancy has been involved with the medical world for over two decades as a caregiver and patient. Nancy's daughter Kathryn was diagnosed with high-risk acute lymphoblastic leukemia when she was three years old. Nancy supported and advocated for Kathryn during two years of intensive treatment. Kathryn is now eleven years old.

Nancy's first book, *Childhood Leukemia: A Guide for Families, Friends & Caregivers*, blends technical information with stories from over 50 parents, children with cancer, and their siblings. Her second book, *Your Child in the Hospital: A Practical Guide for Parents*, now in its second edition, helps parents physically and emotionally prepare their child for hospitalization. Her third book, *Working with Your Doctor: Getting the Healthcare You Deserve*, takes an in-depth look at the doctor-patient relationship and provides suggestions on how to solve everyday health and communication problems. She is now working on a book about late effects of treatment called *Childhood Cancer Survivors: A Practical Guide to the Future*, with Kathy Ruccione and Wendy Hobbie.

Nancy lives in Washington state and is busy writing and raising her two daughters. She spends her limited free time volunteering in school, talking with parents (in person, over the phone, and on the Internet) of children newly diagnosed with cancer, reading an eclectic mix of books, and dreaming of travel.

Honna and Nancy are two of the first five people appointed as patient advocates to the Children's Cancer Group (CCG), a research organization consisting of pediatric cancer specialists from Canada, the United States, and Australia. They attend CCG meetings and facilitate communication between CCG investigators and the patient community.

You can reach the authors care of O'Reilly & Associates, Inc., by mail or email (*patientguides@oreilly.com*).

Colophon

Patient-Centered Guides are about the experience of illness. They contain personal stories as well as a mixture of practical and medical information. The faces on the covers of our Guides reflect the human side of the information we offer.

The cover of *Childhood Cancer: A Parent's Guide to Solid Tumor Cancers* was designed by Edie Freedman using Adobe Photoshop 5.0 and QuarkXPress 3.32 with Onyx BT and Berkeley fonts from Bitstream. The cover photo is from Rubberball Productions, and is used with that company's permission. The cover mechanical was prepared by Kathleen Wilson.

The interior layout for the book was designed by Alicia Cech, based on a design by Nancy Priest and Edie Freedman. The interior fonts are Berkeley and Franklin Gothic. The text was prepared by Edie Freedman and Mike Sierra using QuarkXPress 3.32 and FrameMaker 5.5. Illustrations were created by Martha Deller, Rhon Porter, Chris Reilley, and Robert Romano using Adobe Photoshop 5.0 and Macromedia FreeHand 8.0. The text was copyedited by Lunaea Hougland and proofread by Sarah Jane Shangraw. Maureen Dempsey, Colleen Gorman, and Claire Cloutier LeBlanc provided quality assurance. The index was written by Kate Wilkinson. Interior composition was done by Sarah Jane Shangraw.

Whenever possible, our books use RepKover™ or Otabind™ lay-flat binding. If the page count exceeds the limit for lay-flat binding, perfect binding is used.

Some of the photographs in Appendix A are reprinted with permission from the following: Glamour Shots, Portland, Oregon; House of Photography, Livingston, Tennessee; Rehor Studio, Seward, Nebraska.

Nancy Keene's photo is © Donette Studio, Bellingham, Washington. Honna Janes-Hodder's photo is © Rostotski Studio Limited, St. John's, Newfoundland.

Patient-Centered Guides™

Questions Answered
Experiences Shared

We are committed to empowering individuals to evolve into informed consumers armed with the latest information and heartfelt support for their journey.

When your life is turned upside down, your need for information is great. You have to make critical medical decisions, often with what seems little to go on. Plus you have to break the news to family, quiet your own fears, cope with symptoms or treatment side effects, figure out how you're going to pay for things, and sometimes still get to work or get dinner on the table.

Patient-Centered Guides provide authoritative information for intelligent information seekers who want to become advocates of their own health. They cover the whole impact of illness on your life. In each book, there's a mix of:

- **Medical background for treatment decisions**
  We can give you information that can help you to intelligently work with your doctor to come to a decision. We start from the viewpoint that modern medicine has much to offer and also discuss complementary treatments. Where there are treatment controversies we present differing points of view.

- **Practical information**
  Once you've decided what to do about your illness, you still have to deal with treatments and changes to your life. We cover day-to-day practicalities, such as those you'd hear from a good nurse or a knowledgeable support group.

- **Emotional support**
  It's normal to have strong reactions to a condition that threatens your life or changes how you live. It's normal that the whole family is affected. We cover issues like the shock of diagnosis, living with uncertainty, and communicating with loved ones.

Each book also contains stories from both patients and doctors — medical "frequent flyers" who share, in their own words, the lessons and strategies they have learned when maneuvering through the often complicated maze of medical information that's available.

We provide information online, including updated listings of the resources that appear in this book. This is freely available for you to print out and copy to share with others, as long as you retain the copyright notice on the print-outs.

http://www.patientcenters.com

Other Books in the Series

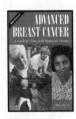

Advanced Breast Cancer
A Guide to Living with Metastatic Disease
By Musa Mayer
ISBN 1-56592-522-X, Paperback 6" x 9", 542 pages, $19.95

"An excellent book...if knowledge is power, this book will be good medicine."

—David Spiegel, MD
Stanford University
Author,
Living Beyond Limits

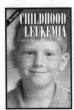

Working with Your Doctor
Getting the Healthcare You Deserve
By Nancy Keene
ISBN 1-56592-273-5, Paperback, 6" x 9", 382 pages, $15.95

"Working with Your Doctor fills a genuine need for patients and their family members caught up in this new and intimidating age of impersonal, economically-driven health care delivery."

—James Dougherty, MD
Emeritus Professor of Surgery,
Albany Medical College

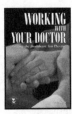

Childhood Leukemia
A Guide for Families, Friends, and Caregiver, 2nd Edition
By Nancy Keene
ISBN 1-56592-632-3, Paperback, 6" x 9", $24.95, 564 pages

"What's so compelling about Childhood Leukemia is the amount of useful medical information and practical advice it contains. Keene avoids jargon and lays out what's needed to deal with the medical system."

—The Washington Post

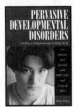

Pervasive Developmental Disorders
Finding a Diagnosis and Getting Help
By Mitzi Waltz
ISBN 1-56592-530-0, Paperback, 6" x 9", 592 pages, $24.95

"Mitzi Waltz's book provides clear, informative, and comprehensive information on every relevant aspect of PDD. Her in-depth discussion will help parents and professionals develop a clear understanding of the issues and, consequently, they will be able to make informed decisions about various interventions. A job well done!"

—Dr. Stephen M. Edelson
Director,
Center for the Study of Autism,
Salem, Oregon

Patient-Centered Guides
Published by O'Reilly & Associates, Inc.
Our products are available at a bookstore near you.
For information: **800-998-9938 • 707-829-0515 • info@oreilly.com**
101 Morris Street • Sebastopol • CA • 95472-9902

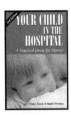
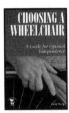
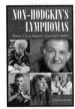
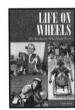

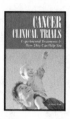

Cancer Clinical Trials
Experimental Treatments and How They Can Help You
By Robert Finn
ISBN 1-56592-566-1, Paperback, 5" x 8", 216 pages, $14.95

"I highly recommend this book as a first step in what will be for many a difficult, but crucially important, part of their struggle to beat their cancer."
—From the foreword by Robert Bazell
Chief Science Correspondent for NBC News
and author of *Her-2: The Making of Herceptin, a Revolutionary Treatment for Breast Cancer*

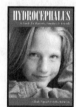

Hydrocephalus
A Guide for Patients, Families & Friends
By Chuck Toporek and Kellie Robinson
ISBN 1-56592-410-X, Paperback, 6" x 9", 384 pages, $19.95

"Toporek, a medical editor, and wife Robinson, a writer and hydrocephalus patient, fill a void of information on hydrocephalus (water on the brain) for the lay reader. Highly recommended for public and academic libraries."
—Library Journal

"In this book, the authors have provided a wonderful entry into the world of hydrocephalus to begin to remedy the neglect of this important condition. We are immensely grateful to them for their groundbreaking effort."
—Peter M. Black, MD, PhD
Franc D. Ingraham Professor of Neurosurgery,
Harvard Medical School
Neurosurgeon-in-Chief,
Brigham and Women's Hospital,
Children's Hospital,
Boston, Massachusetts

Patient-Centered Guides
Published by O'Reilly & Associates, Inc.
Our products are available at a bookstore near you.
For information: **800-998-9938** • **707-829-0515** • **info@oreilly.com**
101 Morris Street • Sebastopol • CA • 95472-9902